MODERN TRENDS

IN

PSYCHOLOGICAL MEDICINE
2

Edited by

JOHN HARDING PRICE
M.D. (Lond.), D.P.N., A.K.C.

Consultant Psychiatrist, St. John's Hospital and The Lawn, Lincoln and Scunthorpe War Memorial Hospitals; Visiting Professor, Lovelace Foundation, Albuquerque, New Mexico; Physician in Charge, Electroencephalography Department, Lincoln Hospitals

LONDON

BUTTERWORTHS

ENGLAND: BUTTERWORTH & CO. (PUBLISHERS) LTD.
                LONDON: 88 Kingsway, W.C.2

AUSTRALIA: BUTTERWORTH & CO. (AUSTRALIA) LTD.
                SYDNEY: 20 Loftus Street
                MELBOURNE: 343 Little Collins Street
                BRISBANE: 240 Queen Street

CANADA: BUTTERWORTH & CO. (CANADA) LTD.
                TORONTO: 14 Curity Avenue, 374

NEW ZEALAND: BUTTERWORTH & CO. (NEW ZEALAND) LTD.
                WELLINGTON: 49/51 Ballance Street
                AUCKLAND: 35 High Street

SOUTH AFRICA: BUTTERWORTH & CO. (SOUTH AFRICA) LTD.
                DURBAN: 33/35 Beach Grove

Suggested U.D.C. Number 616·89
Suggested Additional Number 615·851

ISBN 0 407 31201 3

Printed in Great Britain Page Bros. (Norwich) Ltd., Norwich & London

MODERN TRENDS

IN

PSYCHOLOGICAL MEDICINE

CONTENTS

v

PREFACE

The task of this volume, to span the gap of years since the appearance of the earlier edition, has been formidable. Psychiatric medicine, which for so long lagged behind the other medical sciences, has now gathered momentum and kept pace with the advances made in other medical specialties.

This volume reflects those parts of the subject in which there is much authoritative agreement and thus most of the practice set forth has stood the tests not only of the clinician, but also of the statistician and time.

Treatment has altered radically and this has, in turn, affected the pattern of care of patients and more slowly of public attitudes. Illness can now be more easily hidden in the massive conglomerations of society—indeed that society can itself generate tensions and illness. However, mental illness is no easier for the patient to bear whilst living in society than while in the hospital and indeed it may be much more difficult for his relatives.

It is the responsibility of the psychiatrist to assess and evaluate the results of current therapy upon the patient. Thus it is not sufficient to give the depressed patient antidepressive drugs and presume that they will be effective. The acceptance by the patient and his relatives of the treatment available is not an indication that this is the best available. Furthermore, modern powerful drugs (particularly when pharmacological antagonisms are considered) demand closer liaison between the hospital doctor and the general practitioner. This contrasts with the character disorders because psychopathy is no problem to the patient but an increasing burden to society.

It is hoped that this volume will make a helpful and individual contribution to the series. It has not been possible to include all the subjects which consultants have asked us to incorporate. One is always grateful to colleagues for indicating those parts of clinical medicine which they feel require further clarification.

JOHN HARDING PRICE

CHAPTER 1

THE CONTRIBUTION OF CYTOGENETICS TO CLINICAL PSYCHOLOGY

L. S. PENROSE

PSYCHOLOGY AND GENETICAL DISEASES

Among the most difficult problems met with in human genetics are those which concern the influence of hereditary factors on mental functioning. It is clear from the systematic study of families and of twins that, besides intelligence and special abilities, character traits and temperaments have genetical determiners. However, the genetical influence on mental characters is only partial and the modes of inheritance of the factors involved have not been elucidated. This ignorance is usually concealed by the statement that the hereditary mechanisms are multifactorial or polygenic. There are, however, a few striking examples of mental diseases and defects which have clearly definable genetical causes.

SINGLE GENE DEFECTS

In a number of instances, the genetical defect has a specific biochemical origin and the result is a disorganization of mental functioning which can be associated with either mental deficiency or abnormal behaviour.

Defects produced by amino-acidurias, such as phenylketonuria, homocystinuria, cystathioninuria and arginosuccinicaciduria, are predominantly intellectual; they range from gross idiocy to mild retardation, but they are not typically associated with behaviour disorders other than those which can be directly attributed to intellectual failure. For example, in phenylketonuria, all grades of defect have been found in untreated cases, almost invariably accompanied by docile temperament unless the severity is such that the patient is unable to achieve more than minimal contact with his environment. In the severe cases peculiar hyperkinetic mannerisms of the hands are noticeable (*see also* Cowie[14]).

Diseases which are rapidly progressive, such as the cerebromacular degenerations (amaurotic idiocies) and Hurler's disease (gargoylism), are not noticeably associated with behavioural problems because neurological change or deterioration of mental functioning predominates. In Wilson's disease, however, the neurological manifestations, incoordination and tremor, are usually accompanied by

1

euphoric and childish mentality. All these recessively inherited metabolic disorders differ from the rare dominant (heterozygous) conditions, Huntington's chorea and Alzheimer-Pick disease, which develop in late adult life and in which the neurological defects are liable to be associated with psychotic reactions. It has also been observed that mild psychotic states can develop in later life in heterozygous carriers of the phenylketonuria gene.

In true microcephaly, which is recessively inherited, the biochemical basis is unknown but, again, intellectual deficit is the chief mental sign. In epiloia, a disease with dominant transmission and obscure pathology, severe epilepsy may complicate mental retardation.

From the point of view of the present discussion, the critical factor in all these diseases is that the error is a specific peculiarity inherited in a Mendelian manner and caused by a change in the DNA instructions at one location on one particular chromosome. The change, which must have arisen initially by mutation, is of exceedingly small physical dimensions. The defect cannot be demonstrated visually even with the most powerful magnification of nuclear material. The location of the change, somewhere on the chromosome map, is inferred from the mode of inheritance of the disease. Theoretically, allocation to a specific point on a given chromosomal pair can be achieved by linkage studies. At the present time the only abnormal genes, whose chromosomal positions are approximately known, are those on the sex chromosomes. This is possible because of the phenomenon of sex-linkage.

AUTOSOMAL ABERRATIONS

Introduction

Improvement of cytological techniques, which took place during the years 1952 to 1956, enabled the human chromosomes to be seen clearly and classified. There is one pair of sex chromosomes: the female two are similar (homologous) and are termed XX; the male are disparate and are termed X and Y. The remaining 22 pairs are termed autosomes.

The commonest kind of aberration observed is an alteration in the number of chromosomes; for example, a complement of 45 or 47, instead of the normal 46, in every cell examined. If one chromosome is missing the affected pair is said to be monosomic. If there is an extra chromosome, and one of the pairs has become a triplet, the state is described as trisomic.

The best known example of autosomal trisomy occurs in mongolism, or Down's syndrome. Here the trisomic state affects one of the smallest pairs which belong to the group named G (i.e. No. 21 or No. 22). Though mortality is high compared with normal, the expectation of life at birth in Down's syndrome is now nearly 20 years. Thus there is plenty of opportunity for mental characteristics to be studied in these patients. In the other, clearly defined, types of autosomal trisomy, it is extremely rare to find an affected child who has survived more than the first few months of life. Thus, apart from the knowledge that they are severely handicapped mentally at birth, there is little to record about their behaviour. To some extent this lack of information can be made good by studying cases of mosaicism, that is, conditions in which the trisomy (or other aberration) only occurs in a proportion of the cells of an individual. In such instances a partial or modified form of the syndrome can be produced and, from the study of such people, the nature of the fully developed condition can be inferred.

Besides trisomics and monosomics there are innumerable chromosomal peculiarities which are compatible with life and a great many of them have been found to be associated with diminished mental functioning. Many aberrations, however, are found in normal subjects. Balanced reciprocal translocations occur after double chromosomal breakage and incorrect rejoining. They are of genetical importance in that they may increase the risk of abnormal offspring, but are not, in themselves, harmful in any way to mental health. The same applies to minor peculiarities such as enlargements of the ends of certain chromosomes so that they appear, under the microscope, to have abnormally large attachments or satellites. A relatively common aberration, harmless to the individual but dangerous to the offspring, is the DG translocation or fusion; in this aberration two chromosomes, from different pairs and normally separate, are combined into one chromosome and there are, in each cell, only 45. So long as the total amount of relevant information carried by the chromosome complement is unimpaired, no harm results in the individual who carries the peculiarity in his cells. Even small extra chromosomes are sometimes found in perfectly normal people and they must be assumed to contain almost functionless material.

On the other hand, there are examples known of aberrations which disturb the genetical programme and which produce gross malformations and marked mental changes. For instance, the deletion of a portion of an autosome in the B group (No. 4 or No. 5) produces a type of mental defect accompanied by some physical peculiarities, known as the 'cat cry syndrome' because affected infants emit weak high-pitched sounds. Occasionally, in consequence of reciprocal

3

chromosomal translocation in a parent, a child is born which has too much of one kind of chromosome and too little of another. That is to say, it is partially trisomic for one pair and partially monosomic for another pair. There are many such types already described and, almost invariably, mental impairment, often of a severe degree, accompanies anatomical anomalies.

Down's Syndrome (Mongolism)

The characteristic mentality of the patient who has the morphological signs of mongolism has been commented upon frequently since Langdon Down[39] first clearly demarcated the condition. Intellectual defect is always present, but it is subject to a considerable range of variation. In the most unfavourable cases the child never learns to speak though he can learn to walk and to feed himself. At the other extreme, the mongol child can learn to read and to write quite efficiently and to cooperate in all ordinary household affairs. The intelligence level, measured by the Stanford-Binet scale, hardly ever exceeds six and a half years, though Dunsdon, Carter and Huntley[19] recorded one boy of 17, with a mental age of 10, among 390 cases. There is a block which seems to be associated with the process of generalization and which prevents them from being able to master abstract ideas. This is specially noticeable in their failure at arithmetical manipulation of even the simplest kind. Rote memory may enable them to say that twice three are six or twice four are eight, but they cannot understand the principles of addition or of multiplication. Consequently they have great difficulty in using money except under close supervision. They readily appreciate and recognize quite complex stimuli, like stories, scenes or social incidents, but cannot analyse them into components. They appreciate differences, but have great difficulties in making any generalizations. Their perceptual senses are good and so also is memory when it concerns concrete objects like people and places; but they are weak in memory of times, distances and everything quantitative.

Two important sources of variation in the mental levels of mongols have been repeatedly noted. The first is that, very frequently and possibly invariably, a fall in mental capacity takes place in the early years. That is to say, the I.Q. is assessed, on the average, to be between 40 and 50 during the first two or three years of life, but by the age of about eight years it has fallen to between 30 and 40 and, for the average adult patient, it is between 20 and 30. The second source of variation is concerned with educational and social opportunities. It has been reported often that the I.Q.s of mongol patients under hospital care have a lower average than that of those who stay at home. This difference is widely attributed to the superior opportunities for training afforded by home surroundings. Alternatively, it can be the result of selection of less amenable, less healthy and less intelligent cases for training at residential schools or hospitals. Probably both factors contribute to the effect and the question can only be satisfactorily answered when children of the same initially measured I.Q. levels are followed up over a considerable number of years in different environments. Shipe and Shotwell[58], for example, followed two groups of children from the age of two to seven years in a hospital, and reported that those reared at home in early life had a mean I.Q. ten points higher than those admitted to institutions at birth. However, the state of these infants at birth was not recorded nor were the intelligence levels of their families investigated. Another source of variation was examined by Gibson and Gibbins[29] who attempted to show that the more 'mongolian' stigmata the patient possessed the better he was at intelligence tests.

A common feature of the Down's syndrome mentality is a capacity for imitation. Mimicry of both adults and other children gives them much pleasure; it can be a social asset, but it is superficial and unsystematic so that it may give a false impression of intellectual achievement. This ability can be exploited in devising methods of training and education. The vocabulary can be, in rare cases, of normal dimensions although the precise use of words is imperfectly appreciated. According to Dunsdon, Carter and Huntley[19], if the I.Q. is above 45, mongol children profit by attendance at schools for the educationally subnormal.

Down's syndrome carries a strong impression of stereotyped personality[18] though some psychologists have been unable to demonstrate this objectively. The noticeable features, common to the great majority of these cases, include friendliness and cheerfulness, combined with rather obstinate and repetitive behaviour pattern. Fondness for music is almost universal. Mongol children, as well as adults, like to be the centres of attention in a manner normal for children aged two years. They are usually tidy, clean and methodical if well trained. They enjoy jokes, especially of the kind which involve mischance to someone else. On the whole, temperament in mongols is such that these patients, if treated in a friendly manner, are able to respond cooperatively. They can never fend for themselves and they always require close supervision, but they repay their guardians or parents with affection and personal charm.

In general, the emotional life of a mongol is similar to that of a a child of two to four years. The feelings are probably not as deep as those of normals though this is difficult to assess. Langdon Down[40] noted that they were not passionate nor strongly affectionate. Some patients, however, have temperaments which depart from the usual pattern. Menolascino[49] found 11 out of 86 children to be emotionally disturbed. Some are irritable, mute, uncooperative and destructive and may be considered to be psychotic. Among neuropsychiatric symptoms in mongolism, epilepsy has been occasionally observed, though it is usually not severe[45], but catatonia has been observed more frequently and Earl[20] has drawn attention to psychotic mannerisms and to waxy flexibility. The marked discrepancy between reasoning ability and the compulsive acquisition of verbal knowledge, lists of names for example, shown by some relatively intelligent patients might also be regarded as a psychotic symptom. Even in those cases who are recognizably psychotic, however, there is no tendency to violence although destructiveness is common. It is usual for patients with Down's syndrome, when they are in hospital, to be among the most well-adapted and happiest of the residents. They have no tendency towards antisocial conduct and they radiate an infectious cheerfulness.

Miscellaneous Defects

As previously mentioned, apart from mongols, few cases with standard types of autosomal aberration survive long enough for accurate observations to be made about their mental conditions. An exceptional case of trisomy of one of the large acrocentrics (D group, i.e. Nos 13, 14 or 15) was reported by Marden and Yunis[47]. The patient, a girl aged ten years, could sit up, but was unable to walk without help though she was not paralysed. She used a sound and gesture language, but no words. Her I.Q. was estimated to be less than 20.

In other cases the inference has to be made that, because the child is very weakly at birth, does not react normally to stimuli, such as light or touch, and does not make normal movements of limbs and mouth, it would be demonstrably severely mentally retarded should it survive. This applies to the condition associated with trisomy of chromosome No. 18 and also to a great number of infants who die soon after birth and whose chromosomes are found to be grossly abnormal.

One special condition requires attention, namely that in which one of the B chromosomes, No. 4 or No. 5, has suffered a deletion with loss of part of the shorter arm. The effect is fairly characteristic clinically and the patients may be healthy and reach adult life. The oldest reported was a male, 33 years of age[4]. His mental age was just below two years, he was of a friendly disposition but excitable. He could express himself, very indistinctly, in words, could feed himself but not dress himself, and was clean in his habits. Although the syndrome has been characterized by the fact that, in infancy, such children have a high-pitched cry, the voice of this patient, and that of other adults who have been studied, is not unusual. Most patients with this syndrome, described in the literature, have been children and their 'developmental quotients' have varied between 10 and 45 with an average, in eight cases, of about 25. As compared with mongols, their mental powers may be somewhat weaker and in temperament, though friendly and usually cheerful, they tend to be more excitable and hyperactive.

Another condition is known, in which there is absence of part of a G chromosome or, occasionally, the whole of it. When this occurs the chromosome may form a ring because both ends have lost fragments by simultaneous fracture and have then joined together. Ring chromosomes are unstable and may disappear from some or all cells in the course of development. To some extent, the condition produced by G chromosome deficiency may be considered to be physically the opposite of mongolism, but in respect of the mental state this is not so. Such patients tend to be retarded mentally, though to a lesser degree than in Down's syndrome. The patient described in 1962 (J. L. German and A. G. Bearn. Unpublished) was not obviously retarded mentally at the age of six, though she was quiet and very timid and she was found to have an I.Q. of 65. On the other hand, the girl aged three and a half, described by Al-Aish and colleagues[1], was seriously retarded. She was considered to have a developmental quotient of 25 to 30 and was specially handicapped in motor skills. Most of the other cases found to fall into this not very homogeneous category of 'anti-mongolism' have been too young and too physically feeble for their mental capacities to have been closely studied, but they have all been considered to have some degree of mental defect. Absence of part of one of the D chromosomes (large acrocentrics) has not been found to be associated with any noticeable degree of mental retardation and does not, in any strict sense, produce the opposite condition of the D trisomy[41].

The presence in the body cells of an extra chromosome, not identifiable as a member of one of the normal pairs, is likely to produce mental changes; but this is not always the case. A girl, who had a small extra chromosome with very peculiar morphology[22], suffered, at the age of 13, from frequent epileptic attacks and was intellectually backward though she had a good command of language. In temperament she was affectionate but liable to be spiteful. However, a very similar extra chromosome was found (R. A. Pfeiffer, 1956. Unpublished observations) in a somewhat dwarfed girl of five, without

7

mental defect, whose mother and maternal grandmother both carried the same peculiarity and were mentally normal.

Such examples can be multiplied because a great deal of morphological variation of chromosomes exists in the normal population. It may, thus, be supposed that some small regions are less important than others in the chemical messages which they transmit. Duplication or loss of chromosomal material, which is inactive, can give rise to slightly abnormal appearances in chromosomes and may yet be of little consequence to the individuals in whom they occur.

The group of anomalies which arise in consequence of breakage and rejoining of chromosomes so as to produce 'balanced' translocations do not appear, in themselves, to damage the individual, but a predisposition is engendered for offspring to be abnormal. Thus, the parent who carries a translocation which involves a G chromosome is likely to be perfectly healthy although his or her child can suffer from Down's syndrome. Many other types of balanced translocation have been described and, although the parents are unaffected, there is serious risk that their children will have unbalanced chromosomes, with excess and deficit of material, and suffer from marked mental and physical debility. In a family reported by Edwards and colleagues[21], a brother and sister were of low mental capacity and dysplastic appearance with unbalanced chromosomes whereas their father, who carried a balanced translocation of chromosomes No. 4 and No. 9, was normal. At the same time these writers reported a boy of four years, with unbalanced chromosomes and multiple minor malformations, whose developmental quotient was between 33 and 50, with a normal father who had a balanced translocation of chromosomes Nos 1 and 6. In another family[61] there were three brothers with multiple malformations not characteristic of mongolism, whose mother, maternal grandfather, two sisters and other normal relatives carried a balanced translocation of chromosome No. 18 and a G chromosome. In none of these cases, however, has any detailed study of the mentalities of the abnormal children been made.

The instances quoted of intellectual defect associated with chromosomal aberrations leave no doubt that an autosomal anomaly, visible microscopically, which implies excess or deficit of material, nearly always causes mental defect and, as a general rule, the greater the magnitude of the error the more serious is the retardation.

SEX CHROMOSAL ERRORS

Introduction

In contradistinction to the effects produced by autosomal aberrations, those which result from peculiarities in the sex chromosomes are not very closely associated with intellectual impairment. As with autosomal aberrations, however, the more striking the peculiarity the more likely is the mental capacity to be lowered. The commonest peculiarity is a disturbance of number, that is to say, there are too few or too many sex chromosomes associated with a normal set of autosomes. With the best known types of sex chromosomal errors, single-X females (Turner's syndrome), XXX females, XXY males (Klinefelter's syndrome) and XYY males, the patients are more likely to come to the attention of the physician on account of emotional disturbances or disorders of personality than on account of intellectual defect. Consequently, the disturbance of intellectual function produced by the chromosomal error can best be demonstrated by comparing the incidence of such patients in mental deficiency hospitals, clinics or other psychiatric institutions, with the incidence of the chromosomal peculiarities, which characterize them, in the general population or at birth. It has to be shown that the frequency of the condition is greater in a particular hospital or prison population than would be expected on chance sampling. Then the risk that the type of patient will suffer from the particular condition, with which a given institution is concerned, can be estimated.

Turner's Syndrome

The frequency at birth of the aberration, in which only one sex chromosome, an X, is present instead of two, can be ascertained by testing all females for negative sex chromatin. The sex chromatin test, derived from the work of Barr and Bertram, originally on nerve cells in cats, enables the number of X chromosomes in the tissues to be estimated. Normally females, with XX sex chromosomes, are positive, which means, in practice, that a Barr body (or chromatin body) has been found at the periphery of the nucleus in epithelial cells taken from a scraping of the mucous membrane on the inside of the cheek. Males with XY sex chromosomes are negative in this respect: so also are single-X females. The frequency of chromatin negative females, in the surveys summarized by Court Brown[12], is 14 in 40,096 births, or 0·03 per cent; and all of these can be expected to develop into cases of Turner's syndrome.

The clinical aspects of Turner's syndrome include an oedematous state, which subsides with age, shortness of stature, webbing of the neck, circulatory weakness, diminution of development of secondary sexual characters, amenorrhoea and complete infertility. The mental condition is usually not noticeably abnormal. Patients tend to be quiet, unobtrusive, industrious, reliable and of average intellectual ability.

The study of samples of females in mental deficiency hospitals indicates, according to Court Brown's summary of published surveys, that the incidence of Turner's syndrome there is 5 in 8,882, or 0·06 per cent which is double that in females at birth. Hence, there is a slight, though far from statistically significant, excess of Turner's among mentally retarded females. It is not, therefore, surprising to find that, in groups of Turner patients where mental states have been carefully examined, most have been found to have normal intelligence although a few have been rated as subnormal. The mean I.Q. of 44 cases reported by Lindsten[43] was 98 on the CVB scale of intelligence tests and 94 on the SRB scale. The mean Wechsler I.Q. of 16 patients studied by Money and Alexander[51] was 101, with verbal I.Q. 112 and performance I.Q. 87. These patients showed some deficiency in space–form perception and in numerical manipulation. Three cases studied by Mellbin[48], between the ages of 28 and 57, had measured I.Q.s of 75, 85 and 121, respectively, and a fourth was considered to have a 'normal' I.Q. Two patients[5], however, showed intellectual defect and the I.Q. of one of them was 51.

A striking feature of the mentalities of many cases of Turner's syndrome is their liability to develop certain kinds of mental illness. The cases, described by Mellbin, all had neuropsychiatric disorders. Two had infantile dispositions, one was emotionally unstable and self-centred and the other had epilepsy and was subject to hallucinatory psychotic episodes. Moreover, depression and obsessional tendencies are not uncommon reactions in Turner patients.

In consequence of the fact that these patients have only one X chromosome, as do normal males, they are liable to have defects or illnesses which occur almost exclusively in males because of sex-linked or X-linked inheritance. Colour-blindness has a frequency of about four per cent in the male population, but is extremely rare in normal females, about 1 in 2,000. In Turner's syndrome, it is as common as in the male population. For the same reason Turner patients, unlike normal females, can suffer from severe sex-linked physical diseases, such as muscular dystrophy and haemophilia. Some types of deafness and certain unusual neuropsychiatric disturbances, like those described by Blanc, Bourgeois and Fontange[5], which have been found with Turner's syndrome, may have genetical origins related to the presence of only one X chromosome. However, making allowance for poor health, short stature and other physical defects, it is remarkable how well adjusted mentally the majority of patients with Turner's syndrome are found to be.

Triple-X Females

The presence of three X chromosomes, instead of the normal two, in the cells of a female can be detected by examining cells for sex chromatin. If a significant proportion of cells are found to have two Barr bodies, it is probable that there are three X chromosomes in each cell. The inference can then be checked by analysis of leucocyte or skin fibroblast cultures. According to the summarized figures given by Court Brown[12], among 36,454 female births, 23 were found to have double sex chromatin. This implies that the incidence in the female general population of XXX types is 0·06 per cent. Higher values had formerly been accepted[38], but they were based upon much smaller samples.

The majority of triple-X females are of normal physical appearance, they are healthy, they are fertile and they are rarely obviously abnormal in their behaviour. Most adult cases have been identified on account of some degree of social inadequacy which brings them in touch with a hospital. Surveys of the populations of mentally ill patients have indicated that females with double sex chromatin occur much more frequently in such groups than in the general population. According to Court Brown's[12] summary, this phenomenon has been found in 43 out of 8,421 females in subnormality hospitals, an incidence of 0·51 per cent which is some eight times as great as that in the general population at birth. However, not all the surveys summarized are homogeneous and the chromatin test is only a quick screening method. The number of actually proved cases of XXX females in the hospital surveys is lower than the number scored as having doubly positive chromatin. Nevertheless, it is clear that triple-X females have a higher risk than XX females of being diagnosed as mentally subnormal, a risk between four and eight times as high.

In one study[38] 22 triple-X females, found among the patients in mental deficiency hospitals, were compared with other defective females with the same mean age (46 years). The only pronounced difference between the two groups was that the XXX patient suffered especially from psycho-social inadequacy. In both groups about half of the patients were considered to be psychotic.

No systematic survey of the intelligence levels in XXX patients seems to have been made. The proportion of the female general population which comes under medical scrutiny on account of mental deficiency and social inadequacy is not easy to estimate, but it probably does not exceed three per cent. If the risk for XXX females is about five times the average, 15 per cent of them may come under

11

observation in this way so that five-sixths of them, at least, live un-
noticed among their neighbours. Furthermore, it is interesting to
find that, although theoretically they are liable to have daughters
who have XXX chromosomes, no one has yet recorded this.

Other phenomena, closely related to triple-X, are quadruple- and
quintuple-X females. These are exceedingly rare conditions and every
case, so far described, has suffered from rather marked mental defect.
Carr, Barr and Plunkett[10] discovered two women, one aged 13 with
I.Q. 30 and the other aged 32 with I.Q. about 50, both of whom had
XXXX sex chromosomes with the normal complement of 44 autosomes, i.e. 48 chromosomes altogether. The physical appearance and
sexual development were, in both cases, satisfactory. A patient of the
same type[17] had an I.Q. of 50, but manipulative ability was less
retarded than speech. In cases of females with five X chromosomes,
49 chromosomes altogether, mental retardation has been apparent
and Brody, Fitzgerald and Spier[7] estimated that, in their case, at
29 months of age, the mental age was 12 months.

Klinefelter's Syndrome

The condition which is cytologically the converse of Turner's
syndrome, a female with too few X chromosomes, is the syndrome of
Klinefelter, a male with too many X chromosomes. Physically, male
patients with this condition tend to have a somewhat feminine build
though they may be tall. The body hair is diminished, the voice is
rather high-pitched and the testes are small. They are completely
infertile.

The incidence of the condition at birth can be found by chromatin
tests. Using the figures summarized by Court Brown[12], out of 41,688
males tested, 71 were found to be chromatin positive. This represents
an incidence of 0·17 per cent for Klinefelter's syndrome.

In consequence of their sexual incapacity, many cases come under
observation at fertility clinics and these are mostly of normal mental
ability. A noticeable proportion of cases, however, have been
identified in hospitals for mental subnormality, by chromatin tests,
and a summary of published figures indicates that the incidence
among such patients, of Klinefelter types, is 126 among 13,349, or
0·94 per cent. This figure is more than five times that for the general
population. By the argument already used for the triple-X females,
this figure suggests that some 15 per cent of Klinefelter patients of all
kinds are definitely mentally inferior. It should be noted that there
are types of Klinefelter cases with more than one extra X chromosome. For example, Jancar[36] described two cases, each with XXXXY
sex chromosomes, that is, with 49 chromosomes altogether, who had

I.Q. levels of 19 and 22. These are extremely rare types, but, since their mental abilities seem to be cumulatively impaired by each excessive X chromosome which they carry, they are not so rarely found in mental deficiency hospitals; the frequencies of the three types XXY, XXXY and XXXXY in such institutions are as 25 : 5 : 1, respectively. In chromatin surveys, they will all be included among cases scored as positive, so that the estimate of mean I.Q. 89·5 for 23 positive males[50], may be a little lower than the mean I.Q. for typical XXY cases. The average I.Q. for 47 'true' Klinefelter males[59] was 91·9 with standard deviation 16·4. Court Brown estimates that XXY males are almost four times as frequently diagnosed mentally deficient as are members of the general population.

An important feature of Klinefelter's syndrome is a tendency to unstable or even psychotic behaviour; compared with other patients of the same level of intelligence, they tend to show defensive reactions; they are not aggressive and they have inferiority feelings in sexual matters[8]. Some of them show signs of schizophrenia[2] but it is doubtful how far this is a characteristic reaction though it was diagnosed in 11 out of 30 mental hospital Klinefelter patients in a survey[46]. Chronic psychosis, with paranoia, hallucinations or delusions of grandeur, was noted frequently by Hambert[30], but homosexuality was uncommon. Hunter[33] described 13 XXY males and one XXXY who had been apprehended for delinquency; childhood behaviour problems, sexual misdemeanours and larceny were features of some of their histories. On the whole, the evidence available indicates that behaviour peculiarities are more important than low intelligence in Klinefelter cases who come under observation on account of their mental condition.

Double-Y Males

Much attention has recently been focused upon males who have two Y chromosomes. In the standard case, there are the usual 44 autosomes but XYY, instead of XY, sex chromosomes. The incidence at birth or in the adult general population is difficult to determine because there is no simple test for the presence of an extra Y chromosome; it is necessary to culture cells every time and to look at the chromosomes. Present evidence suggests that the true incidence is about one per thousand males (0·1 per cent)[13].

The main physical characteristic of XYY males is increased stature, which is over 5 ft 10 in (178 cm) in most adult cases. They are healthy, normal in appearance and fertile. The problem of estimating their intelligence distribution is bedevilled by the peculiarity that they have strong tendencies towards psychopathic behaviour. The incidence of these patients in hospital for the mentally defective is low, perhaps no greater than that in the general population. However, the incidence in special hospitals for criminal or psychopathic defectives is remarkably high; surveys have indicated that it lies between one and two per cent. Thus, Price and Whatmore[56] studied nine among 315 criminal defectives and Welch, Borgaonkar and Herr[63] found one among 464 defective delinquents, that is ten out of 779. Since these psychopathic patients represent a relatively small and uncertain proportion of all subnormals, the increased incidence of XYY cases among all subnormals might be about only three-fold, rather more than Turner's but less than Klinefelter's. This is equivalent to assuming a mean I.Q. for all cases of a little above 90. The lowest I.Q. recorded, at the present time, has been 71[64] and the highest 116[27].

It is in relation to behaviour characteristics that the XYY males are of particular interest. This became evident from the finding of seven cases among 197 patients in a criminal mental hospital[35]. Other surveys have confirmed this finding; for example, Bartlett and colleagues[3] found two cases among 204 male inmates of a security prison. Many other surveys have been carried out, usually making use of the fact that XYY cases are concentrated among the prisoners of tall stature. For example, Nielsen[52] found three cases in the forensic psychiatric ward of a state hospital in Denmark by testing patients over 180 cm tall. Of particular interest is the survey of tall males in an Australian prison[64]. Four XYY cases were identified, one of whom had been sentenced to death for committing murder[9]. He had been reprieved, after a fierce popular outcry, on account of his obvious signs of mental instability although he was neither technically insane nor mentally defective.

The general problem of a characteristic temperament associated with the XYY karyotype is of extreme interest. At present the information available strongly indicates that there is a behaviour stereotype. When the condition is diagnosed before puberty, anti-social traits may already be observed, as in the boy described by Cowie and Kahn[15]. Moreover, first offences of prisoners with XYY chromosomes have been earlier in life (mean age 13 years) than those for other prisoners (mean age 18 years)[57]. The crimes of which such patients tend to be convicted are not always those of violence although attacks of compulsive aggression seem to be common. Arson[52] and larceny may be characteristic. Some disorder of personality seems to be present in almost every case, but this may not amount to more than childish irritability when frustrated, inability to settle at any work, liability to alcoholism and having difficulty in maintaining normal personal relationships. It also appears that the lower the intelligence level, the more likely is criminal behaviour to develop. It is possible also that their unusual stature may be a factor in facilitating their apprehension as criminals.

In the male prison population altogether, the incidence of XYY patients is roughly one per cent which is but ten times that in the general population; consequently, the over-all risk of being apprehended for committing a crime is increased, in these cases, by a factor of 10. Nevertheless, the majority of XYY men will probably not be considered as abnormal and will only be diagnosed accidentally —as was the case described by Hauschka and colleagues[31] and in several recent reports[27, 44, 60].

The combination of the double-Y aberration with another error can lead to a condition in which two syndromes are combined. Thus, a very rare type of patient with XXYY sex chromosomes tends to have the usual features of Klinefelter's syndrome with increased stature and antisocial behaviour in addition. One patient[23], aged 44, 6 ft 5 in in stature and with an I.Q. of 44, had been repeatedly charged with theft and was homosexually orientated but was of a reliable and friendly disposition. Gibson and Martin[28] described an XXYY male of similar stature, who was mentally retarded and not antisocial, and Jancar[37] recorded another such patient with I.Q. 62, amiable and polite but subject to manic depressive episodes. Casey and colleagues[11], however, found seven XXYY cases among 742 males at a state hospital for defective patients who required special security precautions. Their behaviour disorders were, nevertheless, not distinguishable from those of XXY Klinefelter males in the same institution. It is probable that XXYY males are invariably below average in their intelligence, as are XXXX females.

BIOLOGICAL ASPECTS

General Principles

The great majority of the conditions connected with chromosomal aberration and discussed here arise spontaneously by some accident which can, in a wide sense, be termed mutation: they have no hereditary background and their parents are normal. It has, moreover, been shown that the autosomal aberrations cause more marked physical defects than those of sex chromosomes. Further, the mental changes in the autosomal aberrations are, in the main, concerned with loss of intellectual function, which may be associated with cerebral malformation, whereas the sex chromosomal errors predominantly affect temperament and behaviour[54] and malformation of the nervous system has not been shown to be a characteristic feature.

There is, nevertheless, a tendency for all the sex chromosomal errors to reduce the intelligence more or less proportionately to the quantity of the deviation from the normal karyotype. The amount of

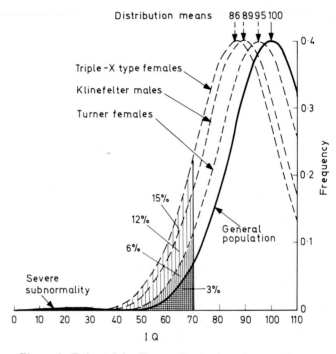

Figure 1. *Estimated intelligence distributions for sex chromosal aberrations (broken outlines) compared with the general population (continuous outline). The assumption is made that each I.Q. distribution is approximately Gaussian with standard deviation 16 points to which the same non-Gaussian tail or extension, representing severe subnormality, is added (solid black area). The estimated I.Q. means for triple-X females, Klinefelter's, Turner's and normals are 86, 89, 95 and 100, respectively*

variation in mental ability within each group, Turner's, Klinefelter's, etc., is about the same as in the general population but the mean value is reduced. The effect of this is to increase the proportion of cases in each aberrant group which fall below the level considered to separate the mentally defective or subnormal from the normal. For the general population this lies at the I.Q. of 70, or at a point approximately twice the standard deviation below the mean (100). According to American estimates the I.Q. standard deviation is 16 points; this means that three per cent of the general population is mentally subnormal if the distribution is Gaussian. A population, like that of patients with Turner's syndrome, with twice as large a proportion (six per cent) subnormal, has a mean intelligence level of about 95. Correspondingly, Klinefelter's, with about four times the general proportion of cases below I.Q. 70, that is, about 12 per cent, have a mean intelligence level of just below 90. These approximations are shown in *Figure 1*.

A point of interest is the fact that sex chromosomal errors are found mainly among high grade defectives, that is, mildly subnormal patients, in particular those with I.Q. above 40. The patients with intelligence levels below 40 are almost exclusively what Lewis[42] called 'pathological' cases, that is, they suffer from specific diseases which may be hereditary defects, like epiloia or phenylketonuria, diseases caused by injury or infection or diseases caused by auto-somal aberrations. Sex chromosomal errors are occasionally co-incidental with conditions which cause severe subnormality. Mongols with Klinefelter's syndrome[26] are known and so also are triple-X female mongols[16] and double-Y mongols[62]. These conditions are all extremely rare and, considering the enormous numbers of Down's syndrome cases which have been karyotyped, are probably not more frequent than would be expected by chance coincidence. In their mental processes, these patients with additional errors, moreover, have not been noticeably different from uncomplicated cases of Down's syndrome.

The question of the origin of the variations in intelligence level, in cases of the same type of chromosomal error, is a matter which can be directly investigated by studying the families of these patients. In Court Brown's[13] small material there is a significantly positive correlation between stature of XYY patients and statures of their brothers. The same is almost certainly true of intelligence, not only for XYY males but for Klinefelter's and other sex chromosome aberrations also. It seems probable that most of the variation is caused in the same way as natural variation in the general popula-tion and that superimposed on this is an independent effect of the aberration which diminishes intelligence. The intelligence level in Down's syndrome is probably related to the mental abilities of the parents though no convincing data on this question have been pub-lished. However, it has been shown[32] that, although finger-print patterns are distorted in mongolism, they nevertheless have strong similarities to the patterns on the fingers of normal parents and sibs.

17

Comparable origins of variation in dermatoglyphic phenomena can be postulated in cases of sex chromosome anomaly[55].

A question which, at the present time, has received little attention is how the chromosomal aberrations produce their distorting effect on mental ability and behaviour. In the case of mongolism, the mechanism must be related to the simplification in cerebral architecture and the reduction of brain size which are characteristic of the condition. The reason for this malformation, as for other malformations connected with autosomal aberrations, is unknown. In view of the fact that disturbance of the fluid balance in the tissues of the embryo is known to occur as a consequence of abnormal chromosome complement in amphibia as well as in plants, such an explanation has to be considered as a possible source of malformation in human aneuploidy, especially since foetal oedema has been established in Turner's syndrome.

In sex chromosomal errors, with the exception of Turner's syndrome, physical development is much less grossly affected than in autosomal errors. It is widely believed that disturbances of sex hormones may be significant factors, not only in adolescence but in an early period of embryonic life. With respect to the XYY character peculiarities, it is natural to enquire if an excess of male hormone could be responsible. At present, opinions are divided on this point. There is evidence which indicates that urinary testosterone levels are increased in XYY and decreased in XXY males[34], but there is much natural variation in normal males from day to day and methods of estimation may not always be reliable. Disturbance of urinary gonadotrophin excretion in XYY males has been reported by Papanicolau, Kirkham and Loraine[53]. It would be of great interest and practical value if it could be shown that hormonal disturbances were responsible for the behaviour problems in these groups of cases.

Mosaic Types

Not all chromosomal errors affect every cell in the body. The commonest type of mosaicism occurs when a proportion of cells is aberrant and a proportion normal. This peculiarity may sometimes be associated with a relatively mild manifestation of a standard syndrome. In mongolism, for example, when a substantial proportion of cells in fibroblast cultures, say more than 15 per cent, is normal, the condition is ameliorated, physical signs are less marked and the I.Q. approaches normal limits. The presence of normal cells in the blood is of less significance from this point of view. Mosaicism is not uncommon in Turner's and Klinefelter's syndromes, but there is no evidence as to its effect on the intelligence. One might suppose that the bizarre combination of some XYYY cells with XYY cells, found in the reprieved murderer mentioned earlier[64], may have increased his liability to psychopathic behaviour.

Some cases of mosaicism are of quite peculiar interest. Among these are mosaic triploids. Typically, in these patients, about half the cells in the solid tissues of the body are normal and half have 69 chromosomes, a triplet in each group instead of a pair. The leucocytes in the blood are usually all normal. The male described by Böök and Santesson[6] had XXY sex chromosomes in the triploid cells and he did not have any signs of mongolism although half his cells had their G chromosomes tripled. Triploid cells are, in some respects, balanced but, nevertheless, they do not function quite normally. If all cells are triploid in an infant, it cannot survive and such a foetus almost always miscarries at an early stage. The mosaic cases, however, are not necessarily unhealthy though they are liable to be physically asymmetrical and are mentally retarded. Böök and Santesson's[6] case was severely subnormal and muscularly weak. A girl with comparable karyotype[24] had a higher intelligence level. Her I.Q., at the age of ten, was stated to be 73. She was backward in speech, suffered from epileptiform attacks and was of timid disposition. Cases on record, with a smaller proportion of triploid cells, have been also found to have intelligence much diminished. The boy described by Ferrier and colleagues[25] at the age of ten, had a mental age of only $3\frac{1}{2}$ years and, again, was physically weak. Only eight per cent of his body cells were triploid and the blood, as usual, was normal. This case emphasizes the lack of any close relationship between the proportion of abnormal cells found in a mosaic patient and the degree of mental disturbance and other clinical signs. Moreover, the uncertainty of the mental effects of mosaicism serves to show the enormous field for researches which has opened for the clinical psychologist on account of cytological discoveries of the last ten years.

REFERENCES

1. Al-Aish, M. S., de la Cruz, F., Goldsmith, L. A., Volpe, J., Mella, G. and Robinson, J. C. (1967). 'Autosomal Monosomy in Man. Complete Monosomy G in a Four-and-one-half-year-old Mentally Retarded Girl'. *New Engl. Med. J.* **277**, 777
2. Anders, J. M., Jagiello, G., Polani, P. E., Giannelli, F., Hamerton, J. L. and Lieberman, D. M. (1968). 'Chromosome Findings in Psychotic Patients'. *Br. J. Psychiat.* **114**, 1167

3. Bartlett, D. J., Hurley, W. P., Brand, C. R. and Poole, E. W. (1968). 'Chromosomes of Male Patients in a Security Prison'. *Nature, Lond.* **219,** 351

4. Berg, J., Delhanty, J. D. A., Faunch, J. A. and Ridler, M. A. C. (1965). 'Partial Deletion of Short Arm of a Chromosome of the 4–5 Group (Denver) in an Adult Male'. *J. ment. Defic. Res.* **9,** 219

5. Blanc, M., Bourgeois, M. and Fontange, X. (1966). 'Syndrome de Turner et Troubles Neuropsychiatriques'. *Annls méd.-psychol.* **2,** 346

6. Böök, J. A. and Santesson, B. (1960). 'Malformation in Man Associated with Triploidy (69 Chromosomes)'. *Lancet* **1,** 858

7. Brody, J., Fitzgerald, M. G. and Spiers, A. S. D. (1967). 'A Female Child with Five X Chromosomes'. *J. Ped.* **70,** 105

8. Burnand, G., Hunter, H. and Hoggart, K. (1967). 'Some Psychological Test Characteristics of Klinefelter's Syndrome'. *Br. J. Psychiat.* **113,** 1091

9. Burns, C. (1962). *The Tait Case.* Parkville, Victoria: Melbourne University Press; London: Cambridge University Press

10. Carr, D. H., Barr, M. L. and Plunkett, E. R. (1961). 'An XXXX Sex Chromosome Complex in Two Mentally Defective Females'. *Can. med. Ass. J.* **84,** 131

11. Casey, M. D., Segall, L. J., Street, D. R. K. and Blank, C. E. (1966). 'Sex Chromosome Abnormalities in Two State Hospitals for Patients Requiring Special Security'. *Nature, Lond.* **209,** 641

12. Court Brown, W. M. (1969). 'Sex Chromosome Aneuploidy in Man, its Frequency and with Special Reference to Mental Subnormality and Criminal Behaviour'. *Int. Rev. exp. Path.* **7,** 31

13. — (1968). 'The Development of Knowledge about Males with an XYY Sex Chromosome Complement'. *J. med. Genet.* **5,** 341

14. Cowie, J. (1968). 'Psychological Considerations in the Treatment of Inborn Errors of Metabolism'. *Brain Damage by Inborn Errors Metabolism.* Haarlem: de Erven F. Bohn N.V.

15. — and Kahn, J. (1968). 'XYY Constitution in Prepubertal Child'. *Br. med. J.* **1,** 748

16. Day, R. W., Wright, S. W., Koons, A. and Quigley, M. (1963). 'XXX 21-Trisomy and Retinoblastoma'. *Lancet* **2,** 154

17. de Grouchy, J., Brissaud, H. E., Richardet, J. M., Repéssé, G., Sanger, R., Race, R. R., Salmon, Ch. and Salmon, D. (1968). 'Syndrome 48, XXXX Chez une Enfant de Six Ans Transmission Anormale du Groupe X$_g$'. *Annls Génét.* **11,** 120

18. Domino, G., Goldschmid, M. and Kaplan, M. (1964). 'Personality Traits of Institutionalized Mongoloid Girls'. *Am. J. ment. Defic.* **68,** 498

19. Dunsdon, M. I., Carter, C. O. and Huntley, R. M. C. (1960). 'Upper End of Range in Intelligence in Mongolism'. *Lancet* **1,** 565

20. Earl, C. J. C. (1934). 'The Primitive Catatonic Psychosis of Idiocy'. *Br. J. med. Psychol.* **14,** 230

21. Edwards, J. H., Fraccaro, M., Davies, P. and Young, R. B. (1962). 'Structural Heterozygosis in Man: Analysis of Two Families'. *Ann. hum. Genet.* **26,** 163

22. Ellis, J. R., Marshall, R. and Penrose, L. S. (1962). 'An Aberrant Small Acrocentric Chromosome'. *Ann. hum. Genet.* **26, 77**

23. — Miller, O. J., Penrose, L. S. and Scott, G. E. B. (1961). 'A Male with XXYY Chromosomes'. *Ann. hum. Genet.* **25,** 145

24. — Marshall, R., Normand, I. C. S. and Penrose, L. S. (1963). 'A Girl with Triploid Cells'. *Nature, Lond.* **198,** 411

25. Ferrier, P., Ferrier, S., Stalder, G., Bühler, E., Bamatter, F. and Klein, D. (1964). 'Congenital Asymmetry Associated with Diploid–Triploid Mosaicism and Large Satellites'. *Lancet* **1,** 80

26. Ford, C. E., Jones, K. W., Miller, O. J., Mittwoch, U., Penrose, L. S., Ridler, M. A. C. and Shapiro, A. (1959). 'The Chromosomes in a Patient Showing both Mongolism and the Klinefelter Syndrome'. *Lancet* **1,** 709

27. Forssman, H., Åkesson, H. O. and Wallin, L. (1968). 'The YY Syndrome'. *Lancet* **2,** 779

28. Gibson, A. L. and Martin, L. (1968). 'Aggression and the XXYY Anomaly'. *Lancet* **2,** 870

29. Gibson, D. and Gibbins, R. J. (1958). 'The Relation of Mongolian Stigmata to Intellectual Status'. *Am. J. ment. Defic.* **63,** 345

30. Hambert, G. (1966). *Males with Positive Sex Chromatin.* Göteborg: Scandinavian University Books

31. Hauschka, T. S., Hasson, J. E., Goldstein, M. N., Koepf, G. F. and Sandberg, A. A. (1962). 'An XYY Man with Progeny Indicating Familial Tendency to Non-disjunction'. *Am. J. hum. Genet.* **14,** 22

32. Holt, S. B. (1968). *The Genetics of Dermal Ridges.* Springfield, Ill.: Charles C. Thomas

33. Hunter, H. (1968). 'Klinefelter's Syndrome and Delinquency'. *Br. J. Criminol.* **8,** 203

34. Ismail, A. A. A., Harkness, R. A., Kirkham, K. E., Loraine, J. A., Whatmore, P. B. and Brittain, R. P. (1968). 'Effect of Abnormal Sex-chromosome Complements on Urinary Testosterone Levels'. *Lancet* **1,** 220

35. Jacobs, P. A., Brunton, M., Melville, M. M., Brittain, R. P. and McClemont, W. F. (1965). 'Aggressive Behaviour, Mental Subnormality and the XYY Male'. *Nature, Lond.* **208,** 1351

36. Jancar, J. (1964). 'Mentally Defective Males with XXXXY Chromosomes'. *Proceedings of the International Copenhagen Congress on the Scientific Study of Mental Retardation* **1,** 179

37. — (1968). 'XXYY with Manic-depression'. *Lancet* **2,** 970

38. Kidd, C. B., Knox, R. S. and Mantle, D. J. (1963). 'A Psychiatric Investigation of Triple-X Chromosome Females'. *Br. J. Psychiat.* **109,** 90

39. Langdon Down, J. (1866). 'Observations on an Ethnic Classification of Idiots'. *Lectures Rep. Lond. Hosp.* **3,** 259

40. Langdon Down, J. (1887). *Mental Affections of Childhood and Youth*. London: Churchill
41. Lele, K. P., Penrose, L. S. and Stallard, H. B. (1963). 'Chromosome Deletion in a Case of Retinoblastoma'. *Ann. hum. Genet.* **27**, 171
42. Lewis, E. O. (1933). 'Types of Mental Deficiency and their Social Significance'. *J. ment. Sci.* **79**, 298
43. Lindsten, J. (1963). *The Nature and Origin of X Chromosome Aberrations in Turner's Syndrome*. Stockholm: Almquist and Wiksell
44. Lisker, R., Zenzes, M. T. and Fouesca, M. T. (1968). 'YY Syndrome in a Mexican'. *Lancet* **2**, 635
45. MacGillivray, R. C. (1967). 'Epilepsy in Down's Anomaly'. *J. ment. Defic. Res.* **11**, 43
46. Maclean, N., Court Brown, W. M., Jacobs, P. A., Mantle, D. J. and Strong, J. A. (1968). 'A Survey of Sex Chromatin Abnormalities in Mental Hospitals'. *J. med. Genet.* **5**, 165
47. Marden, P. M. and Yunis, J. J. (1967). 'Trisomy D_1 in a 10-Year-Old Girl. Normal Neutrophils and Fetal Hemoglobin'. *Am. J. Dis. Childh.* **114**, 662
48. Mellbin, G. (1966). 'Neuropsychiatric Disorders in Sex Chromatin Negative Women'. *Br. J. Psychiat.* **112**, 145
49. Menolascino, F. J. (1965). 'Psychiatric Aspects of Mongolism'. *Am. J. ment. Defic.* **69**, 653
50. Money, J. (1964). 'Two Cytogenetic Syndromes: Psychologic Comparisons'. *J. Psychiat. Res.* **2**, 223
51. — and Alexander, D. (1966). 'Turner's Syndrome: Further Demonstration of the Presence of Specific Cognitional Deficiencies'. *J. med. Genet.* **3**, 47
52. Nielsen, J. (1968). 'The XYY Syndrome in a Mental Hospital'. *Br. J. Criminol.* **8**, 186
53. Papanicolau, A. D., Kirkham, K. E. and Loraine, J. A. (1968). 'Abnormalities in Urinary Gonadotrophin Excretion in Men with a 47, XYY Sex Chromosome Constitution'. *Lancet* **2**, 608
54. Penrose, L. S. (1966). 'The Contribution of Mental Deficiency Research to Psychiatry'. *Br. J. Psychiat.* **112**, 747
55. — (1967). 'Finger-print Patterns and the Sex Chromosomes'. *Lancet* **1**, 298
56. Price, W. H. and Whatmore, P. B. (1967). 'Criminal Behaviour and the XYY Male'. *Nature, Lond.* **213**, 815
57. — — (1967). 'Behaviour Disorder and Pattern of Crime Among XYY Males Identified at a Maximum Security Hospital'. *Br. med. J.* **1**, 533
58. Shipe, D. and Shotwell, A. M. (1965). 'Effect of Out-of-home Care on Mongoloid Children: A Continuation Study'. *Am. J. ment. Defic.* **69**, 649
59. Šipová, I. and Raboch, J. (1960). 'Mental Level in 47 Patients with "True" Klinefelter's Syndrome'. *Ces. Lek. Cesk.* **99**, 682

60. Thorburn, M. J., Chutkan, W., Richards, R. and Bell, R. (1968). 'XYY Sex Chromosomes in a Jamaican with Orthopaedic Abnormalities'. *J. med. Genet.* **5,** 215

61. Uchida, I. A., Wang, H. C., Laxdal, O. E., Zaleski, W. A. and Duncan, B. P. (1964). 'Partial Trisomy-deficiency Syndrome Resulting from a Reciprocal Translocation in a Large Kindred'. *Cytogenetics* **3,** 81

62. Verresen, H. and van den Berghe, H. (1965). '21-Trisomy and XYY'. *Lancet,* **1,** 609

63. Welch, J. P., Borgaonkar, D. S. and Herr, H. M. (1967). 'Psychopathy, Mental Deficiency, Aggressiveness and the XYY Syndrome'. *Nature, Lond.* **214,** 500

64. Wiener, S., Sutherland, G., Bartholomew, A. A. and Hudson, B. (1968). 'XYY Males in a Melbourne Prison'. *Lancet* **1,** 150

CHAPTER 2

THE EFFECTS OF AGEING ON PROFESSIONAL PILOTS

JACEK SZAFRAN

INTRODUCTION

Although the title of this chapter suggests something like a general survey, its real theme is a group of airline, military and test-pilots, ranging in age from the mid-twenties to the early sixties, who had elected to participate on a voluntary basis in an interdisciplinary study of the possible effects of ageing, sponsored since 1962 by the United States Public Health Service at the Lovelace Foundation for Medical Education and Research. It is hoped that this particular case may convey more than an equivalent amount of general speculation. The chapter is based on material presented in greater detail in several previous publications[42-46], but some new data are also included. Earlier work in the same general area has been reviewed extensively by McFarland[29].

It should be explained at the outset that the measurement and analysis of progressive age changes in this occupational group have been undertaken for two reasons. In the first place, because their profession demands high standards of bodily and mental fitness, the pilots appear to offer certain obvious advantages for the important differentiation between the effects of ageing *per se* and those of cumulative pathology. In the second place—and this is possibly of greater interest to the readers of this volume—the problem of early detection of deteriorative trends in flying personnel in command of high-performance aircraft has become a major cause for concern among the aviation medical consultants. The older pilot, like other employees, is commonly defined as one who approaches a conventionally fixed age limit, a practice which may be totally misleading. Indeed, some years ago, the age limit of 60 for airline pilots proposed by the medical division of the International Civil Aviation Organization was strongly criticized by the United Kingdom delegation on the grounds that not enough is known in the medical field to lay down any strict standards. On the other hand, particularly on this side of the Atlantic, pessimistic statements have been made from time to time about 'premature ageing' in pilots at the age of 40 or 50. Clearly, then, in an exercise of this kind the investigators are to some extent obliged to steer a course midway between the purely academic and frankly applied considerations.

The object of the investigation as a whole is to elucidate the extent to which, given the chronological age of an individual, it would be feasible to evaluate, from the standpoint of the disciplines of cardiovascular and pulmonary physiology as well as of experimental psychology, his position regarding the traditionally expected impairment of capacities in later adult life. Averaging, so to speak, over all possible cases of this type, it becomes at once clear that the answer could at best be only a very heavily qualified one. Nevertheless, it does not seem too unreasonable to expect that such an inquiry might succeed at least in developing a working technique of prediction of tolerance limits and range of constancy of the relevant functions and skills. It was recognized from the very beginning of the effort that, as ever, there were bound to be many problems of technique and interpretation in assessing, in the necessarily 'reduced' situations afforded by the laboratory, the subtle variations in capacity occurring through adulthood with advancing years. In spite of these limitations, however, it is hoped that when the initial cross-sectional comparison can eventually be supplemented by the necessary longitudinal data, the work might conceivably help to provide a rational basis for adopting a retirement policy for flying personnel.

METHODS

It is not easy in a short space to give an adequate idea of the range of assessments made in a single day on a volunteer subject participating in the study. For the present purpose it will be sufficient to note that between 7 a.m. and noon, ultra low frequency ballistocardiogram stroke volume recorded before and after exercise[36], electrical impedance plethysmograph, pulse wave velocity and radioisotope determination of blood flow, as well as oxygen uptake and heart rate at maximum effort[28] are investigated, followed by psychological appraisal from 1 p.m. till 5.30 p.m.

Among the many possible investigations that might have been undertaken from the standpoint of psychology, the programme of laboratory experimentation outlined below acknowledges the well established findings on age changes in the resolving power of sensory detectors, efficiency of access to information near the time of its input and the speed of response[6, 50]. This investigation also draws upon the important guidelines established by the theory of human skill[2, 13, 14, 24]. From this point of view, a man performing a skilled task is an element in a system—an 'information transducer', and the relationship between input and output is an 'information transfer function'. The characteristics of this function are of interest to psychologists and physiologists, as well as to those physicians who speculate about what may be going on, and going wrong, in their patients' heads[47]. All this is, of course, to be understood in the sense of 'as if'; within a certain field of discourse; it is as if the brain were a channel along which information flows. Among the various approaches to the study of the integrative functions of the central nervous system, the attempts to estimate the rate at which intelligence is processed through it are of great importance, even though it is not easy at present to envisage the transmission of information in concrete neurophysiological terms.

The over-all design of the psychological experiments is intended to reflect the particular feature that flying requires, *inter alia*, making high-speed decisions and detecting low probability and low intensity signals, as well as an ability to receive and retain significant amounts of information in the course of routine control procedures. In the theory of the human operator of control systems the concept of 'channel capacity' is held to be fundamental, since the efficiency of coding and decoding operations performed by the brain must be assumed to depend very intimately on the entropy of messages in time being less than the overall capacity of the system. This formulation has in turn suggested the desirability, in principle, of evaluating 'reserve channel capacity' in the face of 'information overload' and reduced signal-to-noise ratio. The pilot of modern aircraft has become progressively less concerned with continuous manual monitoring and correspondingly more concerned with the interpretation of a large variety of signals for action that may originate from different sources simultaneously or in rapid succession. Insofar as control in this sense must involve transfer of information, the emphasis is on sustained readiness for quite complex judgments and decisions, many of which have to be made within very restricted time limits if they are not to become antiquated in relation to a rapidly changing display.

Rate of Gain of Information, 'Reserve Channel Capacity' and Central Intermittency

Information theory deals with the entire ensemble of possible signals for action which can be dealt with by the human operator in a skilled task, and the ways in which the signals must be encoded so as to convey the messages as fast as possible, given certain levels of unwanted disturbance and error tolerance. The amount of information in events is assessed in terms of the uncertainty which they resolve when they do actually happen. Different messages are, of course, likely to contain different amounts of information, but what is of interest is the average amount of information that can be gained. The novelty of this approach lies in the treatment of the whole set as relevant even though only one event occurs on any particular occasion. Experimentally, if the signals are arranged in a random sequence the average response latency is found to be approximately proportional to the logarithm of the number of equivalent choices or, in other words, to the minimum quantity of information that must be extracted from the input to identify it[25]. Consequently, the experiment which is concerned with the timing aspects of high-speed sequential decisions takes the form of recording in all the necessary detail (i.e., in μs (microseconds), together with error rates, employing the SETAR[51]) latencies of responses in serial choice tasks of known information content and observing their altered characteristics under various conditions of increased task load. The technique consists of introducing subsidiary tasks and measuring their effects on the performance of the concurrent main task, so that a comparison of average rates of gain of information, with and without overload, can yield an estimate of 'reserve channel capacity'. Except for certain unimportant details of instrumentation, the primary task is a conventional one in which the subject is presented with a random sequence of visual signals, generated by an automatic programmer, is required to identify them and then to operate an appropriate control, of the microswitch type, with the maximum of speed and minimum of error; the inter-signal intervals vary randomly over the range 0·5 to 5·0 s, in runs of some 300 in length, each signal having an equal probability of occurrence in ensembles of different number of alternatives, from three to eight. With some subjects, particularly test-pilots and senior airline pilots, data are also obtained for a 12-choice task. In addition, whenever the time schedule allows, supplementary information on central intermittency is also sought[13, 49]. The experimental procedure in this case consists of recording response latencies to sequences of random signals, about 200 in length, arranged in sets of two to eight equivalent choices, the intersignal intervals ranging from 100 to 2250 μs. After excluding the few unavoidable errors in recording resulting from an occasional overlap between successive events exceeding the capacity of the buffer storage of the SETAR, some 25 response times to the second signal at each interval are available for estimating the rate of gain of information.

The 'overload' tasks are designed to tax the subject's short-term memory and his ability to tolerate an interference with the aural monitoring of speech. Specifically, one such task (sub-task M) requires the subject to watch a succession of symbols (letters and numbers) projected onto the centre of the primary task display (each presentation lasting some 4 s) and to recall the material presented two stages earlier. This task is included because of the importance that is attached to sequential recall in the psychological literature on skill and ageing[50]. The other type of subsidiary task (sub-task DF) requires the subject, in addition to executing the manual responses in the primary task, to describe the successive characteristics of display and control, using a few simple code words; something approaching a 'stress' situation is imposed by arranging for a delay of 0·18 s in the auditory feedback from the subject's speech production[27]. This task has been introduced because it is felt that in present day flying the voice link with the ground control stations constitutes an important part of the pilot's job and from certain points of view could be suspected of being at least potentially capable of interfering with the main task of keeping the aircraft under control. Although there are many other possibilities for the selection of subsidiary tasks, it is assumed that the two actually employed are reasonably suitable for the purpose of gauging the extent to which an increase in information load may 'swamp' the man whose skill should on general grounds be susceptible to the effects of ageing.

Sensory Perception and Signal Detection Strategy

In the sensory perception studies the following procedures are employed on a routine basis:

(1) Measurement of visual accommodation, using the Costenbader Accommodometer. For some subjects an independent clinical assessment of this parameter is available in which Prince's Rule is used.

(2) Determination of the critical flicker fusion frequency (CFF) and the minimum perceptible inter-flash interval (IFI); in both cases the Grass PS 2 Photo-Stimulator is used, with a circular test area subtending an angle of 0·2 degree and the luminance reaching the level of 20 mL; flash duration is fixed at 10 μs and independent of frequency.

(3) Recording of the course of dark adaptation, employing the Goldmann-Weekers Adaptometer and their recommended test standards, i.e., light pre-adaptation at 2500 lx, brightness of test field at 6 lx, and a striped test figure with 100 per cent contrast. Recently the 'photostress test' has also been included in the procedure, in the light of the work of Severin, Tour and Kershaw[40], who, in the course

of an investigation of flash blindness have arrived at a possibly important method of studying early changes in macular function associated with ageing. They have succeeded in demonstrating that in the dark adapted eye the recovery from the after-effects of an intense flash of light is markedly slower for individuals over 40 years of age, as compared with younger adults. The procedure adopted in the present investigation consists of re-testing the subject, at the end of the afternoon schedule, with the Goldmann-Weekers Adaptometer up to the alpha-point threshold (i.e. five minutes of dark adaptation), and the measurement of the latencies (employing the SETAR) in recovery of the pre-flash threshold of the dark-adapted cones following each of a series of six consecutive flashes (25 J (joules) or 1.7×10^4 lm (lumens); flash duration 1 μs), presented at approximately 1·3 min intervals.

In addition, tachistoscopic recognition thesholds, using a three channel electronically controlled instrument (Scientific Instrument Prototype Co.), and fluctuations of auditory thresholds, employing Bekesy's[4] method and the Grason-Stadler Type E 800-4 Audiometer, are investigated in some detail, particularly with regard to what might be called 'threshold resistance' in the presence of deliberately introduced noise or under conditions of divided attention.

(4) In the case of Bekesy audiometry, the subject sits in a double-walled sound-proof room (IAC, 1201A), listens through TDH-39 earphones, and is required to 'track' his threshold over the range of frequencies 250–8000 Hz (at an attenuation rate of 2·5 dB/s). Initially threshold fluctuations of a pulsed tone (with an interruption rate of 2·5/s and a rise-decay time of 25 μs) are recorded for each ear; an additional tracing, employing a continuous tone, is obtained for the 'worse' ear, i.e., the one showing more hearing loss. Following this conventional procedure, noise audiometry is investigated in the following manner: for the 'better' ear. i.e., the one showing less hearing loss, the subject is required to retrace his pulsed-tone thresholds when 50 dB and 80 dB SPL wide-spectrum white noise is presented to the contralateral ear; for the 'worse' ear only the 80 dB SPL level of white noise is employed and the tone is a continuous one. In addition, for the 'worse' ear, fixed-frequency pulsed-tone tracings are obtained for that part of the range which shows the most pronounced hearing loss. The audiometric tracings, each run lasting approximately 7 min, are interspaced with other tests so as to minimize the effects of practice and transfer. Following Bekesy's[4] original recommendation, threshold values are interpolated between peaks and troughs in the tracings, i.e., the 'just not heard' and the 'just heard' tones, respectively.

(5) In the case of the tachistoscopic perception studies, recognition thresholds are obtained at exposure of $0.2\,\mu s$, with field luminances being held constant at approximately 10 mL, and the display—consisting of shapes, numbers, letters and words—subtending a visual angle of about 2 degrees (control condition). On some occasions, 'visual noise' patterns of the type described by Julesz[23] are exposed for the same duration as the signal card and immediately following it, in an attempt to 'erase' some of the information contained in the after-image (condition VN). In other runs the subject is required to monitor a subsidiary auditory task of the 'vigilance' type; he listens to two tones of different frequencies, one of which is occasionally interrupted, and has to acknowledge the occurrence of this event by operating an appropriate hand switch (condition DA). In all three conditions input information varies between groups of 10 cards from 2·8 to 76·5 binary units of information (bits) per symbol, the subject being told in advance about the relevant characteristics of each symbol group. To simplify computer analysis, information transmitted is assessed only at certain points of input entropy—low (i.e., 3 and 5 bits/symbol), intermediate (about 18 bits/symbol), and high (some 46 bits/symbol).

The data from the different experiments are punched on IBM cards and all further quantitative analyses are carried out with the aid of a Burroughs 5500 computer.

It will be appreciated that the above is not a complete description as much as an outline of the essential features of the methods employed, an outline which the author hopes is as informative as a limited presentation can be.

RESULTS

Taking a critical glance across the data so far accumulated, the most characteristic and striking trends are, again in outline, as follows below. The experimental details have been somewhat restricted in order to keep the central themes uncluttered. It should be noted that the number of subjects referred to in the different experiments is unequal because not all of the necessary equipment was available at the time the main study was initiated.

Sensory Perception: Vision

Visual Accommodation $(N = 198)$—The expectation of a reduced ability of the older eye to focus sharp images on the retina at short viewing distances has been fully sustained in the present study. In line with the classical results of Duane[16], the correlation coefficient between age and amplitude of accommodation, as measured by the appearance of first blurred image, is found to be of the order of $r = -0.75$, $p < 0.001$. As already mentioned, for about one-third of the subjects an independent clinical assessment is available in which the Prince's Rule was employed. In spite of certain minor discrepancies, due in part to a different criterion (disappearance of image), the two sets of data are essentially similar ($r = 0.80$, $p < 0.001$). In agreement with other studies[11], the mean values for the younger half of the sample are about six dioptres, for the older half about four dioptres.

Theories of presbyopia usually emphasize the diminished elasticity of the crystalline lens and anatomical changes in the ciliary muscle, but there are suggestions that genetic, dietetic and climatic factors may also be implicated[37]. Even so, it seems exceedingly doubtful—particularly in the light of other data accumulated in the present study—whether anything of further importance could be extrapolated from these variations in the refractive power of the lens to provide an 'index of ageing' in the visual pathway[48].

CFF and IFI (*N = 228 and N = 217*)—For this again only a few words are needed. Although temporal discrimination is necessarily limited by intensity discrimination, the data on CFF and IFI (intercorrelated at the level of $r = -0.44$, $p < 0.001$, which have been interpreted by some investigators in a similar manner to that of the findings on visual accommodation, fail to confirm convincingly the expected change of threshold with age. The values of correlation coefficients are very small indeed: $r = 0.01$, $p < 0.90$ for the CFF, and $r = 0.14$, $p < 0.05$ for the IFI. For about one-quarter of the subjects these estimates of the temporal resolution of the visual system are also available employing a version of the classical psychophysical method, after the manner of the technique of Bekesy[4] for the continuous recording of auditory threshold fluctuations. Although the variance tends to increase somewhat in this case, the correlation between average values obtained by the conventional and the 'tracking' methods is of the order of $r = 0.80$ ($p < 0.001$) for the CFF and $r = 0.60$ ($p < 0.001$) for the IFI.

Unfortunately, because of technical limitations, it was not possible to vary systematically the levels of light time in the flicker cycle[31], and to this extent the present evidence can perhaps be regarded as not fully conclusive.

Dark Adaptation (*N = 286*)—The determination of threshold energies in the course of dark adaptation confirms the expected correlation with age at both alpha and terminal points ($r = 0.22$, $p < 0.001$ and $r = 0.41$, $p < 0.001$ respectively). However, since the data also reveal somewhat lower average values for the pilots than those quoted for the general population employing the same adaptometer[17], it seems permissible to assume that as an occupational group they are better observers and consequently may be able to extract information more efficiently even at very low levels of signal-to-noise ratio. Furthermore, as shown in *Figure 1*, in the 'photo-stress test'

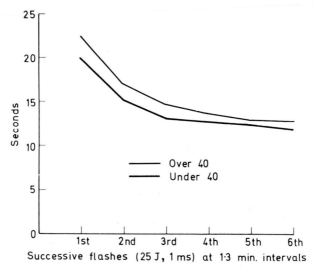

Figure 1. Latency of recovery of pre-flash threshold in the dark-adapted eye (alpha point)

(N = 107) the duration of experimentally induced scotomata following each of the consecutive flashes is progressively reduced. Although the average latency of recovery from blindness produced by the first flash is correlated with age at the level of $r = 0.20$, $p < 0.01$, the latencies following the last three flashes are not significantly greater for the older subjects ($r = 0.08$, $p < 0.10$), suggesting that perhaps no special significance need be attached to the presumptive change in macular function with age in individuals free of eye pathology. Surprisingly, the values of threshold at the alpha point during the dark adaptation test are negatively correlated with those for the latency of recovery of the pre-flash level during the 'photostress test' ($r = -0.27$, $p < 0.01$; $r = -0.35$ when age is held constant), indicating that different retinal mechanisms may be involved (i.e., receptive and transmission systems, respecively).

It is instructive to reflect in this connection, that although the classical theory of vision relates sensitivity of the eye to concentration of rhodopsin—leading to explanations of age changes in dark adaptation in terms of slower regeneration of the visual purple— newer theories postulate constant efficiency of the retina and a 'variable gain' mechanism acting as an amplifier between retinal receptors and optic nerve fibres[1]. In the case of dark adaptation it may be supposed that time is required to 'reset' the gain mechanism to its maximum value, the gradual improvement in seeing following the increase in amplification[38]. On this view of visual discrimination it is tempting, but perhaps rash, to expect that the more experienced an observer, e.g. a professional pilot, the less amplification would be needed to present the information to the brain.

On general grounds, as well as within the framework of any particular theory of ageing, it should be borne in mind that measurements of the resolving power of the sensory systems must inevitably reflect not only the properties of the peripheral detectors, but also the intelligent use of perceptual skills[48, 50].

Tachistoscopic Recognition Thresholds (N = 101)—In the tachistoscopic experiments it is found that the channel capacity curves are remarkably near perfect transmission of information up to about 20 bits. They drop by some 20 to 25 per cent in the presence of 'visual noise' and there is a similar change of the order of up to 20 per cent under conditions of division of attention. This trend is in line with other findings, which suggest that diverting attention away from a high-information signal is likely to produce an effect resembling a reduction in its intensity[10]. The relevant data are summarized in *Figure 2*, from which it will be seen that there is some lowering of performance with increasing age at the higher levels of information input, reflecting the well established fact that the ageing eye, because of miosis and lenticular yellowing, requires more light[48] (as could be expected from this, the data for dark adaptation and tachistoscopic perception are intercorrelated at the level of $r = 0.28$, $p < 0.01$). The individual differences in this respect are, however, larger than group differences and none of the correlation coefficients attain the level of statistical significance: $r = -0.17$, $p < 0.10$ in the control condition; $r = -0.01$, $p < 0.90$ in the 'visual noise' condition; and $r = -0.07$, $p < 0.20$ in the divided attention condition. Paradoxically, a comparison of information transfer functions in the presence of 'visual noise' suggests that it is the younger pilots, i.e. under 40 years of age, who may be more embarrassed by this reduction of the signal-to-noise ratio. They show a relative loss of the order of up to 25 per cent as compared with that of up to only 20 per cent for the over 40 age group. In other words, the older pilots appear to adopt a more efficient strategy for signal detection and one which outweighs at least some of the limitations imposed by the peripheral end of the visual pathway. Their capacity to deal with the equivocal odds under conditions of divided attention is lower than that of the younger group essentially for the same reason, but very likely also because this involves short-term retention and recall (up to 20 per cent relative loss, as compared with about 15 per cent for the younger pilots; on the other hand, the proportion of signals missed in the

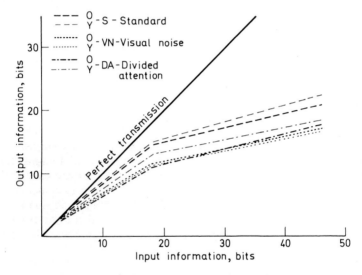

Figure 2. Channel capacity curves for recognition of shapes, numbers, letters and words at 0·2 ms exposure

subsidiary auditory task, of the order of 10 per cent on the average, is not related to age: $r = 0·12$, $p < 0·30$). In spite of these disadvantages, however, the differential values for information transfer under the 'visual noise' and divided attention conditions, as compared with the control, do not reveal any decline with age ($r = -0·24$, $p < 0·05$).

A relationship can probably be traced between these data and the statistical theory of sensory thresholds[20] which assumes, unlike conventional psychophysics, that shifts in the 'criterion' which the human observer of faint signals must employ in arriving at a decision about the input may be promoted by training and further enhanced by experience. It is of further theoretical interest that these results are not inconsistent with those reported by Gregory[21]. In a carefully controlled experiment designed to test the hypothesis of Barlow[1] and

Rose[38] that 'noise' in the optic pathway limits its sensitivity, the evidence suggested that 'retinal noise' is not likely to increase with age, whereas 'neural noise' at a more central level might. Similarly, in a study of information intake and discrimination in relation to age, Crossman and Szafran[15] have felt obliged to conclude from their data showing easily discriminable signals to be relatively more affected than difficult ones—each category defined quantitatively in terms of a 'confusion function'—that changes in performance with age should be attributed to an elevated level of 'neural noise' in the perceptual mechanisms. They offer the speculation that in physiological terms the noise might be an increasing rate of spontaneous firing of neurones, or a greater likelihood for neighbouring neurones to excite one another by non-synaptic pathways. It follows from their argument that differential thresholds are likely to be much less affected by ageing than absolute ones.

Sensory Perception: Hearing

Bekesy Audiometry $(N = 287)$—In the auditory perception studies the important feature of more efficient use of perceptual skills by professional pilots, as compared with the general population, becomes once again apparent. *Figure 3* contrasts the average hearing threshold levels at four frequencies observed in the Lovelace Study with the corresponding estimates for the 'better' ear reported in several large scale surveys in the U.S.A.[32]. There has been some question as to whether or not Bekesy thresholds, assessed conventionally by mid-points between audibility and inaudibility, are in fact strictly comparable to those obtained by traditional audiometric techniques; some investigators have argued that the mid-point estimates may be too high, the inaudibility points giving a better fit[12]. If so, the comparison would be even more in favour of the pilots.

As in the National Health Survey[32], the left ear shows more pronounced hearing loss than the right ear in a greater proportion of cases, and the dissimilarity between the two ears becomes more striking for the higher tones. The reason for this trend, depicted in Table 1, is not clear, however.

It is of considerable theoretical interest that the older pilots, as compared with the younger, do not show the traditionally expected more severe change of the 'effective threshold' in the presence of white noise input to the contralateral ear. Signal detection under these unfavourable circumstances appears to be surprisingly efficient and, in spite of increased presbyacusis, there is no evidence of any disproportional loss in auditory discrimination with advancing age

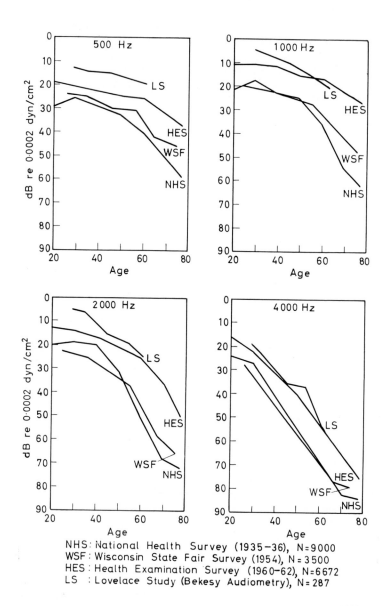

NHS: National Health Survey (1935–36), N=9000
WSF: Wisconsin State Fair Survey (1954), N=3500
HES: Health Examination Survey (1960–62), N=6672
LS : Lovelace Study (Bekesy Audiometry), N=287

Figure 3. Comparison of average hearing thresholds by age at 500, 1000, 2000 and 4000 Hz for the 'better' ear

$(r = -0.01, p < 0.80$ to $r = -0.05, p < 0.50)$. By way of illustration, the average differences between the pulsed tone thresholds in quiet and in noise for the 'better' ear are shown in *Figure 4* for three age groups. The corresponding values for the continuous tone in the 'worse' ear reveal essentially the same pattern. The precise significance of this paradoxical trend cannot as yet be assessed with any

TABLE 1

Proportion of Subjects with Threshold Differences ($\Delta > 5$ db) Between the Two Ears: National Health Survey (N = 6672) and Lovelace Study (N = 283) Data

Frequency (Hz)	National Health Survey (Standard audiometry)		Lovelace Study (Bekesy audiometry)	
	Right ear 'Worse' (percentage)	Left ear 'Worse' (percentage)	Right ear 'Worse' (percentage)	Left ear 'Worse' (percentage)
250	—	—	20·6	10·5**
500	15·9	11·5	16·9	11·5
750	—	—	14·9	12·8
1000	10·7	9·8	13·5	14·9
1500	—	—	17·2	19·3
2000	13·2	17·6	15·9	29·1**
3000	14·7	22·1	18·6	37·8***
4000	18·0	23·6	20·3	38·9***
6000	23·1	27·1	25·7	36·5*
8000	—	—	24·3	33·8*

* Difference significant at 5 per cent level
** Difference significant at 1 per cent level
*** Difference significant at 0·1 per cent level or better

degree of confidence, but it is noteworthy that it seems to be in line with other reports that older pilots can deal quite efficiently with auditory inputs in the presence of noise[8, 30]. Whether the concept of critical bandwidths[18] could satisfactorily account for these effects is conjectural, for much more rigorous control would be required than has proved feasible in the present study. An explanation in terms of shortening of the loudness scale has to be carefully considered before the one in terms of varying level of random neural activity can be preferred. However, detailed analysis of the small discrepancies between mean levels for the appearance and disappearance of continuous and pulsed signals in the 'worse' ear, reveals that the average threshold values for the older subjects, as compared with those for the younger, do not favour an explanation in terms of recruitment phenomena, proposed by some investigators[30]. Moreover, the threshold difference is negatively correlated with age ($r =$

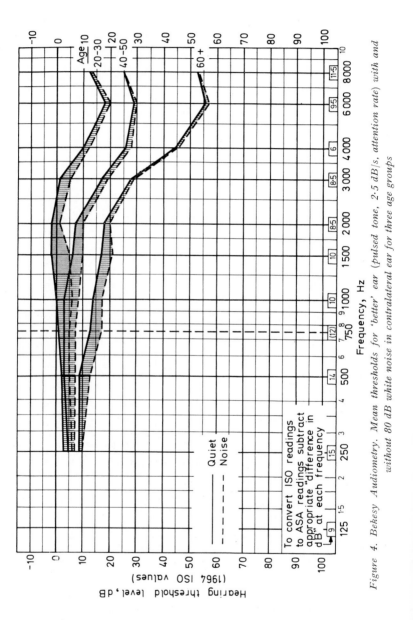

Figure 4. Bekesy Audiometry. Mean thresholds for 'better' ear (pulsed tone, 2·5 dB/s, attention rate) with and without 80 dB white noise in contralateral ear for three age groups

$-0.23, p < 0.001$) Furthermore, if we accept the original suggestion of Bekesy that a reduced amplitude of tracing is likely to be observed where loudness recruitment is present, such differences as can be discerned between the pulsed and continuous signals over the critical range of frequencies showing hearing loss (i.e. 3,000–8,000 Hz) reveal again a negative correlation with age ($r = -0.28, p < 0.01$). On the average, the width of the tracings for the younger subjects is of the order of 9 dB in the case of pulsed tone and 7dB in that of a continuous one. For the older subjects the corresponding values are around 8 dB in both cases. Clinical studies suggest that whereas the normal envelope of the Bekesy audiogram is about 7–10 dB, in cases of recruitment it is less than 5 dB wide[35]. The evidence adduced here is in line with that of Yantis[53] who has questioned whether recruitment occurs in conjunction with presbyacusis.

What is even more surprising, and could not have been predicted from the classical data on binaural masking, is that the difference between the fixed frequency tracings obtained under quiet and 85 dB SPL white noise conditions ($N = 134$; age range 29–61), in favour of the latter, appears to be positively correlated with age ($r = 0.35. p < 0.01$). Some representative individual records are shown in *Figure 5*. The understanding of this finding is far from easy, particularly since very little is known about the nature of high-tone deafness. A conventional theory, based on clinical and pathological findings, is that there may be two types of presbyacusia: one in which the lesion is in the organ of Corti at the basal turn; and another in which a partial atrophy of the nerve supply, again at the base of the cochlea, is more marked. The reason why ageing processes should selectively affect the basal end of the cochlea is not understood at present[39]. Detailed comparison of air and bone conduction thresholds suggests that the changes characteristic of ageing may also involve the connective tissues of the middle ear[33]. An unusual point of view is that nerve deafness might be caused by raised level of 'neural noise' associated with damage to the hair cells[21]. This would tend to lower the signal-to-noise ratio and consequently produce the effect of high levels of externally introduced noise having relatively less impact on the hearing threshold[50].

Although further experimental studies are needed, it is perhaps possible to view these unexpected findings in the light of the suggestion that amplification of ambient sensory inflow may, in the case of older adults, increase the 'gain' of the mechanisms upon which the high-information signal impinges[9]. The increase in 'gain' might correspond to a higher level of 'vigilance'[22] or 'arousal'[23]. On the other hand, since the 'threshold resistance' data for audiometry and those

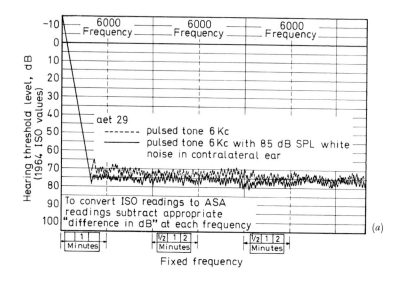

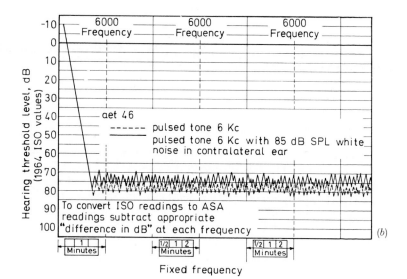

Figure 5. Bekesey audiometry: fixed frequency tracings in quiet and with white noise in the contalateral ear. (a) Subject age 29; (b) subject aged 46.

TABLE 2

Rate of Gain of Information. Regression Analysis of Individual Performance
Records for Five Age Groups

Baseline Condition

Age groups	Choice reaction time $= a + b \log_2 n$	t-test on the slope constant	Rate of gain of information (bits/s)	Standard deviation of the rate (bits/s)
20–29·5 Mean Age 27·6 N = 49	0·289+0·077	54·09***	5·03	0·44
30–39·5 Mean Age 34·0 N = 133	0·272+0·083	103·71***	5·01	0·51
40–49·5 Mean age 44·8 N = 130	0·293+0·080	97·94***	4·89	0·44
50–59·5 Mean Age 53·2 N = 59	0·287+0·089	66·21***	4·91	0·41
60+ Mean age 60·5 N = 25	0·282+0·084	38·00***	4·88	0·46

Overload Condition

Twenties	0·382+0·089	33·45***	3·93	0·56
Thirties	0·394+0·088	53·00***	3·89	0·50
Forties	0·435+0·089	43·23***	3·62	0·43
Fifties	0·468+0·083	27·61***	3·59	0·33
Sixty and over	0·444+0·093	18·52***	3·56	0·42

Correlation Coefficient r (N = 396)

	Baseline	Overload	Difference between baseline overload
Comparison with Age			
Intercept constant (a)	0·02	0·26***	0·24**
Slope constant (b)	0·09	−0·02	0·08
Rate of gain of information (R)	−0·10	−0·35***	0·28***

Comparison Between Tasks

Rate of Gain of Information:
Baseline × Overload   r = 0·68***
Overload × Sub-task 'M'   r = 0·83***
Overload × Sub-task 'DF'   r = 0·88***
Sub-task 'M' × Sub-task 'DF'   r = 0·73***

** Significant at 1 per cent level.
*** Significant at 0·1 per cent level or better.

for tachistoscopic recognition are inter-correlated ($r = 0.44$, $p < 0.001$), the alternative hypothesis which deserves consideration is that an important change of 'strategy' in detecting distorted signals may occur as a cumulative effect of prolonged experience and that this change can be relatively immune to the adverse effects of ageing in selected individuals.

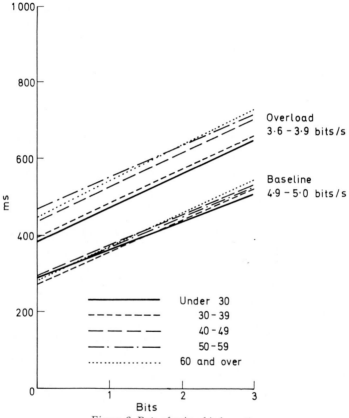

Figure 6. Rate of gain of information

High-speed Sequential Decisions

Rate of Gain of Information ($N = 396$)—A perusal of Table 2 and *Figure 6* makes it quite clear that estimates of 'channel capacity' in the baseline condition are not significantly related to age and that therefore to this extent the traditional association between advanced age and slowing of decision has to be challenged. Although the slope constant shows some unimpressive tendency to increase with age, basically the regression lines for the higher age decades are displaced upward, changing the intercept constant. This feature is essentially preserved in the results for the 'overload' conditions, which, however, also indicate a small but consistent negative correlation with age.

On the average, the amount of error made in the primary and subsidiary tasks (of the order of 5 per cent and 15 per cent respectively) is too small to be suggestive of any changes in perceptual grasp and thus at this stage of the analysis, for the sake of brevity, it may well be disregarded. It is particularly in the short-term memory subsidiary task that age and error are correlated at the level of $r = 0.16$ ($p < 0.05$). Bearing this in mind, it can perhaps be concluded that older pilots are likely to be relatively more susceptible than the younger to the effects of information overload if this involves short-term recall when some other activity intervenes during the period of retention. It is not clear, however, whether the inference that, to this extent, they may be said to possess less 'reserve mental capacity' than the young is really forced upon us by the data. The paramount difficulty is that of deciding whether a difference of the order of 0.3 bits/s in the rate of gain of information can be regarded as a compelling indication of loss.

These general trends are reflected in the pattern of results for a higher degree of choice than those employed in the main study. For some 52 subjects, the only differences approaching, but not quite reaching, an acceptable level of statistical significance are with respect to the initial and total rate under conditions of information overload; in line with other results[15], the incremental rate remains essentially unaltered.

The over-all reliability of the procedure of estimating the rates of gain of information appears to be satisfactory. For some 50 subjects retested after an interval of approximately one year, the correlation coefficients for the baseline and overload conditions are of the order of $r = 0.70$ ($p < 0.001$) and $r = 0.60$ ($p < 0.01$) respectively. One-half of these subjects have recently been examined for the third time and the correlation coefficients between the second and third year results are of the order of $r = 0.70$ ($p < 0.001$) for the baseline and $r = 0.80$ ($p < 0.001$) for the overload conditions. Since this group of pilots constitutes the nucleus of a longitudinal study, it will be imperative to check further whether these preliminary indications are not misleading.

It might be of interest to consider briefly the possibility that

43

cerebral ambilaterality, as indicated by hand dominance and family history of left-handedness, may render an individual relatively more susceptible to the effects of stress[54], here defined as 'information overload'. An examination of the comparative data for left-handed and right-handed pilots reveals a difference of the order of 0·10 bits/s in the rate of gain of information under conditions of overload, which does not reach the level of statistical reliability. However, the incidence of 'dysphasic episodes' in the verbal sub-task, with the auditory monitoring of speech delayed, is quite substantially higher for the sinistrals (incidence of some 30 per cent compared with about 10 per cent for the dextrals, $p < 0.001$). One may perhaps interpret this trend as indicating that the left-handed individuals are indeed more vulnerable in the face of information overload but that they are so only in the language sphere. Apparently they are able to compensate for what may be an embarrassment to them in such a way as to maintain fully adequate performance in the principal perceptual-motor task. These are, of course, only vague assertions and it should be borne in mind that the precise significance of this trend, if genuine, for aviation cannot be easily assessed because of the numerous imponderable factors involved[19]. Clearly, even if fully substantiated, a generalization of this type would necessarily have to be interpreted with great caution in almost any practical situation.

Although further experimental and theoretical inquiry is obviously needed to discover the limits within which these inferences are justifiable, it is clear that, insofar as skill proficiency can be gauged at all outside the flying situation itself, the routine aspects of the professional pilot's skill are, on the present evidence, unlikely to be seriously affected by ageing over the usual span of normal working life.

Central Intermittency ($N = 48$; *age range: 20's–50's*)—When, in psychological experiments, the subject is required to respond as rapidly as possible to a signal closely following another, an increase in response latency is observed. It has become customary to refer to this aspect of high-speed sequential performance as the 'psychological refractory period', on analogy with changes in threshold of neurones, following the propagation of impulses, where the recovery is divisible into an absolute and a relative phase. Welford[49] has argued that the slowing of response to the second of two successive signals is due not to a temporary reduction of sensitivity in the cerebral mechanisms subserving the 'computing process' but rather to the feature that 'no two central organizing times can overlap'. The theory postulates that if the central mechanisms are already analysing a signal, or are occupied by the feedback from a response, when a second signal arrives, the processing of it is delayed until the organization of the first has been completed, for 'new sensory impulses entering the brain while the central computing process is going on would disturb it'[13]. Some experiments suggest, however, that the delays observed may be due not to the start of the processing of the second signal being prevented, but to the decision mechanism

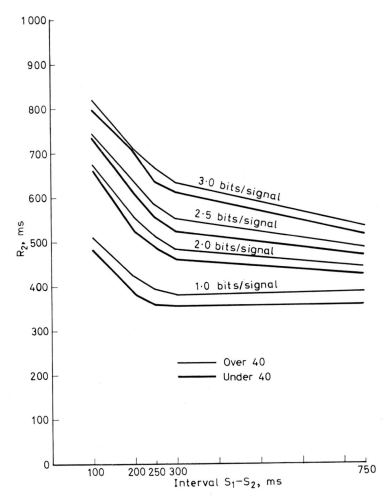

Figure 7. Mean response latency R_2 at five intervals S_1–S_2 for 2, 4, 6 and 8-choice tasks

45

operating less quickly for a short time after it had again become free to deal with signals[9]. Such an interpretation, if correct, implies that the analogy with physiological refractoriness is more exact than commonly assumed. Possibly it is important to distinguish between an 'absolute phase', in which signal analysis is held up until the central processes already begun have ended, and a 'relative phase' during

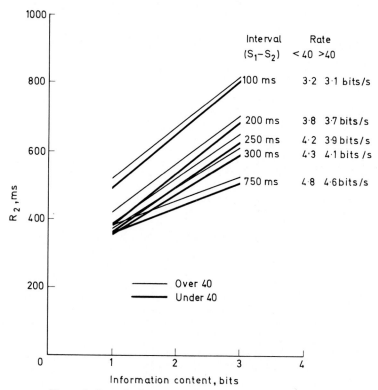

Figure 8. Central refractoriness and rate of gain of information

which the speed of decision is lowered, the duration of both phases being in part a function of signal probability. This distinction, if valid, is of some interest in relation to the question of central intermittency in continuous performance, when the size of the ensemble of possible signals varies.

It seems fairly evident from an analysis of response times to the second signal (R_2) at the different intervals between successive signals (S_1–S_2), summarized in *Figures 7* and *8*, that what can at present be inferred from the slopes does not point to any adverse change with age in either of the two hypothetical components of the refractory phase with increase in information content. Although some presumptive evidence of a longer 'sampling time' for incoming information can be discerned ($r = -0.17$, $p < 0.05$ on a one-tailed test), none of the age differences in the rate of gain of information attain an acceptable level of statistical reliability. The possibility of an increase in central intermittency is of considerable interest, however, because of its relevance for the theory of a varying with age level of random fluctuations in nerve-impulse frequency. The extended duration over which information could be integrated would increase the signal-to-noise ratio and thus allow the input to be more easily distinguished from the system noise[21]. A strategy of this kind, if adopted by the brain, might conceivably enhance the selective responsiveness of central mechanisms to high information signals.

DISCUSSION

This brief glance across the results of an investigation still in progress suggests certain preliminary conclusions, some of which may be of general import for psychological medicine as applied in the field of aviation.

In the first place, there is some evidence, at present suggestive rather than conclusive, that a trend in the combined cardio-pulmonary and psychological data for the pilots, who (needless to say, are in perfect health from the clinical standpoint) can be discerned. Comparing the efficiency of cardiac output—as assessed on the basis of ballistocardiogram stroke volume and of heart rate recorded after exercise—and the magnitude of reduction in the speed of decision under conditions of information overload, a negative correlation of the order of $r = -0.23$ was obtained [42, 44, 45], and found to be statistically reliable at the level of $p < 0.01$. Furthermore, the results of the pulmonary physiology studies under conditions of maximum effort were also found to be in line with this trend in that the maximal oxygen pulse, a ratio measure based on oxygen uptake and heart rate, was correlated with the difference in the rate of gain of information between baseline and overload at the level of $r = -0.20$ ($p < 0.01$). However, in view of the relatively low magnitude of these coefficients, the substantial increase in the size of the sample has since then required a much more sophisticated statistical analysis, employing the method of step-wise regression, the results of which regrettably are not yet available. Assuming that the agreement between the psychological and cardio-pulmonary tests observed

47

during the earlier stages of the study is not misleading, it is difficult to dismiss the possibility that the intriguing and no doubt complex relationship which it suggests might imply that the analytical operations performed by the brain in a high-grade skill are more likely to depend on the efficiency of the lung–heart system than upon age *per se*.

Although it would not be profitable at present to attempt to formulate a theory in strictly physiological terms, and therefore the hypothesis must be regarded as too sketchy, this interpretation has nevertheless the advantage of linking the psychological and physiological data accumulated in a number of studies[7, 34, 41], including the present one. If the idea that 'neural noise' within the central nervous system increases with age is at all feasible, it does not seem unreasonable to suppose that a reduced rate of cerebral blood flow may contribute to the hypothetical random activity in brain cells. Some qualified support for this contention can be found in studies which report that an important factor underlying EEG changes with age is a reduction of cerebral oxygen uptake[34]. There are reasons to believe that oxygen uptake probably parallels cardiac output, although much of this relationship is inadequately understood at present.

In the second place, as already mentioned, even though the slowing with age observed in the face of additional information challenge is formally equivalent to a somewhat lower 'channel capacity', it does not unequivocally suggest a reduced reserve capacity, for example, for adequate responses to sudden emergencies. It may mean that the forms of code transformations of the information entering the central nervous system are adjusted to the characteristics of the available channel according to the nature of prevailing input and the weight assigned to other inputs. At these high neural levels, the information transfer could be taking place in terms of detection of gradients of activity in the channel, rather than by the detection of maxima[52]. Such a process would have the advantage of being able to operate efficiently in a noisy system and there is some direct neurophysiological evidence that neurones in the auditory pathway may indeed have the properties required by the theory[52]. It must be borne in mind, however, that more detailed interpretation of these findings would be desirable, particularly with regard to the characteristics of short-term storage and retrieval of information. On the other hand, a number of features of sensory perception commonly investigated in studies of ageing appear, in the light of the present material, quite unremarkable. Thus, for example, even though the amplitude of accommodation is reduced in later adulthood, and in spite of the fact that less and less light reaches the retina, Weale[48] is correct in questioning the justification for inferring from variations in ocular refraction or pupil diameter any 'law of physiological ageing'[5] governing visual performance. It would appear from the data adduced here that it might be more pertinent to reflect on how effective the increased visual and auditory thresholds are in unfavourable circumstances, in which case we need not necessarily be pessimistic. Indeed, a critical review of the literature on high-grade skill bears out the impression that under a wide range of different forms of stress, as in conditions of fatigue and organically based age changes, the central nervous system is able to maintain the very high efficiency of its integrative action[3].

In the third place, the evidence reviewed here, together with other cases reported in the literature, conclusively demonstrate that many of the characteristics allegedly suggestive of 'relative functional loss' are not a necessary feature of the performance of a professionally successful and healthy middle-aged or older individual. Possibly, in sketching the 'ageing profile' of capacities from a physiological and psychological standpoint, considerations of reserve channel capacity and signal detection strategy may eventually introduce important qualifications to the doctrine of 'wear-and-tear', a commonly preferred 'model' of the ageing processes. For the time being, however, this broad question must remain a controversial issue on which more experimental detail would be welcome. At least in the case of professional pilots, their impressive ability to guard against the very subtle shift with the passage of time in the direction of 'chronic fatigue' is probably a combination of a specific capacity to adapt rapidly to changing requirements and conditions and of a general willingness to plan the effort so as to maximize the likelihood of sustained performance in the skills which provide their *raison d'être*[2, 3, 24] In some ways it is unfortunate that the theory of the human operator of control systems is only of limited value in handling a quality of this kind, for it undoubtedly deserves to be taken fully into account when discussing the effects of ageing on flying personnel. The evidence adduced here makes it possible to argue that at least in this profession, age *per se* could not necessarily be equated with decline, nor should it be considered a sufficient reason for retirement. In suggesting these conclusions, however, it must be recognized that, as always, there is room for other views.

ACKNOWLEDGEMENTS

The investigation reported in this paper was supported by the United States Public Health Service Research Grant No. HD-0518 from the

National Institutes of Health. The late Dr W. Randolph Lovelace, II, had been closely associated with the work from its inception. Thanks are also due to the late Professor Sir Frederic Bartlett, C.B.E., F.R.S., Professor J. E. Birren, Professor H. Kay and Dr J. H. Price for comment and criticism; to Dr N. T. Welford and E. E. Fletcher for help with the instrumentation; to A. Pavlos, V. Bogo, A. Almagro, Mrs J. Massey, Miss C. Baca and Mrs J. Hicks for assistance in the testing of subjects; and to J. Paden, Mrs B. Sklower and Mrs M. Elrick for help with the computer analysis of the data.

REFERENCES

1. Barlow, H. B. (1956). 'Retinal Noise and Absolute Threshold'. *J. opt. Soc. Am.* **46,** 634
2. Bartlett, Sir F. C. (1947). 'The Measurement of Human Skill'. *Br. med. J.* **1,** 835, 877
3. — (1962). 'The Outlook for Flying Personnel Research'. In *Human Problems of Supersonic and Hypersonic Flight.* Ed. by A. B. Barbour and H. E. Whittingham. London: Pergamon Press
4. Bekesy, G. von (1947). 'A New Audiometer'. *Acta oto-lar.* **35,** 411
5. Bernstein, F. and Bernstein, M. (1945). 'Law of Physiologic Ageing as Derived from Long Range Data on Refraction of Human Eye'. *Archs Ophthal.* **34,** 378
6. Birren, J. E. (1964). *The Psychology of Ageing.* Englewood Cliffs, N. J.: Prentice-Hall
7. — Butler, R. N., Greenhouse, S. W., Sokoloff, L. and Yarrow, M. R. (1963). *Human Ageing.* Washington, D. C.: U.S. Department of Health, Education and Welfare
8. Bragg, V. C. and Greene, J. W. (1963). 'Speech discrimination in Senior Naval Aviators'. *U.S. Naval School, Aviation Medical Research Report.* August 1963
9. Brebner, J. and Szafran, J. (1961). 'A Study of the Psychological Refractory Phase in Relation to Ageing'. *Gerontologia* **5,** 241
10. Broadbent, D. E. and Gregory, M. (1963). 'Division of Attention and the Decision Theory of a Signal Detection'. *Proc. R. Soc. (B)* **158,** 222
11. Bruckner, R. (1958). 'Uber Methoden Longitudinaler Alterforschung am Auge'. *Ophthalmologica* **138,** 59
12. Corso, J. (1956). 'Effects of Testing Methods on Hearing Thresholds'. *A.M.A. Archs. Otolar* **63,** 78
13. Craik, K. J. W. (1947). 'Theory of the Human Operator in Control Systems'. *Br. J. Psychol.* **38,** 56, 142
14. Crossman, E. R. F. W. (1964). 'Information Processes in Human Skill'. *Br. med. Bull.* **20,** 32
15. — and Szafran, J. (1956). 'Changes with Age in the Speed of Information Intake and Discrimination'. *Experientia* (Suppl.) **4,** 128

16. Duane, A. (1922). 'Studies in Monocular and Binocular Accommodation with their Clinical Application'. *Am. J. Ophthal.* **5**, 865

17. Fankhauser, F. and Schmidt, T. (1957). 'Die Untersuchung der Funktionen des Dunkeladaptierten Auges mit dem Adaptometer Goldmann-Weekers'. *Ophthalmologica* **133**, 264

18. Fletcher, H. (1940). 'Auditory patterns'. *Rev. mod. Phys.* **12**, 47

19. Gerhardt, R. (1959). Left-handedness and Laterality in Pilots'. In *Medical Aspects of Flight Safety.* London: Pergamon Press

20. Green, D. M. and Swets, J. A. (1966). *Signal Detection Theory and Psychophysics.* New York: John Wiley

21. Gregory, R. L. (1957). 'Increase in "Neurological Noise" as a Factor in Ageing'. *Proceedings of the Fourth International Congress on Gerontology*, **1**, 314. Merano, 1957

22. Head, Sir H. (1926). *Aphasia and Kindred Disorders of Speech.* London: Cambridge University Press

23. Hebb, D. O. (1955). 'Drives and the CNS'. *Psychol. Rev.* **62**, 243

24. Hick, W. E. (1951). 'Man as an Element in a Control System'. *Research* **4**, 112

25. —— (1952). 'On the Rate of Gain of Information'. *Q. Jl exp. Psychol.* **4**, 11

26. Julesz, B. (1961). 'Binocular Depth Perception and Pattern Recognition'. In *Information Theory.* Ed. by C. Cherry. London: Butterworths

27. Lee, B. S. (1950). Effects of Delayed Speech Feed-back'. *J. acoust. Soc. Am.* **22**, 824

28. Luft, U. C. (1967). 'Early Detection of Deteriorative Trends in Pulmonary Function'. In *The Art of Predictive Medicine.* Ed. by W. L. Marxer and G. R. Cowgill. Springfield, Ill.: Charles C. Thomas

29. McFarland, R. A. (1953). *Human Factors in Air Transportation,* New York: McGraw-Hill

30. —— and O'Doherty, B. M. (1959). 'Work and Occupational Skills'. In *Handbook of Ageing and the Individual.* Ed. by J. E. Birren. Chicago: Univeristy of Chicago Press

31. —— Warren, A. B. and Karis, C. (1958). 'Alterations in Critical Flicker Frequency as a Function of Age and Light–Dark Ratio. *J. exp. Psychol.* **56**, 529

32. National Health Survey (1965). *Hearing Levels of Adults by Age and Sex. U.S.* 1960–62. Washington, D.C.: U.S. Department of Health, Education and Welfare

33. Nixon, J. C., Glorig, A. and High, W. S. (1962). 'Changes in Air and Bone Conduction Thresholds as a Function of Age'. *J. Lar. Otol.* **76**, 288

34. Obrist, W. D. (1965). 'Electroencephalographic Approach to Age Changes in Response Speed'. In *Behavior, Ageing and the Nervous System.* Ed. by A. T. Welford and J. E. Birren. Springfield, Ill.: Charles C. Thomas

35. Palva, T. (1956). 'Recruitment Tests at Low Sensation Levels'. *Laryngoscope* **66**, 1519
36. Proper, E. (1968). 'Age-related Changes in Professional Pilots as Defined by the Klensch-Schwarzer Ultra-low Frequency Ballisto-cardiogram'. *Bibl. Cardiol.* **20**, 50
37. Rambo, V. C. and Sangal, S. P. (1960). 'A Study of the Accommodation of the People of India'. *Am. J. Ophthal.* **49**, 993
38. Rose, A. (1948). 'The Sensitivity Performance of the Human Eye as an Absolute Scale'. *J. opt. Soc. Am.* **38**, 196
39. Schuknecht, H. F. (1955). 'Presbycusis'. *Laryngoscope* **65**, 402
40. Severin, S. L., Tour, R. L. and Kershaw, R. H. (1967). 'Macular Function and Photo-stress Test'. *Archs Ophthal., N.Y.* **77**, 2
41. Spieth, W. (1965). 'Slowness of Task Performance and Cardiovascular Diseases'. In *Behavior, Ageing and the Nervous System*. Ed. by A. T. Welford and J. E. Birren. Springfield, Ill.: Charles C. Thomas
42. Szafran, J. (1963). 'Age Difference in Choice Reaction Time and Cardiovascular Status Among Pilots'. *Nature, Lond.* **200**, 904
43. — (1964). 'Prospects in Psychological Research on Ageing'. In *Age with a Future*. Ed. by P. F. Hansen. Copenhagen: Munksgaard
44. — (1965). 'Decision Processes and Ageing'. In *Behavior, Ageing and the Nervous System*. Ed. A. T. Welford and J. E. Birren. Springfield, Ill.: Charles C. Thomas
45. — (1966). 'Age Differences in the Rate of Gain of Information, Signal Detection Strategy and Cardiovascular Status Among Pilots'. *Gerontologia* **12**, 6
46. — (1968). 'Psychophysiological Studies of Ageing in Pilots'. In *Human Behavior and Ageing: Recent Advances in Research and Theory*. Ed. by G. A. Talland. New York: Academic Press
47. Thomas, E. L. (1964). 'Information and Eye Movements'. *Fifth IBM Medical Symposium*. New York. 1964
48. Weale, R. A. (1963). *The Ageing Eye*. London: Lewis
49. Welford, A. T. (1952). 'The Psychological Refractory Period and the Timing of High-speed Performance'. *Br. J. Psychol.* **42**, 2
50. — (1958). *Ageing and Human Skill*. London: Oxford University Press
51. Welford, N. T. (1952). 'An Electronic Digital Recording Machine–the Setar'. *J scient. Instrum.* **29**, 1
52. Whitfield, I. C. (1967). *The Auditory Pathway*. London: Edward Arnold
53. Yantis, P. A. (1955). 'Locus of the Lesion in Recruiting Ears'. *Archs Otolary* **62**, 625
54. Zangwill, O. L. (1960). *Cerebral Dominance and its Relation to Psychological Function*. Edinburgh: Oliver and Boyd

CHAPTER 3

SLEEP, DREAMS AND DRUGS

IAN OSWALD

The practical applications and limitations of the electroencephalo-gram (EEG) in clinical psychiatry have slowly become defined. In an earlier period of research most attention was paid to the EEG during wakefulness. Recently, however, there has been a quickening of interest in sleep. The recent sleep research has not had much practical application to individual patients, but has contributed basic know-ledge of importance to the psychiatrist.

The papers of Dement and Kleitman[20, 21] provided the impetus for a new approach to the study of dreaming and human sleep. They reported that about every one and a half hours the EEG of human nocturnal sleep changed from one of high voltage slow waves and sleep spindles (the latter being bursts of wave sat about 14 c/sec) to a low voltage record of faster rhythms (though less fast than waking) accompanied by the trace of frequent rapid jerky movements of the eyeballs. These last appearances persisted on average for about 20 min and would recur four or five times a night. When volunteers were wakened from these 'rapid eye movement' periods and asked if they had just been dreaming they replied affirmatively on 80 per cent of occasions and gave relatively detailed accounts. When wakened from sleep with EEG spindles and slow waves they only recalled dreams on 7 per cent of occasions.

TWO KINDS OF SLEEP

The two states of sleep were first thought to be 'deep' or non-dreaming sleep and 'light' or dreaming sleep, respectively. It is now, however, generally accepted that they do not represent different phases of a continuum but that they are *two qualitatively different kinds of sleep*[55, 83] having physiological characteristics which sharply differentiate the one from the other (*Figure 1*).

The two states have now been described in all of a very large number of mammalian species and in some marsupials and birds. There seem only minor inter-specific differences among mammals in

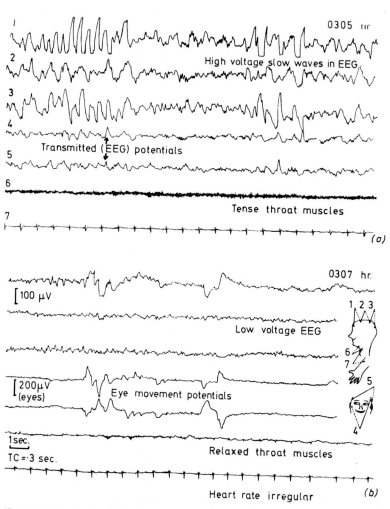

(Reproduced from Oswald (1963) by courtesy of The Editor of the *British Medical Bulletin*).

Figure 1. Some of the commonly recorded features of human sleep. (a) Orthodox (NREM) sleep; (b) two minutes later, paradoxical (REM) sleep. In orthodox sleep the EEG shows large slow waves and faster sleep spindles, the eyes are not moving, considerable muscle tone is revealed and the heart is regular. In paradoxical sleep the EEG is of low voltage and in the first channel, just before the first eye movement burst, a few 'saw-tooth' waves at 2–3 c/sec are visible. In the same channel a few muscle spikes, so common in this phase, are also visible. The eyes jerk around, the muscles are relaxed and the heart rate irregular

the characteristics of the two states which are now generally known as slow wave, NREM (non-rapid eye movement) or orthodox sleep and REM (rapid eye movement) or paradoxical sleep. Many reviews of the features of these two states exist; for example (and in order of increasing technicality of writing) there are the books of Oswald[87], Hartmann[48], Kales[56] and Kety, Evarts and Williams[64].

Paradoxical sleep differs from orthodox sleep in the EEG appearances, which in man include some characteristic 'saw-tooth' waves of 2–3 c/sec occurring briefly for two or three seconds, usually just before a burst of rapid eye movements[9]. Also during paradoxical sleep there is not merely much greater relaxation of many skeletal muscles, but virtual paralysis, with active inhibitory impulses descending to the spinal anterior horn cells[52, 98]: lesions of the anterior cervical cord in man can prevent the descending inhibition of reflexes[107]. Despite the greater relaxation, brief muscular twitches are common in the face and limbs and brief major body movements interrupt paradoxical sleep with greater frequency than orthodox sleep[94]. The blood pressure, respiration and heart rate are irregular in paradoxical sleep[109]. In animals, the total electrical activity of brain cells is diminished in orthodox sleep, but in paradoxical sleep it equals that of wakefulness, though the patterns of firing are different[28]. Brain blood flow[103] considerably exceeds waking levels in feline paradoxical sleep. In man, the penis is erect during paradoxical sleep[32].

DEPRIVATION EXPERIMENTS

When a normal man falls asleep he always passes first into orthodox sleep and only after about an hour switches into paradoxical sleep. Consequently, if an individual is deliberately awakened whenever the EEG machine indicates the onset of paradoxical sleep, he will always return to orthodox sleep and so become progressively deprived of paradoxical sleep. Dement[19] first showed that this procedure led, as nights progressed, to increasingly frequent onset of paradoxical sleep (and more frequently necessary awakenings) and to an excess percentage of paradoxical sleep on a subsequent night when undisturbed sleep was allowed. Frequent wakenings from orthodox sleep did not have this effect. Dement's original paper suggested that psychotic manifestations could result, owing to a 'need to dream'. In more recent publications, however, he has not sustained the last proposition and others who have repeated the experiments, and confirmed the effect on sleep, have not observed frank psychological abnormalities (e.g. Kales and colleagues[58]; Vogel and Traub[115]). However, it is only to be expected that deprivation of this physiological state will be discovered to cause adverse psychological effects when more sophisticated techniques become available for their detection. In the cat, excessive and indiscriminate sexual behaviour, overeating and abnormalities in brain sensory processing have been demonstrated after selective deprivation of paradoxical sleep[23, 25], while in man there is some evidence from psychological testing to suggest disorder of emotional life—'an increase in need and feeling intensity with a drop in certain ego-control functions'[14].

Total deprivation of sleep has been the subject of many reports and is of interest to the psychiatrist owing to the fact that, after two or three successive nights without sleep, a proportion of subjects develop intermittent psychotic manifestations of 'organic' type with visual illusions and hallucinations, some auditory hallucinations of elementary type (e.g. of dogs barking) and paranoid delusions[8, 12, 73, 111, 118]. Efficiency in skilled performance is impaired by sleep loss and the individual cannot *sustain* his attention, so that the effects are most noticeable where prolonged, continuous tasks are involved, and are less marked in the case of tasks of an intermittent and self-determined rate of working[123]. Appropriate testing can reveal the deficits after a single night where less than five hours sleep was obtained[121]. If sleep is lost for one whole night, the subsequent night's sleep of up to 13 hours does not fully restore normal capacity[120].

Chronic partial deprivation of sleep, generally believed to foster irritability, has been little studied. A former student of mine, now Dr P. Woodings, conducted an experiment[84] in which he stayed awake on alternate nights and slept unrestrictedly on the intervening nights. He suffered no ill-effects and after a month felt practically normal on a regular 11 hours of sleep every 48 hours. Meddis[76] repeated the experiments in more detail over a two month period. His subjects never fully adjusted to the regime. Although they totalled much less than normal sleep, they suffered no ill-effects. An EEG recording of all-night sleep revealed an abnormal distribution of paradoxical sleep, which occurred mainly at the start of the sleep period (whereas it is normally at a minimum in the first two hours of sleep). This finding is of importance as Hartmann[48] and Snyder[108] have reported that severely depressed patients suffer prolonged sleep deficiency and that their sleep is also abnormal with a relative excess of paradoxical sleep immediately after sleep onset. The experiments of Meddis suggest that the latter abnormality in the sleep of depressives could be a non-specific one, secondary to over-all sleep lack.

DREAMING

The original report of Dement and Kleitman concerning the association of dreaming and paradoxical sleep has been repeatedly confirmed. Goodenough and colleagues[40] showed that even persons who believed they never dreamed would describe dreams if wakened from paradoxical sleep. A great deal of evidence has accumulated to suggest that although dreams may occupy at least a couple of hours of the night, they are rapidly forgotten, consistent with the evidence of sleep-learning experiments that the memory or storage of new information during sleep is very poor[69]. There has been a tendency to refer to paradoxical sleep as 'dreaming sleep', but the work of Foulkes[33, 34] especially has demonstrated that mental life, sometimes having the characteristics of 'dreaming', can be present at any time during sleep. Apart from its lack of precision, the term 'dreaming sleep' is unfortunate since paradoxical sleep recurs during the sleep of decerebrate animals[113] in which dreaming cannot be inferred.

In his research, Foulkes[33] did not waken subjects and ask, 'Have you been dreaming?' but instead, 'Was anything going through your mind?' Nearly 90 per cent of awakenings from paradoxical sleep led to a description of mental life, but so did over 70 per cent of awakenings from orthodox sleep. There was a complete overlap in the types of mental life reported from the two states, but on statistical analysis the paradoxical sleep reports were significantly more 'dream-like', containing more emotional and sensory features. Furthermore, Monroe and colleagues[81] found that when independent but experienced judges were presented with a large number of reports of mental life given after awakenings throughout the night, they were able to discriminate between reports from the two different states with a very high degree of accuracy.

At a time when paradoxical sleep and dreaming were often equated it was worth emphasizing that dreaming occurs at sleep onset[84]. The further studies of Foulkes and Vogel[36] have shown the frequency of these sleep-onset dreams, similar in content to dreams of the later night, and especially likely to be reported by persons with 'greater social poise', who are 'more self-accepting' and 'less rigidly conforming to social standards'[37]. Although dreams often occur at sleep onset there is evidence that the longer sleep has lasted, the more vivid, the more out-of-contemporary-context, and the more emotional, is the dream[112].

The fact that mental life having the quality of dreaming is not confined to paradoxical sleep periods indicates that the duration of the latter cannot be taken as a sole criterion of the 'amount' of dreaming, nor of 'need' for dreaming. The original proposal by Dement[19], developed by Fisher and Dement[31], was that there was a need to dream, consistent with the Freudian view that dreams serve definite psychic functions, particularly satisfaction of the imperious impulses arising in the unconscious, the dream-work making possible their disguised fulfilment.

The neonate spends a very large part of his time in paradoxical sleep, before he could be said to have developed any psychic structure or to be possessed of wishes which could be satisfied through the utilization of memory traces of sufficient stability to allow their re-evocation as the hallucinatory events of dreaming. Again the 'pontine' animal preparation continues to manifest apparent sleep, in which there occur regular periods of paradoxical sleep. Selective deprivation of the latter is followed by subsequent compensation[55]. The 'pontine' animal could not be said to possess a need to dream. Certain pharmacological manoeuvres can promote paradoxical sleep in man in the absence of any prior evidence of dream lack, for example, administration of tryptophan[27, 49, 95] and LSD[82]. The concept of 'need to dream' has proved unable to cope with all the evidence. A physiological concept of 'need for sleep' is more generally inclusive, but, given that the physiological concept be allowed primacy, I believe it would be wrong to dismiss as improper the psychological concept of a need for dreaming. We have waking needs of a psychological nature—a need to feel secure, to feel important and so on—we may well have also psychological needs while asleep. Problems arise if one tries to devise an experiment to test the purely psychological hypothesis.

It may be interpolated here that studies which have explored the possibility of a link between the psychotic thinking of the dream and paradoxical sleep on the one hand, and the psychotic thinking of schizophrenia on the other, have been disappointing and have failed to demonstrate any clear link between paradoxical sleep and schizophrenia[114]. The report by Zarcone and colleagues[126] that selective deprivation of paradoxical sleep in the chronic schizophrenic is followed by a uniquely high rebound was not confirmed by Vogel and Traub[115]. Luby and Caldwell[72] imposed total sleep deprivation on schizophrenics and compared their subsequent recovery nights with those reported for normal volunteers[8]. The schizophrenics failed to show the normal marked increase of Stage 4 orthodox sleep. The work has yet to be confirmed.

The fact that one may be reasonably certain a person is dreaming during paradoxical sleep has given us a method for the study of dreams which renders obsolete many older reports. It used to be claimed, for example, that dreams did not occur after leucotomy, but my colleague, J. I. Evans, woke a number of leucotomized patients from paradoxical sleep periods and obtained dream reports despite a generally poor level of co-operativeness. Swanson and Foulkes[110] have shown the variation in dream content with the hormonal state or at least with the menstrual cycle. Judges rated manifest sexuality in women's dream reports and scored it highest during menstruation, at a time when the subjects themselves rated waking sexual desire as low, but rated dream unpleasantness and overt hostility as maximal. Hartmann[47] found the percentage of sleep spent in the paradoxical phase to be at a maximum on the final nights before menstruation.

It is a common clinical observation that unpleasant dreams are described by patients who are anxious or unhappy by day. Beck and Hurvich[6] reported that independent judgment of such themes as rejection, humiliation, and disappointment showed these higher in dreams of depressed patients and Kramer and colleagues[66] found elements of anxiety and hostility decreased during imipramine treatment of depression, while heterosexual and 'motility' features of dream content increased with clinical improvement.

Other experimenters have looked for effects on dream content of pre-sleep emotion. An important point is made by Whitman and colleagues[119] that when dreams are collected in a laboratory situation their content may be influenced by the setting. They found indications of anxiety about the laboratory setting in a third of 111 dreams. Male volunteers were considered to betray castration anxiety in their dreams and female volunteers dreams of sexual exploitation. Despite the fact that thousands of dreams have been collected from college males, dreams accompanied by orgasm and seminal emission have rarely been encountered. Only three reports appear in the literature, cases of Fisher[30], Karacan and colleagues[63] and of Evans (illustrated in Oswald[86]). Domhoff[26] reports a comparison of 120 dreams obtained from a home environment with 120 dreams of the same subjects in the laboratory. Laboratory dreams appeared retarded by the environmental anxieties. Home dreams had more aggression, more sexual interactions, more misfortunes, more friendliness, success and failure . They were spicier.

Although 32 children aged 6–12 studied by Foulkes and colleagues[38] gave 72 per cent dream reports from 249 paradoxical sleep awakenings, I know of no studies of the effect on children's dreams of, for example, exciting television films. Young adults were, however, shown two films on different evenings by Foulkes and Rechtschaffen[35], one containing much violence, the other being non-violent. Dreams from paradoxical sleep awakenings after the violent film were more imaginative, vivid and emotional, though not more unpleasant or violent than after the non-violent film. Witkin and Lewis[124] also showed films to men prior to sleep. One was of an Australian aboriginal ceremony of sub-incision of the penis. The incision into the penis and scrotum is made with a sharp stone and the bleeding organ is seen being held over a fire while the faces of the initiates clearly reflect their anguish. The other, in colour, was a medical film of the birth of a baby. The dreams later in the night contained many striking features suggesting disguised incorporation of events in, or anxiety aroused by, the films (e.g. after the first ' . . . the barrel of the gun pointing directly at me . . . the gunsight on top and two winglike projections . . .'). Unfortunately this particular study, though I find it convincing, was not designed to allow independent judgment, or statistical analysis, of any incorporations.

A more carefully designed study by Berger[7] showed clear evidence of incorporation of external auditory stimuli into dreams, with again disguise or transformation on the basis of assonance especially. Judgment of incorporation into the dreams that Berger had collected was made by myself. I did not know when making the judgments which of four possible auditory stimuli had been used during any particular paradoxical sleep period, but was able correctly to judge the actual stimulus significantly better than chance would allow. As an example, the stimulus 'Robert, Robert, Robert' was followed by a dream report about a film of a 'rabbit' which looked 'distorted'. Rechtschaffen and Foulkes[100] studied subjects whose eyes had been glued open prior to sleep. Various visual stimuli were presented during sleep, but no evidence of their incorporation into dreams could be detected.

Visual imagery in dreams has been thought to be related to the rapid eye movements of paradoxical sleep. Roffwarg and colleagues[101] claimed a close and often exact relation between the rapid eye movement direction and the direction of expected eye movements had the dream events been real. Their study has been criticized on the ground that the judgments of congruence were not made 'blind' and because the factor of the degree of 'activity' was not controlled. 'Active' dreams of events which, had they occurred in real life, would be accompanied by profuse eye movements, are closely correlated with 'active' paradoxical sleep periods having profuse eye movements[9, 22]. My colleagues and I at one time reported that, whereas men who had been blind for only a few years still had visual imagery and rapid eye movements in sleep, other men who had been blind all their lives had no visual imagery and no rapid eye movements during their periods of paradoxical sleep[10]. However, this last apparent finding was incorrect. In many cases of congenital blindness the corneo-retinal potential is absent, so that the usual method of recording eye movements can fail to demonstrate their presence. Gross, Byrne and Fisher[45], using a strain-gauge on the eyeball, demonstrated that rapid eye movements do indeed occur in the congenitally blind, a fact I have since confirmed by recalling one of our former congenitally-blind subjects and filming his eye movements during sleep (courtesy of B.B.C. Television).

The action of drugs on paradoxical sleep will be outlined subsequently, but apart from reducing the proportion of sleep spent in the paradoxical phase, the barbiturates also reduce the number or profusion of rapid eye movements per minute during the paradoxical sleep period[3, 94]. As mentioned above there is a relation between this profusion of eye movements and the dream content. Pivik and Foulkes[97] showed that selective deprivation of paradoxical sleep led not only to subsequent rebound increase in its percentage, as Dement had shown, but to more vivid dream content and to a profusion of eye movements higher than on base-line nights. In other words, increasing the 'pressure' towards paradoxical sleep led not only to more of it, but to greater intensity of one of its features, the eye movements, and to greater intensity of the dream experience.

When barbiturate sleeping pills, nitrazepam, methyprylon, or other drugs which suppress paradoxical sleep, are withdrawn from persons accustomed to their consumption, they often complain of vividly unpleasant dreams and nightmares[57, 70]. Lewis[90] using records of the nitrazepam study of Priest and myself, reported that, after the drug's withdrawal not only was paradoxical sleep abnormally increased, but that there was also a rebound increase in rapid eye movement profusion. Using again the records from the 1965 study by Priest and myself I have compared the final two nights (about three months after any drugs and which may be considered normal nights) with the first and third nights after amylobarbitone withdrawal (up to 600 mg nightly for the previous 18 nights). The number of two second epochs of record containing one or more rapid eye movements (REMs) was scored for each subject.

	With REMs	Without REMs
Withdrawal nights	4857	7983
Control nights	3943	7957

The difference is significant ($\chi^2 = 59 \cdot 4$, $p < 0 \cdot 001$)

This finding that barbiturate sleeping pill withdrawal is associated with increased profusion of rapid eye movements has also been made in Los Angeles (A. Kales. Personal communication). We may conclude that, apart from abnormalities of sleep itself, dream experiences may be made more intense, when sleeping pills are stopped, than would have been the case had they not been given. Since the drugs relieve anxiety, which is probably heightened by their withdrawal, it is not surprising that many of the intensified dreams are fearful ones.

A number of physiological correlates of dream anxiety have been reported. Gottschalk and colleagues[41] had demonstrated a significant correlation between scores of anxiety manifest during five minute periods of waking free association and the concentrations of free fatty acids in plasma. Subsequently other volunteers slept in their laboratory and, at the start of, and again after 15–20 minutes of any period of paradoxical sleep, blood was obtained through an indwelling catheter and the subject awakened and his dream report recorded. These reports were scored for anxiety on the one hand and the change of plasma free fatty acid between the first and second blood samples on the other. It was concluded that anxiety in the dream triggered the release of catecholamines which mobilized free fatty acids from body fat. Shapiro and colleagues[106], significantly, more often got reports of having been asleep and dreaming, and a description of the dream content, when there had been irregular respiration during the paradoxical sleep period. However, reports of having been asleep and dreaming, yet with inability to recall content, were associated with especially extreme irregularity of respiration, permitting the hypothesis that in these last cases dream anxiety was high but repression of the anxiety-provoking content operative.

Penile erection, found to accompany 95 per cent of paradoxical sleep periods by Fisher, Gross and Zuch[32], varies in degree with the anxiety content of the dream. Karacan and colleagues[63] awakened subjects and scored the anxiety level in the dreams. Dreams with high anxiety content were those where there had been no or only partial erection during the paradoxical sleep period prior to awakening. Coitus prior to coming to the laboratory did not affect the sleep erection cycle and in one subject, after a nocturnal seminal emission during the fourth paradoxical sleep period of the night, a full erection occurred in the fifth. Fisher[30] studied 58 dream accounts and attempted blind predictions of the fluctuation of erection during the paradoxical sleep periods concerned. He proved most accurate where sudden detumescence or a sudden increase in tumescence had occurred, the latter tending to be associated with overtly erotic material in the dream and detumescence with anxiety.

SOME COMMON SLEEP DISORDERS

Emphasis has already been laid on the evidence for the continuation of mental life throughout either kind of sleep. Bed-wetting and sleep-walking on rare occasions would be considered within normal limits in any child and persistence of the former at least may be indicative of slow maturation rather than psychopathology. Nevertheless, each of these sleep disorders can become more frequent at times of psychological stress for the child. Both are features of orthodox sleep. Sleep-walking apparently occurs exclusively therein[53, 59] and enuresis nearly always[39, 51]. Rhythmic body rocking (jactatio capitis nocturna) is a comfort response to loneliness and fear in other primates besides the human child and its sudden occurrence *during* sleep must suggest that it is provoked by some unhappy mental life during sleep, of a kind from which the individual long ago learned to seek relief in rhythmic activity. The rocking can interrupt either phase of sleep[39, 85] and the same is true of sleep-talking[2, 85, 101].

The element of paralysis accompanying the fear in nightmares has long been recognized[13]. An explanation of this phenomenon may be seen in the paralysis that characterizes paradoxical sleep. One may suppose that normally we are unaware of the paralysis, but may become so if we are fighting to escape some terrifying fate. Most reports of nightmares recorded from the laboratory have found them to occur in paradoxical sleep[27, 57, 67, 90] though Gastaut and Broughton[39] have described awakenings, in a state of terror, from orthodox sleep also.

Idiopathic narcolepsy includes among its classical features cataplectic attacks, namely sudden brief loss of tone or helpless paralysis provoked by emotion. Usually the emotion is the same one for any given patient, but the responsible emotion varies from patient to patient. In one it may be anger, in another a feeling of triumph (for example, when about to smash at table tennis), in another laughter and another fear. Sleep paralysis is another complaint of the narcoleptic and in the case of both these clinical features it is now suggested that the paralysis may represent a partial manifestation of paradoxical sleep (although in sleep paralysis, the frequent bizarre feeling of, for instance, the presence of headless monsters in the room, may frequently indicate the full manifestation of paradoxical sleep). The new understanding stems from the original observation by Rechtschaffen and colleagues[102] that, unlike the normal person, the narcoleptic will frequently have a paradoxical sleep period at sleep onset (*Figure 2*). Their observation has been repeatedly confirmed. It is only about half the unwanted sleep attacks that are paradoxical sleep episodes and if paradoxical sleep has occurred in the past hour or so the next sleep onset may be into orthodox sleep. Nevertheless, the narcoleptic is exceptional in his extreme liability to paradoxical sleep.

Insomnia

Insomnia is the most widely complained of sleep disorder. Prescriptions for sleeping pills represent about ten per cent of all prescriptions in Britain[79] and 13 per cent in Australia[16]. Prescriptions for barbiturates in Britain doubled between 1954 and 1959[78] doubled in Czechoslovakia between 1958 and 1964[116] and in the U.S.A. 'from 1952 to 1963 the retail sales of sedatives and tranquilizers increased by 535 per cent'[24].

It is among people who complain of neurotic symptoms that insomnia is most often also found as a complaint, and most of all if they are also past middle age[75, 117]. Insomnia is generally assessed by the patients' opinions, by nurses' judgments made at intervals through the night, by motility scores, or, much the most accurately, by the EEG. Nurses' judgments have been used, for example, to show that introverts sleep less than extroverts[17], and the EEG to show that the patient who complains she never sleeps a wink may sometimes sleep the entire night[105].

Insomnia is a normal sequel to an 'over-exciting' or anxiety-provoking day. Baekeland, Koulack and Lasky[5] recorded the all-night sleep of male volunteers (a) after an emotionally neutral film, and (b) after the showing of an emotionally stressful film (of the Australian aboriginal sub-incision rite, previously mentioned). After the latter film there were significantly more awakenings from sleep and these occurred in association with the paradoxical sleep periods, during which also the profusion of rapid eye movements was increased. One may infer that the anxiety provoked before sleep led to vivid dreams as well as excessive awakenings from sleep.

On the other hand, vigorous physical exercise in those accustomed to it, when it occurs in the afternoon leads to what might be considered better sleep, with significantly more time in the extreme stage of orthodox sleep with its very large and slow EEG waves (Stage 4), whereas evening exertions can cause disturbed sleep (as if we need time to 'unwind' before attempting to sleep) as Baekeland and Lasky[4] have shown.

Insomnia is, too, a classical feature of hypomania and mania and of depressive illness of the autonomous ('endogenous') kind. It is often also found in the early stages of acute paranoid schizophrenia and can at other times result from the use of drugs, whether ephedrine

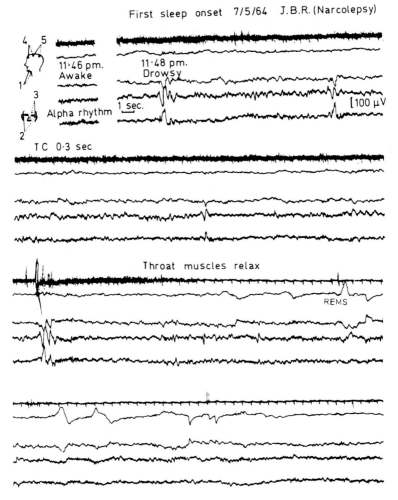

First sleep onset 7/5/64 J.B.R. (Narcolepsy)

Figure 2. Onset of sleep in a narcoleptic patient. At 11·46 p.m. he is awake and has alpha rhythm in his EEG. At 11.48 irregular slow activity is developing as a sign of drowsiness but considerable muscle tension (which makes the top line appear thick owing to a multitude of spikes) is retained. About a minute later the muscle tension in the throat muscles suddenly decreases, after which rapid jerky eye movements begin, while the EEG presents a low voltage picture of irregular 4–6 c/sec activity. He has passed into paradoxical sleep. The excerpts are continuous apart from the break indicated after 11.46 p.m.

for bronchial asthma or dexamphetamine for pep at a party. However, McGhie[74] has shown that psychoneurotic and psychopathic in-patients complain of insomnia as much as depressives. His work has raised the question whether the reputed insomnia of depression is to a large extent a combination of the older age of many such patients, together with a liability to complain the more readily owing to the unpleasantness of the affect and the distressing thoughts experienced in the early hours. On the other hand, EEG studies of the all-night sleep of depressives[44, 48, 77, 94, 108] have all shown that there is indeed an abnormal amount of wakefulness even for their ages.

All-night EEG studies[1, 29, 62] confirm the frequent nocturnal awakenings and short sleep of normal old age. Feinberg's work has shown a correlation too between degree of organic dementia and the degree of sleep disorder. The sleep is most broken in the frankly demented patient, but even among normal persons the impairment of function, which is apparent on tests of cognitive function as age advances, correlated with the frequency of nocturnal awakenings from the thirties onwards.

Although subjective estimates of sleep are usually underestimates[71] when judged by the EEG, one must bear in mind that there may be little-understood features of sleep which may mean that seven hours sleep by EEG criteria may be worth less for one man than for another. Monroe[80] compared young adults who considered themselves 'good' sleepers with others who considered themselves 'poor' sleepers (none were patients). The poor sleepers had more evidence of personality disorder, took longer to fall asleep, got less sleep, woke more often, had less paradoxical sleep and more Stage 2 orthodox sleep, and had higher heart rates and rectal temperature throughout the night. Curiously, they also had higher skin resistance (generally correlated with degree of relaxation). Williams and Williams[122] compared groups of 'restless' and 'quiet' sleepers and then deprived each of sleep. The restless sleepers' performance showed a much greater deficit when subjected to this procedure, suggesting an inherent vulnerability of a global nature.

Another indication of our ignorance about what really constitutes good sleep is to be found in the report by Lester, Burch and Dossett[68]. The galvanic skin response (GSR) is generally taken as an index of emotional arousal following a discrete stimulus. In the course of sleep GSR deflections can be recorded as spontaneous phenomena, especially intense, profuse and random during orthodox sleep Stage 4, with its very large slow EEG waves[91]. Lester and his colleagues, using data from 336 nights from 53 adults, reported that the random spontaneous GSRs were significantly more profuse on nights after day-time stress (such as college examinations). Their report could be interpreted as suggesting a sort of continuing 'excitement' of emotional mechanisms even during profound sleep when there has been day-time stress.

DRUGS AND SLEEP

The action of drugs has not been neglected amidst all the new research into sleep[88]. One result must be a more critical attitude towards the common type of drug trial of hypnotics or sedatives, particularly the assumption that one night or one week is independent of another. There is now evidence that if a patient has a sleeping pill tonight and a placebo tomorrow night, he will sleep badly on the placebo night *because* he had the prior sleeping pill. This indication that the consequences of a 'medium-acting' hypnotic may extend longer than the sleep period must remind us of the paucity of information about how a sleeping pill taken tonight will affect a man's mood or skill tomorrow afternoon, particularly after alcohol at lunch. Kornetsky, Vates and Kessler[65] showed that chlorpromazine 100 mg, or quinalbarbitone 200 mg, given as hypnotics at night, significantly impaired simple skills 14–15 hours later. A variety of authors (e.g. Parsons[96]) have implied that phenobarbitone might just as well be used as a hypnotic as quinalbarbitone. It may be as effective on the first night, but since only 11–23 per cent gets eliminated within 24 hours[11] and since coma following the all-too-common overdose is very much more prolonged, phenobarbitone should never be prescribed as a hypnotic.

When hypnotic drugs are given sleep is altered. There is no foundation for claims that certain drugs are 'euhypnics' promoting 'natural' sleep. The normal alternation of orthodox and paradoxical sleep can be diagrammatically represented as in *Figure 3*. The time of initial sleep onset can be seen from the EEG record, as can the times of shifts from one phase to another. Thus certain measurements can easily be made, including the percentage of whole-night sleep spent as paradoxical sleep.

Many drugs reduce this last percentage. If they are administered for a number of nights (with development of a degree of tolerance) and then withdrawn, a 'rebound' increase in paradoxical sleep occurs. The increase is especially great at the beginning of the night, at which time too the first period of paradoxical sleep may start abnormally soon after first onset of orthodox sleep (as indicated in *Figure 4*).

67

Drugs which cause suppression of paradoxical sleep with subsequent rebound include barbiturates[3, 50, 60, 90, 94], dexamphetamine[3, 89, 99], phenmetrazine[89, 92], diethylpropion[92], alcohol[42, 43, 46, 125], tranylcypromine[18, 67], methyprylon and glutethimide[60], and nitrazepam[90] among non-barbiturate hypnotics.

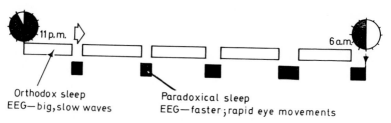

Figure 3. Diagrammatic representation of the alternation of human orthodox and paradoxical sleep through the normal night

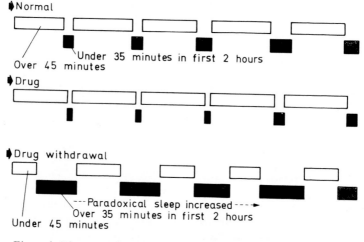

Figure 4. Diagrammatic representation of the alternation of orthodox and paradoxical sleep when affected by a drug of the amphetamine or barbiturate class and the abnormalities which appear when the drug is withdrawn from someone accustomed to it

The rebound is particularly large after drugs are withdrawn from addicts, reaching up to 100 per cent paradoxical sleep in alcoholics entering delirium tremens. In the case of rebound after amphetamine or medium-acting barbiturates, up to two months are required before sleep returns to normal (the drug itself is, of course, eliminated from the body in about 48 hours). One has to suppose that while the drug was present in the brain the cerebral machinery was altered so that something was brought into being which counter-acted the effects of the drug but persisted after it was withdrawn. It is as if the paradoxical sleep releasing mechanisms were 'hypertrophied'. The slowness of the return to normal would imply protein synthesis for the reformation of the paradoxical sleep mechanisms, in accord with modern studies of the role of protein synthesis in the development of the initial drug tolerance itself[88a]. At the time of writing it appears that all drugs of addiction cause, on withdrawal, a rebound in paradoxical sleep[93], usually a rebound increase, though LSD, which causes an initial enhancement of paradoxical sleep is followed by a rebound decrease[82]. My colleagues and I, using ourselves as subjects, have recently demonstrated suppression of paradoxical sleep and subsequent rebound in the case of heroin. The rebound can persist for two months.

The rebound happens to be easily measurable. Other central nervous system functions will doubtless become similarly measurable in the future and further illustrate the naïvety of older distinctions between 'physical' and 'psychological' dependence—it must all depend on how sophisticated are the measuring techniques of 'physical' function. There are other drugs such as phenytoin[15], and fenfluramine[92] which have potent actions on the central nervous system, yet cause neither addiction nor any paradoxical sleep rebound on withdrawal. The action of other drugs has been reviewed elsewhere[88].

Finally, I should like to re-emphasize that EEG sleep research techniques have shown that the drugs so commonly used as hypnotics and simple day-time sedatives, not merely lose their effect after repeated use but, on withdrawal, cause sleep to be shorter, subjectively poorer, and with more unpleasant dreaming, than would have been the case had the drugs never been given. On withdrawal nights patients are at their most inaccurate in their own judgment of sleep duration[71]. It is easy to understand why, once started on sleeping pills, so many patients continue for years and say, quite truthfully, that they now cannot sleep properly without them. It may serve as some explanation of why a quarter of all Scottish middle-aged women regularly take some pharmaceutical preparation with a view to promoting sleep[75]. It would further seem plain that doctors should avoid starting patients on such drugs unless a future point of termination of current anxieties can clearly be foreseen. It would seem desirable that every effort should be made to stop simple sedatives and hypnotics before a patient is discharged from hospital. The ubiquitous prescribing of sedatives and hypnotics in cases of chronic personality disorder seems wholly against the patients' interests, since only temporary relief can be gained, at the price of some inevitable degree of dependence.

REFERENCES

1. Agnew, H. W., Webb, W. B. and Williams, R. L. (1967). 'Sleep Patterns in Late Middle Age Males: An EEG Study'. *Electroenceph. clin. Neurophysiol.* **23,** 168
2. Arkin, A. M. (1966). 'Sleep-talking: A Review'. *J. nerv. ment. Dis.* **143,** 101
3. Baekeland, F. (1967). 'Pentobarbital and Dextroamphetamine Sulfate: Effects on the Sleep Cycle in Man'. *Psychopharmacologia* **11,** 388
4. — and Lasky, R. (1966). 'Exercise and Sleep Patterns in College Athletes'. *Percept. Mot. Skills* **23,** 1203
5. — Koulack, D. and Lasky, R. (1968). 'Effects of Stressful Presleep Experience on Electroencephalograph-recorded Sleep'. *Psychophysiology* **4,** 436
6. Beck, A. T. and Hurvich, M. S. (1959). 'Psychological Correlates of Depression'. *Psychosom. Med.* **21,** 51
7. Berger, R. J. (1963). 'Experimental Modification of Dream Content by Meaningful Verbal Stimuli'. *Br. J. Psychiat.* **109,** 722
8. — and Oswald, I. (1962). 'Effects of Sleep Deprivation on Behaviour, Subsequent Sleep, and Dreaming'. *J. ment. Sci.* **108,** 457
9. — — (1962). 'Eye-movements During Active and Passive Dreams'. *Science* **137,** 601
10. — Olley, P. and Oswald, I. (1962). 'The EEG, Eye-movements and Dreams of the Blind'. *Q. Jl exp. Psychol.* **14,** 183
11. Butler, T. C., Mahaffee, C. and Waddell, W. J. (1954). 'Phenobarbital: Studies of Elimination, Accumulation, Tolerance and Dosage Schedules'. *J. Pharmac. exp. Ther.* **111,** 425
12. Cappon, D. and Banks, R. (1960). 'Studies in Perceptual Distortion: Opportunistic Observations on Sleep. Deprivation During a Talkathon'. *Archs gen. Psychiat.* **2,** 346
13. Cason, H. (1935). 'The Nightmare Dream'. *Psychol. Monogr.* **46,** No. 5
14. Clemes, S. R. and Dement, W. C. (1967). 'Effect of REM Sleep Deprivation on Psychological Functioning'. *J. nerv. ment. Dis.* **144,** 485
15. Cohen, H. B., Duncan, R. F. and Dement, W. C. (1968). 'The Effect of Diphenylhydantoin on Sleep in the Cat'. *Electroenceph. clin. Neurophysiol.* **24,** 401
16. Commonwealth Director General of Health (1966). *Annual Report 1965–66*, Canberra

17. Costello, C. G. and Smith, M. (1963). 'The Relationships Between Personality, Sleep and the Effects of Sedatives'. *Br. J. Psychiat.* **109**, 568

18. Cramer, H. and Ohlmeier, D. (1967). 'Ein Fall von Tranyl-cypromin-und-Trifluoperazine-(Jatrosom)-Sucht: Psychopatholo-gische, Schlafphysiologische und Biochemische Untersuchungen'. *Arch. Psychiat. NervKrankh.* **210**, 182

19. Dement, W. C. (1960). 'The Effect of Dream Deprivation'. *Science* **131**, 1705

20. — and Kleitman, N. (1957). 'Cyclic Variations in EEG During Sleep and Their Relation to Eye Movements, Body Motility and Dreaming'. *Electroenceph. clin. Neurophysiol.* **9**, 673

21. — — (1957). 'The Relation of Eye Movements During Sleep to Dream Activity: An Objective Method for the Study of Dreaming'. *J. exp. Psychol.* **53**, 339

22. — and Wolpert, E. A. (1958). 'The Relation of Eye Movements, Body Motility and External Stimuli to Dream Content'. *J. exp. Psychol.* **55**, 543

23. — Henry, P., Cohen, H. and Ferguson, J. (1967). 'Studies on the Effect of REM Deprivation in Humans and in Animals'. *Res. Publs Ass. Res. nerv. ment. Dis.* **45**, 456

24. Department of Health, Education, and Welfare (1967). *A Report to the President on Medical Care Prices.* Washington, D.C.: U.S. Government Printing Office

25. Dewson, J. H., Dement, W. C., Wagener, T. E. and Nobel, K. (1967). 'REM Sleep Deprivation: A Central-neural Change During Wakefulness'. *Science* **156**, 403

26. Domhoff, G. W. (1969). 'Home Dreams versus Laboratory Dreams.' In *Dream Psychology and the New Biology of Dreaming.* Ed. by M. Kramer. Springfield, Ill.: Charles C. Thomas

27. Evans, J. I. and Oswald, I. (1966). 'Some Experiments in the Chemistry of Narcoleptic Sleep'. *Br. J. Psychiat.* **112**, 401

28. Evarts, E. V. (1965). 'Relation of Cell Size to Effects of Sleep in Pyramidal Tract Neurons'. In *Sleep Mechanisms*, p. 81. Ed. by K. Akert, C. Bally and J. P. Schadé. Amsterdam: Elsevier

29. Feinberg, I., Koresko, R. L. and Heller, N. (1967). 'EEG Sleep Patterns as a Function of Normal and Pathological Aging in Man'. *J. psychiat. Res.* **5**, 107

30. Fisher, C. (1966). 'Dreaming and Sexuality'. In *Psychoanalysis—A General Psychology*, p. 537. Ed. by M. Schur, A. Solnit, R. M. Loewenstein and L. Newman. New York: International Univer-sities Press

31. — and Dement, W. C. (1963). 'Studies on the Psychopathology of Sleep and Dreams'. *Am. J. Psychiat.* **119**, 1160

32. — Gross, J. and Zuch, J. (1965). 'Cycle of Penile Erection Synchronous with Dreaming (REM) Sleep'. *Archs gen. Psychiat.* **12**, 29

33. Foulkes, D. (1962). 'Dream Reports from Different Stages of Sleep'. *J. abnorm. soc. Psychol.* **65,** 14

34. — (1966). *The Psychology of Sleep.* New York: Charles Scribner

35. — and Rechtschaffen, A. L. (1964). 'Presleep Determinants of Dream Content: Effect of Two Films'. *Percept. Mot. Skills* **19,** 983

36. — and Vogel, G. (1965). 'Mental Activity at Sleep Onset'. *J. abnorm. soc. Psychol.* **70,** 231

37. — Spear, P. S. and Symonds, J. D. (1966). 'Individual Differences in Mental Activity at Sleep Onset'. *J. abnorm. Psychol.* **71,** 28

38. — Pivik, T., Steadman, H. S., Spear, P. S. and Symonds, J. D. (1967). 'Dreams of the Male Child'. *J. abnorm. Psychol.* **72,** 457

39. Gastaut, H. and Broughton, R. (1967). 'A Clinical and Polygraphic Study of Episodic Phenomena During Sleep'. *Recent Adv. biol. Psychiat.* **7,** 197

40. Goodenough, D. R., Shapiro, A., Holden, M. and Steinschriber, L. (1959). 'A Comparison of Dreamers and Nondreamers; Eye Movements, Electroencephalograms and the Recall of Dreams'. *J. abnorm. soc. Psychol.* **59,** 295

41. Gottschalk, L. A., Stone, W. N., Gleser, G. C. and Iacono, H. M. (1966). 'Anxiety Levels in Dreams: Relation to Changes in Plasma Free Fatty Acids'. *Science* **153,** 654

42. Greenberg, R. and Pearlman, C. (1967). 'Delirium Tremens and Dreaming. *Am. J. Psychiat.* **124,** 133

43. Gresham, S. C., Webb, W. B. and Williams, R. L. (1963). 'Alcohol and Caffeine: Effect on Inferred Visual Dreaming'. *Science* **140,** 1226

44. — Agnew, H. W. and Williams, R. L. (1965). 'The Sleep of Depressed Patients'. *Archs gen. Psychiat.* **13,** 503

45. Gross, J., Byrne, J. and Fisher, C. (1965). Eye Movements During Emergent Stage 1 EEG in Subjects with Lifelong Blindness'. *J. nerv. ment. Dis.* **141,** 365

46. Gross, M. M., Goodenough, D., Tobin, M., Halpert, E., Lepore, D., Perlstein, A., Sirota, M., Dibianco, H. Fuller, R. and Kishner, I. (1966). 'Sleep Disturbances and Hallucinations in the Acute Alcoholic Psychoses'. *J. nerv. ment. Dis.* **142,** 493

47. Hartmann, E. (1966). 'Dreaming Sleep (the D-State) and the Menstrual Cycle. *J. nerv. ment. Dis.* **143,** 406

48. — (1967). *The Biology of Dreaming.* Springfield, Ill.: Charles C. Thomas

49. — (1967). 'The Effect of l-tryptophan on the Sleep-dream Cycle in Man'. *Psychon. Sci.* **8,** 479

50. — (1968). 'The Effect of Four Drugs on Sleep Patterns in Man'. *Psychopharmacologia,* **12,** 346

51. Hawkins, D. R., Scott, J. and Thrasher, G. (1969). 'Relationship of Enuresis in Children to Level of Sleep'. Personal communication.

52. Hodes, R. and Dement, W. C. (1964). 'Depression of Electrically Induced Reflexes (H-reflexes) in Man During Low Voltage EEG "Sleep"'. *Electroenceph. clin. Neurophysiol.* **17,** 617

53. Jacobson, A., Kales, A., Lehmann, D. and Zweizig, J. R. (1965). 'Somnambulism: All-night Electroencephalographic Studies'. *Science* **148,** 975

54. — Vimont, P., Delorme, F. and Jouvet, M. (1964). 'Étude de la Privation Selective de la Phase Paradoxale de Sommeil Chez le Chat'. *C. r. Séanc. Soc. Biol.* **158,** 756

55. Jouvet, M. (1965). 'Paradoxical Sleep—A Study of its Nature and Mechanisms'. In *Sleep Mechanisms,* p. 20. Ed. by K. Akert, C. Bally and J. P. Schadé. Amsterdam: Elsevier

56. Kales, A. (Ed.) (1969). *Sleep: Physiology and Pathology.* Philadelphia: Lippincott

57. — and Jacobson, A. (1967). 'Mental Activity During Sleep: Recall Studies, Somnambulism, and Effects of Rapid Eye Movement Deprivation and Drugs'. *Expl Neurol. (Suppl.)* **4,** 81

58. — Hoedemaker, F. S., Jacobson, A. and Lichtenstein, E. D. (1964). 'Dream Deprivation: An Experimental Reappraisal'. *Nature, Lond.* **204,** 1337

59. — Jacobson, A., Paulson, M. J., Kales, J. D. and Walter, R. D. (1966). 'Somnambulism: Psychophysiological Correlates'. *Archs gen. Psychiat.* **14,** 586

60. —— Kales, J. D., Marusak, C. and Hanley, J. (1968). 'Effects of Drugs on Sleep'. *Psychophysiology* **4,** 391

61. — Hoedemaker, F. S., Jacobson, A., Kales, J. D., Paulson, M. J. and Wilson, T. E. (1967). 'Mentation During Sleep: REM and NREM Recall Reports'. *Percept. Mot. Skills* **24,** 555

62. — Wilson, T., Kales, J. D., Jacobson, A., Paulson, M. J., Kollar, E. and Walter, R. D. (1967). 'Measurements of All-night Sleep in Normal Elderly Persons: Effects of Aging'. *J. Am. geriat. Soc.* **15,** 405

63. Karacan, E., Goodenough, D. R., Shapiro, A. and Starker, S. (1966). 'Erection Cycle During Sleep in Relation to Dream Anxiety'. *Archs gen Psychiat.* **15,** 183

64. Kety, S. S., Evarts, E. V. and Williams, H. L. (1967). 'Sleep and Altered State of Consciousness'. *Res. Publs Ass. Res. nerv. ment. Dis.* **45,** 1

65. Kornetsky, C., Vates, T. S. and Kessler, E. K. (1959). 'A comparison of Hypnotic and Residual Psychological Effects of Single Doses of Chlorpromazine and Secobarbital in man'. *J. Pharmac. exp. Ther.* **127,** 51

66. Kramer, M., Whitman, R. M., Baldridge, B. and Ornstein, P. H. (1968). 'Drugs and Dreams III: The Effects of Imipramine on the Dreams of Depressed Patients'. *Am. J. Psychiat.* **124,** 1385

67. Le Gassicke, J., Ashcroft, G. W., Eccleston, D., Evans, J. I., Oswald, I. and Ritson, E. B. (1965). 'The Clinical State, Sleep and Amine Metabolism of a Tranylcypromine ('Parnate') Addict'. *Br. J. Psychiat.* **111,** 357

68. Lester, B. K., Burch, N. R. and Dossett, R. C. (1967). 'Nocturnal EEG-GSR Profiles: The Influence of Presleep States'. *Psychophysiol.* **3,** 238

69. Lewis, S. A. (1968). 'Learning While Asleep'. *Bull. Br. psychol. Soc.* **21,** 23

70. — (1968). 'The Quantification of Rapid Eye Movement Sleep'. In *Drugs and Sensory Functions,* p. 287. Ed. by A. Herxheimer. London: Churchill

71. — (1969). 'Subjective Estimates of Sleep: An EEG Evaluation'. *Br. J. Psychol.* **60,** 203

72. Luby, E D. and Caldwell, D. F. (1967). 'Sleep Deprivation and EEG Slow Wave Activity in Chronic Schizophrenia'. *Archs gen. Psychiat.* **17,** 361

73. — Grisell, J. L., Frohman, C. E., Lees, H., Cohen, B. D. and Gottlieb, J. S. (1962). 'Biochemical, Psychological and Behavioural Responses to Sleep Deprivation'. *Ann. N.Y. Acad. Sci.* **96,** 71

74. McGhie, A. (1966). 'The Subjective Assessment of Sleep Patterns in Psychiatric Illness'. *Br. J. med. Psychol.* **39,** 221

75. — and Russell, S. M. (1962). 'The Subjective Assessment of Normal Sleep Patterns'. *J. ment. Sci.* **108,** 642

76. Meddis, R. (1968). 'Human Circadian Rhythms and the 48 Hour Day'. *Nature, Lond.* **218,** 964

77. Mendels, J. and Hawkins, D. R. (1967). 'Sleep and Depression: A Controlled EEG Study'. *Archs gen. Psychiat.* **16,** 344

78. Ministry of Health and Department of Health for Scotland (1961). 'Drug Addiction'. *Report of the Interdepartmental Committee.* London: Her Majesty's Stationery Office

79. Ministry of Health (1964). 'Recent N.H.S. Prescribing Trends', *Reports on Public Health and Medical Subjects No. 110.* London: Her Majesty's Stationery Office

80. Monroe, L. J. (1967). 'Psychological and Physiological Differences Between Good and Poor Sleepers'. *J. abnorm. Psychol.* **72,** 255

81. — Rechtschaffen, A., Foulkes, D. and Jensen, J. (1965). 'Discriminability of REM and NREM Reports'. *J. Personality soc. Psychol.* **2,** 456

82. Muzio, J. N., Roffwarg, H. P. and Kaufman, E. (1966). 'Alterations in the Nocturnal Sleep Cycle Resulting from LSD'. *Electroenceph. clin. Neurophysiol.* **21,** 313

83. Oswald, I. (1962). 'Sleep Mechanisms: Recent Advances'. *Proc. R. Soc. Med.* **55,** 910

84. — (1962). *Sleeping and Waking.* Amsterdam: Elsevier

84a. — (1963). 'The Experimental Study of Sleep'. *Br. med. Bull.* **20,** 60

85.   — (1964). 'Physiology of Sleep Accompanying Dreaming'. In *The Scientific Basis of Medicine Annual Reviews*. Ed. by J. P. Ross. London: Athlone Press

86.   — (1965). 'Some Psychophysiological Features of Human Sleep'. In *Sleep Mechanisms*, p. 160. Ed. by K. Akert, C. Bally and J. P. Schadé. Amsterdam: Elsevier

87.   — (1966). *Sleep*. Harmondsworth, Middlesex: Penguin

88.   — (1968). 'Drugs and Sleep'. *Pharmac. Rev.* **20**, 274

88a   — (1969). 'Human Brain Protein, Drugs and Dreams' *Nature Land.* **223**, 893

89.   — and Thacore, V. R. (1963). 'Amphetamine and Phenmetrazine Addiction: Physiological Abnormalities in the Abstinence Syndrome'. *Br. med. J.* **2**, 427

90.   — and Priest, R. G. (1965). 'Five Weeks to Escape the Sleeping Pill Habit'. *Br. med. J.* **2**, 1093

91.   — Taylor, A. M. and Treisman, M. (1959). 'Further Studies of Response to Stimulation During Sleep'. *Electroenceph. clin. Neurophysiol* **11**, 840

92.   — Jones, H. S. and Mannerheim, J. E. (1968). 'Effects of Two Slimming Drugs on Sleep'. *Br. med. J.* **1**, 796

93.   — Evans, J. I. and Lewis, S. A. (1969). 'Addictive Drugs Cause Suppression of Paradoxical Sleep with Withdrawal Rebound'. In *Scientific Basis of Drug Dependence*. Ed. by H. Steinberg. London: Churchill

94.   — Berger, R. J., Jaramillo, R. A., Keddie, K. M. G., Olley, P. C. and Plunkett, G. B. (1963). 'Melancholia and Barbiturates: A Controlled EEG, Body and Eye Movement Study of Sleep'. *Br. J. Psychiat.* **109**, 66

95.   — Ashcroft, G. W., Berger, R. J., Eccleston, D., Evans, J. I. and Thacore, V. R. (1966). 'Some Experiments in the Chemistry of Normal Sleep'. *Br. J. Psychiat.* **112**, 391

96.   Parsons, T. W. (1963). 'Clinical Comparison of Barbiturates as Hypnotics'. *Br. med. J.* **2**, 1035

97.   Pivik, R. and Foulkes, D. (1966).' "Dream Deprivation": Effect on Dream Content'. *Science* **153**, 1282

98.   Pompeiano, O. (1967). 'The Neurophysiological Mechanisms of the Postural and Motor Events During Desynchronised Sleep'. *Res. Publs Ass. Res. nerv. ment. Dis.* **45**, 351

99.   Rechtschaffen, A. and Maron, L. (1964). 'Effect of Amphetamine on the Sleep Cycle'. *Electroenceph. clin. Neurophysiol.* **16**, 438

100.   — and Foulkes, D. (1965). 'Effect of Visual Stimuli on Dream Content'. *Percept. Mot. Skills* **20**, 1149

101.   — Goodenough, D. R. and Shapiro, A. (1962). 'Patterns of Sleep Talking'. *Archs gen. Psychiat.* **7**, 418

102.   — Wolpert, E. A., Dement, W. C., Mitchell, S. A. and Fisher, C. (1963). 'Nocturnal Sleep of Narcoleptics'. *Electroenceph. clin. Neurophysiol.* **15**, 599

D*

103. Reivich, M., Isaacs, G., Evarts, E. and Kety, S. (1968). 'The Effect of Slow Wave Sleep and REM Sleep on Regional Cerebral Blood Flow in Cats'. *J. Neurochem.* **15,** 301

104. Roffwarg, H. P., Dement, W. C., Muzio, J. N. and Fisher, C. (1962). 'Dream Imagery: Relationship to Rapid Eye Movements of Sleep'. *Archs gen. Psychiat.* **7,** 235

105. Schwartz, B. A., Gilbaud, G. and Fischgold, H. (1963). 'Études Électroencéphalographiques sur le Sommeil de Nuit'. *Presse méd.* **71,** 1474

106. Shapiro, A., Goodenough, D. R., Biederman, I. and Sleser, I. (1964). 'Dream Recall and the Physiology of Sleep'. *J. appl. Physiol.* **19,** 778

107. Shimizu, A., Yamada, Y., Yamamoto, J., Fujiki, A. and Kaneko, Z. (1966). 'Pathways of Descending Influence on H-reflex During Sleep'. *Electroenceph. clin. Neurophysiol.* **20,** 337

108. Snyder, F. (1969). 'Sleep Disturbance in Relation to Acute Psychosis'. In *Sleep: Physiology and Pathology.* Ed. by A. Kales. Philadelphia: Lippincott

109. — Hobson, J. A., Morrison, D. F. and Goldfrank, F. (1964). 'Changes in Respiration, Heart Rate, and Systolic Blood Pressure in Human Sleep'. *J. appl. Physiol.* **19,** 417

110. Swanson, E. M. and Foulkes, D. (1968). 'Dream Content and the Menstrual Cycle'. *J. nerv. ment. Dis.* **145,** 358

111. Tyler, D. B. (1955). 'Psychological Changes During Experimental Sleep Deprivation'. *Dis. nerv. Syst.* **16,** 293

112. Verdone, P. (1965). 'Temporal Reference of Manifest Dream Content'. *Percept. Mot. Skills* **20,** 1253

113. Villablanca, J. (1966). 'Behavioral and Polygraphic Study of "Sleep" and "Wakefulness" in Chronic Decerebrate Cats'. *Electroenceph. clin. Neurophysiol.* **21,** 562

114. Vogel, G. W. (1968). 'REM Deprivation. III. Dreaming and Psychosis'. *Archs gen. Psychiat.* **18,** 312

115. — and Traub, A. C. (1968). 'REM Deprivation. I. The Effect on Schizophrenic Patients'. *Archs gen. Psychiat.* **18,** 287

116. Vondráček, V., Prokupek, J., Fischer, R. and Ahrenbergova, M. (1968). 'Recent Patterns of Addiction in Czechoslovakia'. *Br. J. Psychiat.* **114,** 285

117. Weiss, H. R., Kasinoff, B. H. and Bailey, M. A. (1962). 'An Exploration of Reported Sleep Disturbance'. *J. nerv. ment. Dis.* **134,** 528

118. West, L. J. (1967). 'Psychopathology Produced by Sleep Deprivation'. *Res. Publs Ass. Res. nerv. ment. Dis.* **45,** 535

119. Whitman, R. M., Pierce, C. M., Maas, J. W. and Baldridge, B. J. (1962). 'The Dreams of the Experimental Subject'. *J. nerv. ment. Dis.* **134,** 431

120. Wilkinson, R. T. (1963). 'After Effect of Sleep Deprivation'. *J. exp. Psychol.* **66,** 439

121. — Edwards, R. S. and Haines, E. (1966). 'Performance Following a Night of Reduced Sleep'. *Psychon. Sci.* **5,** 471

122. Williams, H. L. and Williams, C. L. (1966). 'Nocturnal EEG Profiles and Performance'. *Psychophysiology* **3,** 164

123. — Lubin, A. and Goodnow, J. J. (1959). 'Impaired Performance with Acute Sleep Loss'. *Psychol. Monogr.* **73,** No. 14

124. Witkin, H. A. and Lewis, H. B. (1965). 'The Relation of Experimentally Induced Presleep Experiences to Dreams'. *J. Am. psychoanal. Ass.* **13,** 819

125. Yules, R. B., Freedman, D. X. and Chandler, K. A. (1966). 'The Effect of Ethyl Alcohol on Man's Electroencephalographic Sleep Cycle'. *Electroenceph. clin. Neurophysiol.* **20,** 109

126. Zarcone, V., Gulevich, G., Pivik, T. and Dement, W. (1968). 'Partial REM Phase Deprivation and Schizophrenia'. *Archs gen. Psychiat.* **18,** 194

CHAPTER 4

BIOCHEMICAL CHANGES IN THE SCHIZOPHRENIAS WITH SPECIAL REFERENCE TO URINARY PRODUCTS (INDOLEAMINES)

HIROSHI TANIMUKAI
and
HAROLD E. HIMWICH

WHY DO WE PRESUME A BIOCHEMICAL ABERRATION IN THE SCHIZOPHRENIAS?

Since Kraepelin[60] postulated that dementia praecox is a mental disease due to a somatic lesion, a large number of biological studies have been made by many investigators. The abnormalities reported as being specific for this disease have covered the body from head to foot. Most of these findings have not been confirmed by the succeeding investigators or have been forgotten without having been followed by confirmative researches.

Biochemical studies are not exceptions to this unsatisfactory situation and the history of recent biochemical studies in the schizophrenias has been reviewed by Richter[72], Kety[56, 58] and, also, Sourkes[84]. The concept that a biochemical or metabolic disorder is associated with the schizophrenias is based on the results of genetic studies. They include findings on twin patients[55, 81] in which there were significantly higher concordances in monozygotic twins than in dizygotic ones. This concordance is regarded as evidence that schizophrenia is a disease germinated in a hereditary predisposition. Standing on the concept of modern genetics and accepting the 'one gene one enzyme theory', it is quite reasonable to believe that some metabolic aberration may be involved in this disease.

PRECAUTIONS AGAINST ERRORS

Before considering the detailed biochemical data it may be worthwhile discussing why or how the abnormal biochemical findings reported as being characteristic in schizophrenia have not been further pursued, if for no other reason than to prevent reattacking false leads.

First of all, we have to point out that the schizophrenias are not regarded as a single disease arising from a single cause but may be a mixture of mental diseases with different aetiologies. Genetic studies favour this concept. Mitsuda[65] performed a clinico-genetic study of schizophrenia and concluded that the disease generally called schizophrenia today was not homogeneous, but that it could be divided into at least two groups distinguishable from each other not only phenomenally but also genetically. The studies of the prognosis of intrafamilial psychosis endorsed such a conclusion. It is almost impossible from this viewpoint to find a single metabolic aberration specific for schizophrenia and, therefore, the failure to obtain confirmatory results is not surprising. It is not impossible that various scientists dealt with different clinical entities. For a biochemical study, it is obviously better to select a single subgroup from the schizophrenias for investigation or, in lieu of that, to perform longitudinal studies and correlate the biochemical changes with the symptoms of the patient over a long period of time. In this sense, the study on periodic catatonia made by Gjessing[46] should be regarded as an excellent model.

Secondly, we must consider those factors which may influence the biochemical data. They are:

(1) Constitutional. The body build of schizophrenic patients statistically belongs to the leptosomal-asthenic type. If statistical analyses are used, the biochemical data common to the leptosomal-asthenic body build may be erroneously concluded as being specific for this disease.

(2) Physical condition. The influences of long-time hospitalization, malnutrition, complicating infections, hypofunction of the digestive organs (especially hepatic hypofunction and constipation) as well as medical treatments must all be taken into consideration in interpreting data. A good example is an acceleration of N,N-dimethyl-p-phenylenediamine oxidation in the presence of the patients' sera. This phenomenon was confirmed in different laboratories[1, 2, 61] and was once regarded as being a characteristic of schizophrenia, but later it was denied by some investigators[5, 53, 62] who demonstrated that this phenomenon was due to an ascorbic acid deficiency resulting from malnutrition in patients. Chronic schizophrenic patients usually exhibit abulia so that hypoperistalsis increases the absorption of intestinal contents into the blood stream and, therefore, the excretion of the metabolic products of the intestinal flora in the urine. Some findings, such as a high incidence of a positive Millon reaction indicating the presence of indican in urine[48, 75, 78], are now ascribed to constipation[36, 63, 76].

(3) Mental condition. It is known that mental activities, especially emotional stresses, affect endocrine function and bodily metabolism[14, 38, 79]. This factor should be taken into consideration when correlating the data with the aetiology of the disease.

(4) In addition to the above-mentioned factors, dietary precautions must be observed. It is well known, for example, that with increases[59] or decreases[11] of proteins, and especially those containing either tryptophan or methionine, there will be marked changes in the urine. Moreover, if we are to seek psychotogenic indoles or catechols, it is well to eliminate all preformed indoleamines and catecholamines from the diet, largely a matter of the exclusion of higher plants. In the light of the above mentioned criteria, most of the early biochemical studies so far made on patients with schizophrenia are difficult to evaluate.

MODERN TRENDS IN BIOCHEMICAL RESEARCH ON THE SCHIZOPHRENIAS

Recently two series of biochemical researches have appeared which are worthy of mention. One is an immunological study which is based on the hypothesis that schizophrenia is an autoimmune disease. This was theoretically proposed by Burch[27] and is being advanced by Heath and Krupp[49]. Heath's reports have only recently been published, and the subject matter has been reviewed in the *Lancet*[37]. The second biochemical study is based on the transmethylation hypothesis. Based on the structural similarity of a psychotogenic amine, mescaline, to norepinephrine or dopamine, which are the naturally occurring catecholamines in the brain, Osmond and Smythies[67] proposed that catecholamines may be transmethylated to their O-methylated compounds in the body of schizophrenics and that such an O-transmethylated catecholamine may cause mental symptoms. Friedhoff and van Winkle[44] reported the high incidence of 3,4-dimethoxyphenylethylamine (DMPEA) in the urine of schizophrenic patients and the failure of this psychotogenic amine to occur in the urine of normal controls. This finding was regarded as supportive evidence of the transmethylation hypothesis and many experiments confirmed these results[17, 90]. But there were some contradictory results and the present controversial status of this problem has also been reviewed in the *Lancet*[4]. Some investigators are prone to doubt that DMPEA is the substance responsible for the 'pink spot' on the paper chromatogram[10, 15, 16], but that it is one of the substances contained in the 'pink spot' has been indicated by mass spectrographical methods[34].

According to the original transmethylation hypothesis[67], an O-methylated catecholamine was considered as a causal substance for schizophrenia, and this conception is now called the 'catechol-amine hypothesis'. Kety[57], basing his work on the structural similarity of indole psychotogens to serotonin, extended this hypothesis to N,N-dimethylated indoleamines and this is called the 'indoleamine hypothesis'. The main purpose of this chapter is to present and discuss the experimental evidence in regard to the 'indoleamine hypothesis', most of which has been the work of Himwich and his coworkers at the Thudichum Psychiatric Research Laboratory, Galesburg, Illinois.

BIOCHEMICAL EVIDENCE SUPPORTING THE 'INDOLEAMINE HYPOTHESIS'
(With Special Reference to the Research at the Thudichum Laboratory)

Urinary Indoleamines and Indolic Acids and Schizophrenic Behaviour

Brune and Himwich[18] examined the urinary tryptamine and indole-3-acetic acid excretions in schizophrenic patients and compared the biochemical results with the behavioural changes in patients when they were on placebo as well as on reserpine medication. They found that tryptamine rose before the worsening of symptoms, continued at high levels while the symptoms were aggravated and fell with the improvement in behaviour. This was the first report from the Galesburg Laboratory which turned their attention to indole-amine metabolism in the schizophrenias. Brune and Himwich[19, 20], Brune and Pscheidt[23], and Brune, Pscheidt and Himwich[25] continued their experiments on the schizophrenic patients and studying the pharmacologically evoked behavioural worsening, confirmed their own previous data, and concluded that urinary indole-3-acetic acid, 5-hydroxyindoleacetic acid (5-HIAA) and tryptamine rose with the exacerbation of the schizophrenic symptoms and the greatest change was always observed in the tryptamine level and the least in that of 5-HIAA (*Figure 1*). Similar correlations between urinary tryptamine levels and the exacerbation of symptoms were also observed in schizophrenic patients whose behaviour worsened spontaneously[11].

Catecholamines and Steroid Hormones in Urine

With the indoleamines, they also determined urinary catechol-amines and their metabolites as well as steroid hormones. Only when the intensification of psychotic symptoms was accompanied by

81

motor restlessness and increased anxiety were norepinephrine and epinephrine as well as steroids found to be significantly elevated in the urine[13, 18, 19, 23, 25, 64, 71]. They concluded that these three classes of urinary products were more closely associated with the motor activity and/or emotional changes than with the psychopathology of schizophrenia. The Galesburg group has since given greater emphasis to the metabolism of indoleamines than to that of catecholamines in the causation of behavioural worsening in the patients they studied. They, therefore, selectively investigated the simultaneous relationships between indoleamine metabolism and the degree of behavioural activation in their patients.

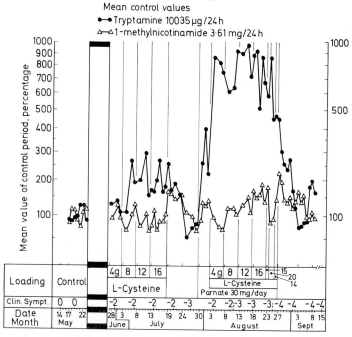

Figure 1(a)

Indole Psychotogens

Apart from the clinical experiments mentioned above, pharmacological experiments concerning psychotogenic amines had been advancing[39, 45, 51, 88, 89]. These studies indicated that all psychotogenic indoleamines possessed a N,N-dimethyltryptamine moiety in their structures. In addition, the structural similarity between psychotomimetic tertiary indoleamines and the naturally occurring primary amines is noted (*Figure 2*).

Axelrod[7, 8] then found an enzyme, the 'non-specific N-methyl-transferase', which catalyses the reactions by which serotonin is transformed to bufotenin and tryptamine to N,N-dimethyltryptamine. The activity of this enzyme was found most potent in the rabbit lung, less so in adrenal gland, kidney, spleen, heart and liver, but was not detected in the brain. Human lung obtained by autopsy

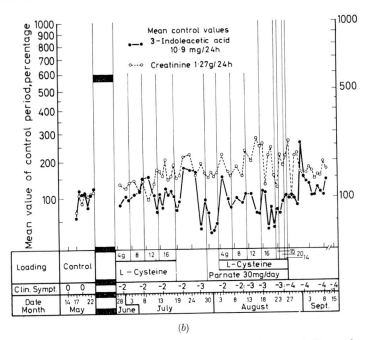

(b)

Figure 1. Simultaneous changes of urinary tryptophan metabolites and creatinine as well as behaviour of the patient. (a) Including the changes in tryptamine and 1-methylnicotinamide; (b) 3-indoleacetic acid and creatinine. The value is expressed as per cent deviations from the means of the values obtained during the control period. Note that the peak excretion of tryptamine occurred prior to the most severe behavioural disturbances as indicated in the column of 'Clinical Symptoms', where O is the usual pattern of behaviour for this patient, and a four point scale from −1 to −4 indicates increasing degrees of severity of the mental symptoms

was reported to exhibit weak activity of this enzyme[8]. If N,N-dimethylated indoleamines occur in considerable amounts in the body, they may affect mental activity and facilitate the intensification of psychotic behaviour in man. Some investigators tried and failed to find psychotogenic N,N-dimethylated indoleamines in the urine of mentally ill patients[41, 73, 86].

83

Effect of Methionine on Schizophrenic Behaviour

Pollin, Cardon and Kety[70] examined the effects of large doses of various amino acids on schizophrenic behaviour and reported that only methionine produced exacerbations of the mental symptoms in some patients when given together with iproniazid, a monoamine oxidase (MAO) inhibitor. The changes in symptoms could be of two different kinds: an acute flare-up of a chronic schizophrenic process or a toxic delirium superimposed upon chronic schizophrenic symptoms.

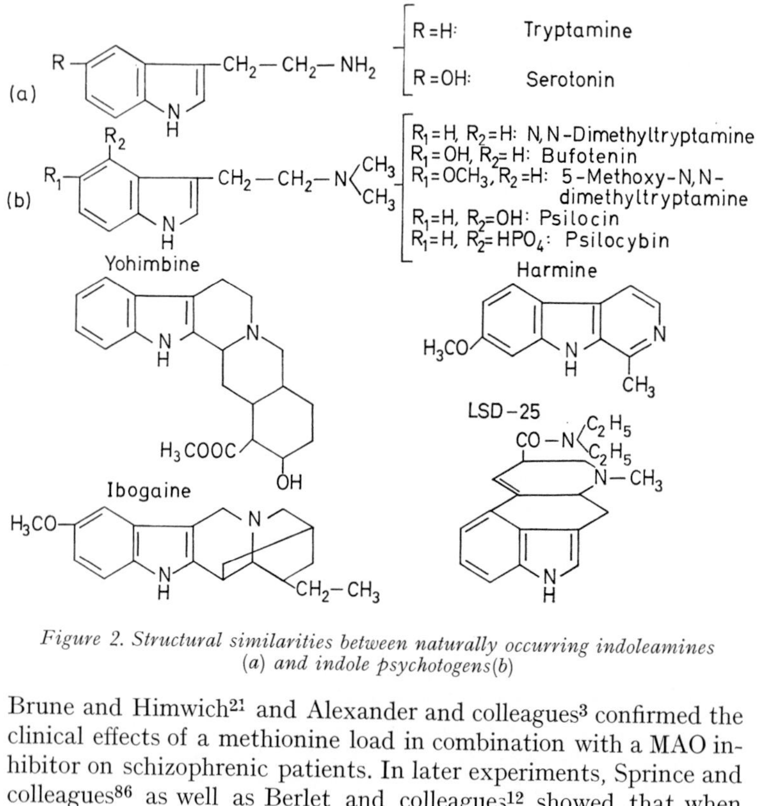

Figure 2. Structural similarities between naturally occurring indoleamines (a) and indole psychotogens(b)

Brune and Himwich[21] and Alexander and colleagues[3] confirmed the clinical effects of a methionine load in combination with a MAO inhibitor on schizophrenic patients. In later experiments, Sprince and colleagues[86] as well as Berlet and colleagues[12] showed that when methionine was given to patients on tranylcypromine, a MAO inhibitor, tryptamine increased in the urine before and during behavioural worsening.

Brune and Himwich[21] suggested that the formation of N,N-dimethylated indoleamines might be facilitated in the body under a methionine load and that these tertiary indoleamines might act as psychotogens to mediate the aggravation of the mental symptoms of schizophrenic patients in the presence of a MAO inhibitor. This hypothetical concept is schematically shown in *Figure 3*.

The finding of Kety's group[70] that methionine at times caused aggravation of the schizophrenic symptoms seemed to support the transmethylation hypothesis because the administration of methionine has been demonstrated to increase the tissue levels of S-adenosylmethionine, an active transmethylating agent[9]. However,

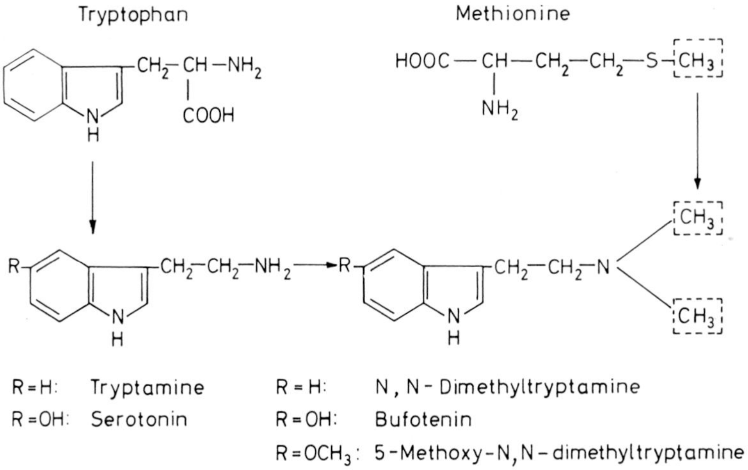

Tryptophan   Methionine

R = H: Tryptamine   R = H: N , N – Dimethyltryptamine
R = OH: Serotonin   R = OH: Bufotenin
                               R = OCH₃: 5 - Methoxy - N, N - dimethyltryptamine

Figure 3. Chemical structures involved in the 'indoleamine hypothesis'

since methionine is concerned not only with transmethylation but other reactions in metabolism as well, this conclusion does not necessarily hold.

Effect of Betaine

In order to check whether or not transmethylation is really involved in the ability of methionine to evoke a schizophrenic reaction, Brune and Himwich[22] examined the effects of betaine, another methyl donor, and observed the same tendency as that displayed by methionine in evoking behavioural changes in schizophrenic patients though the effects of betaine were somewhat weaker.

Effect of Reduced Intake of Methionine and Tryptophan

If N,N-dimethylated indoleamine is formed within the human

body, the indoleamine structure would come from tryptophan, and the methyl group is probably supplied by methionine. If an increase of N,N-dimethylated indoleamines renders schizophrenic symptoms worse, then perhaps the reduced intake of tryptophan and methionine might improve the mental symptoms. This possibility was examined by the Galesburg group. For 12 weeks, Berlet and colleagues[11] gave nine chronic schizophrenic patients a controlled diet in which the tryptophan and methionine contents were reduced to the amounts slightly above the minimal requirement for health. Urinary excretions of indoles, especially of tryptamine, were reduced by this treatment, but no beneficial effects of such diets were observed on the patients' behaviour. This result does not necessarily contradict the transmethylation hypothesis. A minimal requirement of both amino acids was given to the patients because both tryptophan and methionine are essential amino acids, and it was impossible to eliminate them as well as other methyl donors from the diet without causing impairment in the patients' health.

Change in Urinary Creatinine with Behavioural Worsening

The Galesburg group further advanced their experiments when they gave large doses of tryptophan and/or methionine to eight chronic schizophrenic patients either in the absence or in the presence of a MAO inhibitor[12]. In their experiments they not only obtained confirmation of their previous findings on the chemical correlation of tryptophan metabolites and schizophrenic symptoms, but they also noted that urinary creatinine rose as an accompaniment of the worsened behaviour. Berlet and colleagues[12, 13] interpreted these increases of creatinine as being derived from the breakdown of muscle proteins and that this breakdown also yielded tryptophan which was the source of the indole products finally showing up in the urine. The additional tryptamine came from this release of the amino acids.

Effect of Cysteine

Since methionine is a sulphur-containing amino acid the effect of sulphur in producing the intensification of schizophrenic behaviour should be taken into consideration. Spaide and colleagues[85] investigated the effects of large amounts of cysteine on the symptomatology of schizophrenic patients both in the absence and presence of tranylcypromine, a MAO inhibitor. In these experiments, the intensifications of the previous symptoms in the various types of schizophrenia were observed in all four patients when they had received cysteine in combination with a MAO inhibitor. Thus cysteine was added to the amino acids which in large doses can provoke the behavioural worsening of schizophrenic patients. Urinary tryptamine again rose in this experiment as a result of cysteine administration and shortly thereafter the schizophrenic symptoms started to worsen. Such results supported our opinion of the time relationships between the rise of urinary tryptamine and the aggravation of schizophrenic behaviour.

The next question to arise is how cysteine can substitute for methionine since it has no methyl group in its structure. Sprince and colleagues[87] demonstrated in rats that methionine, homocysteine or cysteine inhibited the kynurenine pathway of tryptophan metabolism. If these data were applicable to human beings, we might explain the tryptamine phenomenon in our cysteine study but against this were the experimental facts that though urinary N-methylnicotinamide was lowered in one patient it was raised in two others. But in that case, N-methylnicotinamide, a product of the kynurenine pathway, should decrease in concentration, as it did in one patient. Yet in two others, urinary N-methylnicotinamide rose with the tryptamine suggesting that more of that amino acid was made available in the body during behavioural worsening. Such negative results are not surprising as an important part of the experiments of Sprince and colleagues[87] was the witholding of nicotinic acid from the diet of the animals, which, of course, was impossible in human patients.

The Search for Indole Psychotogens in the Urine of Psychotic Patients

Bufotenin (N,N-dimethylserotonin) was first reported by Bumpus and Page[26] as present in normal human urine, but this finding was not confirmed at first. Some investigators attempted to find N,N-dimethylated indoleamines in the urine of schizophrenic patients, but the results had always been negative until Fischer and colleagues[43], using unidimensional paper chromatography, demonstrated the presence of a bufotenin-like compound occurring only in the urine of schizophrenic patients. Brune, Kohl and Himwich[24], using two-dimensional paper chromatography, confirmed the finding of Fischer and colleagues[43]. Gross and Franzen[47] developed a chemical method for bufotenin determination and, using their method, they reported the presence of bufotenin in the urine as well as in serum of normal subjects. Heller[50] described the presence of bufotenin occurring only in schizophrenic urine and stated that under the favourable influence of tranquillizing drugs, the excretion of bufotenin diminished. In contrast to these reports, other experiments made in various laboratories[41, 54, 66, 69, 73, 74, 80, 91], under carefully controlled conditions, failed to confirm the presence of this psychotogenic indoleamine.

Tanimukai joined the Galesburg group in the midst of their cysteine study and took part in the examination of the psychotomimetic N,N-dimethylated indoleamines. He pointed out that the use of acetone (which had been employed by most of the previous investigators) in the extraction of the substance from the urine might lead to artifactual results[92]. He developed more sensitive and reproducible modifications of paper and thin-layer chromatographic methods for the detection of N,N-dimethylated indoleamines[92]. Using these modifications as well as the recently developed gas–liquid chromatographic methods of Capella and Horning[29], Tanimukai and colleagues[93, 94, 95] examined the urine samples of schizophrenic patients under various experimental conditions at the Thudichum Laboratory. The samples which had been collected during the cysteine study mentioned above were analysed by chromatographic methods. Free and conjugated bufotenin were found in the urine of all four patients when they exhibited the greatest exacerbations of their symptoms[94]. The identification of bufotenin was made by two-dimensional paper and two-dimensional thin-layer chromatography as well as by gas–liquid chromatography using two different stationary phases. The amount of bufotenin excreted increased about two weeks before the behavioural worsening started, remained at high levels as long as the aggravation of mental symptoms continued and returned to the usual level with improvement in behaviour. Using thin-layer chromatography they also disclosed urinary substances suspected of being N,N-dimethyltryptamine and 5-methoxy-N,N-dimethyltryptamine at the time when the patients exhibited their greatest behavioural exacerbations[95, 96]. These findings were confirmed by gas-liquid chromatography (Narasimhachari and colleagues unpublished data). But normal controls, studied under the same conditions, failed to excrete any of these three potentially psychotogenic compounds. In another study[93], using thin-layer techniques, they examined bufotenin in the urine of six schizophrenics and four mentally defective patients from whom all medications had been withheld for at least six weeks. They found free bufotenin in the urine of all patients (six schizophrenics and one mental defective) who exhibited psychotic symptoms, but not in the urine of mentally defective patients who were free of psychotic symptoms. Bound bufotenin, on the other hand, was disclosed in each patient's urine. They suggested, therefore, that only free bufotenin may evoke psychotic reactions and that the conjugation disclosed in each patient's urine represented a detoxication process that neutralized the action of this psychotogenic amine. They excluded from the diet of the patients all known sources of preformed catecholamines and indoleamines but did not put their patients on a plant free diet. Since bufotenin is known to be widely distributed in higher plants[35], the possibility existed that the bufotenin found in these studies had come from exogenous sources. In order to check this possibility in their third series of experiments (Unpublished data), they gave L-tryptophan-2-C[14] together with DL-methionine tritiated at the methyl group to four schizophrenic patients to determine whether or not bufotenin doubly labelled with C[14] and H[3] could be found in the urine. This study, however, has not been completed. Fischer and Spatz[42] recently reported the occurrence of bufotenin in the urine of schizophrenic patients, but again they used acetone for its extraction. Tanimukai. Unpublished data) studied the effects of phenothiazine tranquillizers on the urinary excretion of bufotenin in schizophrenic patients. He could not, however, reach any clear-cut conclusion because of the presence in the urine of many metabolites of the drug which disturbed the thin-layer chromatographic identification of bufotenin.

THE WORK OF THE GALESBURG GROUP

These series of investigations made by the Galesburg group were time consuming, but perhaps they are the shortest way to the goal. They selected chronic male schizophrenic patients with active symptoms and maintained them in a metabolic ward with strictly controlled dietary conditions under the supervision of a research dietitian. In each instance, the patient had been free of tranquillizing drugs before and during the investigation and the influence of intestinal flora was monitored. Urine collections were made on a daily basis and the biochemical data were always interpreted in relation to the simultaneously occurring clinical symptoms which were evaluated by a team of psychiatrists who were unaware of the biochemical results. In this way, the researches made by the Galesburg group met the previously discussed criteria for biochemical studies on the schizophrenias. *They believe that the biochemical change in schizophrenia, if present, should become more prominent at the time of behavioural exacerbations than in the chronic steady state although such changes should be present throughout the course of the illness.* That is, due to a precipitating factor the biochemical disturbance always present in some schizophrenics becomes more severe and in turn gives rise to an activation of the schizophrenic symptoms. Thus they applied, under experimental conditions, a pharmacologically evoked exacerbation of symptoms, as a means of study. Perhaps cysteine is the most effective means, methionine next, and betaine is the least effective among these three amino acids when given with a MAO inhibitor.

Reproduction of Schizophrenic Symptoms or Toxic Reaction?

Pollin, Cardon and Kety[70] who first found the methionine effect on schizophrenia stated

> the extent to which these clinical changes represent a biochemically induced acute flare-up of a chronic schizophrenic process on the one hand, or a toxic delirium superimposed upon chronic schizophrenia on the other, is as yet, uncertain

and claimed in a recent paper[68] that

> in the presently cited three case histories, there are elements in two that are consistent with the diagnosis of a toxic condition: abrupt change in behavior following drug administration (a point that does not help in the present consideration), nausea and dizziness, and the addition of visual hallucinations to previously nonvisual hallucinations. On the other hand, the lack of delirium and the resemblance of behavior to previous disturbances are consistent with the diagnosis of schizophrenic exacerbation. The diagnostic issues in this area are extremely complex, and simple clear-cut interpretations are not readily found.

Kakimoto and colleagues[54], referring to the clinical study made by Asao and Yamano, stated that the symptoms observed in their schizophrenic patients during a methionine load in the presence of isocarboxazid, a MAO inhibitor, were superimposed upon those of intoxication, such as delirium, visual hallucinations, ataxia and other vegetative symptoms. In our opinion, there may occur two kinds of reactions on amino acid loading: one is a toxic reaction and the other a true reproduction or intensification of schizophrenic symptoms. In some cases the toxic reaction may be more prominent and in the other cases the true reproduction is dominant. Many factors, endogenic, exogenic and even psychological factors, may participate in determining which reaction appears more prominent. In the experiments made by Asao and Yamano, a large dosage of methionine was administered from the beginning of the experiment and this acute large dosage might be more likely to evoke toxic reactions than would a gradual increase of a smaller initial dose[20]. In clinical studies using either smaller doses or attaining large doses more gradually, investigators have reported a less prominent delirious state[12]. In our observations[85] many of the mental symptoms each patient had previously shown were reproduced in an exaggerated way. This means catatonic patients became more catatonic and paranoid schizophrenics exhibited more intense delusions. Thus, although care should be taken in the interpretation of the data in relation to the aetiology of the schizophrenias, a method of pharmacological evocation is obviously useful in the research of the biochemical aspect of schizophrenia.

Urinary Products and the Schizophrenias

Urinary tryptamine levels were demonstrated by the Galesburg group as being the most sensitive biochemical indicator, rising before the worsening of the symptoms, continuing at high levels during the symptomatic exacerbations, and decreasing again with the improvement of behaviour. This phenomenon of increases in indoleamine metabolism associated with worsening of the symptoms was observed not only in pharmacologically evoked worsening in behaviour but also in that occurring spontaneously in the course of the illness in schizophrenic patients.

Urinary 5-hydroxyindoleacetic acid (5-HIAA) in the schizophrenic patients was examined by some investigators but their results have not always agreed[6, 28, 30, 100]. This is not strange because the schizophrenias are not a disease entity. Moreover, 5-HIAA is not a sensitive indicator of the symptomatic fluctuations for, unlike tryptamine, it does not derive directly from tryptophan; it is an end product of serotonin metabolism. Bufotenin is also metabolized to 5-HIAA but the bufotenin pathway is negligibly small when compared to the serotonin pathway so that an alteration in bufotenin metabolism cannot significantly influence the urinary levels of 5-HIAA.

The urinary occurrence of bufotenin has long been a controversial subject. We now have more definitive information since our confirmation was made by using two-dimensional paper, two-dimensional thin-layer chromatography, as well as the gas–liquid chromatographic technique with two different stationary phases. The occurrence of this compound is not specific for this mental disease, but our data suggest that the increase of free bufotenin may be related to psychotic behaviour.

THE INDOLEAMINE HYPOTHESIS

The Galesburg group confirmed the urinary excretion of bufotenin, even though it may be only a weak psychotogenic indoleamine. But, as pointed out by Turner and Merlis[98], bufotenin might well exert stronger effects in schizophrenics than in normal controls.

The earlier thin-layer chromatographic findings of N,N-dimethyl-tryptamine and 5-methoxy-N, N-dimethyltryptamine in the urine samples of schizophrenic patients given a large dose of cysteine together with a MAO inhibitor[92, 96] were later confirmed by the gas–liquid chromatographic method (Narasimhachari and colleagues. Unpublished data). These findings strongly suggested that the N-methylating reaction of indoleamines might occur within the human body. This means that psychotogenic indoleamines may be produced within the body, and these amines may in turn evoke psychotic symptoms in some subjects when the formation of such amines is accelerated or their breakdown is inhibited (*Figure 4*).

We do not consider such metabolic aberrations to be characteristic of the schizophrenias but are inclined to correlate psychotogenic

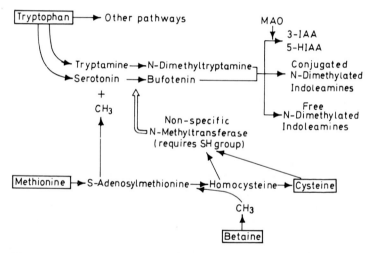

Figure 4. Schema for the 'indoleamine hypothesis' for the pathogenesis of psychotic symptoms. The maintenance of elevated levels of free N,N-dimethylated indoleamines in the body fluids may exacerbate mental and behavioural symptoms of the patient. The levels of these toxic amines are determined by the dynamic balance between the process of their synthesis and detoxication. Tryptophan provides the tryptamine structure which serves as a precursor of tertiary amines, while methionine or betaine may supply methyl groups. Cysteine and methionine may make thiol groups available for the activation of the enzyme catalysing the formation of N,N-dimethyl-ated indoleamines[8]. The amounts of free tertiary indoleamines may also increase when the metabolic breakdown processes are blocked by a MAO inhibitor. Thus all amino acids listed in Figure 4 can reproduce or intensify the identical psychotic symptoms in chronic schizophrenic patients. MAO: monoamine oxidase, 3-IAA: 3-indoleacetic acid, 5-HIAA: 5-hydroxyindoleacetic acid

indoleamines with psychotic behaviour regardless of the nosological diagnosis. Even in non-schizophrenic individuals mental symptoms can occur under certain conditions. An example was seen in Alexander's experiment[3] on a patient with psychoneurosis who exhibited a hallucinogenic reaction with methionine and tranylcypromine. Another example is one of our mentally defective patients[93]. When this patient was transferred to a closed metabolic ward from an open one, he experienced ideas of reference and he then excreted free bufotenin in the urine. Kakimoto and colleagues[54] analysed chemically the urine collected from schizophrenic patients who had been given large doses of methionine together with a MAO inhibitor, and failed to find any psychotogenic catecholamines or indoleamines, nor could they demonstrate an increase of the O-methylation reaction after a methionine load. They found instead that an amino acid imbalance and ionic disturbances took place in the body and interpreted the symptomatic changes in the patients in terms of these biochemical changes. Since the superimposed symptoms of intoxication were more prominent in their cases, as previously discussed, their interpretation does not seem to be applicable to the pharmacological mechanism underlying the reproduction of schizophrenic symptoms. The detection of N,N-dimethylated indoleamines in the urine of the patients showing active psychotic symptoms is compatible with the indoleamine hypothesis which the Galesburg group proposed as shown in *Figure 4*.

Dose–Effect Relationship of Psychotogens

Turner and Merlis[98] doubted the psychotogenic properties of bufotenin and Nishimura and Gjessing[66] pointed out that, if present, the amount of bufotenin was too small to have psychotomimetic effects and they, therefore, questioned the significance of this amine in the pathogenesis of the mental symptoms. It is true that the amounts of psychotogenic indoleamines found in the urine are much smaller than those used in the pharmacological experiments to evoke psychotomimetic effects in human beings[39, 88, 89]. These pharmacological experiments, however, used a single, acute dosage and toxic effects were observed in addition to psychopharmacological ones. It is a well-known fact in pharmacology, however, that the effect of a drug may differ significantly if the administration method is different. Both amphetamine and methamphetamine, on a single acute administration, produce temporary excitation followed by depression. Methamphetamine, after long-term misuse, produces in some addicted individuals chronic psychotic behaviour indistinguishable from the chronic schizophrenias[77]. Connell[33] made a systematic study of individuals with amphetamine addiction and found that the clinical picture is primarily a paranoid psychosis with ideas of reference, delusions of persecution, auditory and visual hallucinations, in a setting of clear consciousness. Long-term abuse of LSD-25, one of the most potent indole psychotogens, is reported to evoke in some individuals a prolonged psychotic state similar to schizophrenia[31, 32, 99], although a single administration of this drug causes temporary mental changes. In a similar way the psychotogenic indoleamines, if they influence the brain over long periods of time, may provoke the symptoms of chronic schizophrenia. In the case of the mentally ill patient, these toxic agents may be synthesized continuously within the body and disturb mental activities even though the amounts of the agents are small. Thus we feel that 'long-term action' of free tertiary amines may evoke psychotic symptoms in mentally ill patients.

As documented above, in regard to urinary bufotenin there have been both positive findings[22, 43, 50] in schizophrenics as well as negative ones[41, 69, 74, 80, 86, 91]. Similarly there have been positive findings[26, 47,] for bufotenin in normals and negative findings[66, 69, 73, 80, 86, 91] in non-schizophrenics. Because of the confused status of this area, we feel that the brief but convincing paper of Faurbye and Pind[40] was all the more welcome. They have shown the excretion of bufotenin in the urine of six of seven schizophrenics and four of six normal controls. Bufotenin, therefore, seems to be a normal metabolic product. This observation is in agreement with the viewpoint of our group, namely that if there is a biochemical aberration in schizophrenia, it is not on a qualitative basis but rather on a quantitative one. Even on this basis, however, there are at least three possibilities for differences between schizophrenics and normals in their reactions to psychotogens.

The first one depends upon the personality structure, i.e., the behavioural reaction of a given individual to the psychotogen. Hoch[52] studying mescaline chiefly, stated that under a psychotomimetic drug, a complete schizophrenic disorganization is much more prominent in schizophrenics and latent schizophrenics than in normal subjects. The experiences of normals are more like organic reactions with some schizophrenic features. On the other hand, in schizophrenics and latent schizophrenics the drug is able to heighten the schizophrenic disorganization of the individual, both emotionally and conceptually. The second factor is concerned with the biochemical reactions of the individual. These may include comparatively impaired detoxicating mechanisms in schizophrenics in contrast with normals. It is also possible that normals, under the same conditions as schizophrenics, may produce smaller amounts of N,N-dimethylated indoleamines. Finally, the form in which the N,N-dimethylated compound exists, whether conjugated or free, should be considered. Tanimukai and colleagues[93] presented evidence suggesting that the free and not the conjugated N,N-dimethylated amines are active psychotomimetically.

The question is larger, however, than the consideration of bufotenin alone but is concerned with the behavioural effects of N,N-dimethylated indoleamines in general. We do not know in what form they exist in the normal control, though for schizophrenics we have some suggestions that not only bufotenin but also N,N-dimethyltryptamine and 5-methoxy-N,N-dimethyltryptamine may exist mainly in the free form[96]. For normals, we have clear-cut results at present only for N,N-dimethyltryptamine. For that compound, there is agreement that it is four times as potent as mescaline[83, 89] in normal controls. For 5-methoxy-N,N-dimethyltryptamine we have no such results on controls, but it has proved to be more potent in animals than N,N-dimethyltryptamine as demonstrated by Gessner and Page[45] and Smythies, Bradley and Johnston[82]. The latter predicted that 5-methoxy-N,N-dimethyltryptamine is a potent hallucinogen on man.

CONCLUSION

The biochemical search for the aetiology of the schizophrenias has had a long history; the way to the goal is still full of difficulties. Honestly, we are not sure whether we are proceeding in the right direction, and the only thing that we say for sure is that we are attempting to converge to the path predicted by Thudichum[97] who stated that

> many forms of insanity are unquestionably the external manifestations of the effects upon the brain substance of poisons fermented within the body, just as mental aberrations accompanying chronic alcoholic intoxication are the accumulated effects of a relatively simple poison fermented out of the body. These poisons we shall, I have no doubt, be able to isolate after we know the normal chemistry to its uttermost detail. And then will come in their turn the crowning discoveries to which our efforts must ultimately be directed, namely, the discoveries of the antidotes to the poisons and to the fermenting causes and processes which produce them.

REFERENCES

1. Abood, L. G., Gibbs, F. A. and Gibbs, E. (1957). 'Comparative Study of Blood Ceruloplasmin in Schizophrenia and Other Disorders'. *A.M.A. Archs Neurol. Psychiat.* **77,** 643

2. Akerfeldt, S. (1957). 'Oxidation of N,N-Dimethyl-p-phenylene-diamine by Serum from Patients with Mental Disease'. *Science* **125**, 117

3. Alexander, F., Curtis, G. C., Sprince, H. and Crosley, A. P. (1963). 'L-Methionine and L-Tryptophan Feedings in Non-psychotic and Schizophrenic Patients With and Without Tranylcypromine'. *J. nerv. ment. Dis.* **137**, 135

4. Annotation (1966). 'The Pink Spot: A Red Herring?' *Lancet* **2**, 848

5. Aprison, M. H. and Grosz, H. J. (1958). 'Ascorbic Acid Level and Lag Time in Oxidation of N,N-Dimethyl-p-phenylenediamine'. *A.M.A. Archs Neurol. Psychiat.* **79**, 575

6. Ashcroft, G. W., Crawford, T. B. B., Eccleston, D., Sharman, D. F., MacDougall, E. J., Stanton, J. B. and Binns, J. K. (1966). '5-Hydroxyindole Compounds in the Cerebrospinal Fluid of Patients with Psychiatric or Neurological Diseases'. *Lancet* **2**, 1049

7. Axelrod, J. (1961). 'Enzymatic Formation of Psychotomimetic Metabolites from Normally Occurring Compounds'. *Science* **134**, 343

8. — (1962). 'The Enzymatic N-Methylation of Serotonin and Other Amines'. *J. Pharmac. exp. Ther.* **138**, 28

9. Baldessarini, R. J. and Kopin, I. J. (1963). 'Assay of Tissue Levels of S-Adenosylmethionine'. *Analyt. Biochem.* **6**, 289

10. Bell, C. E. and Somerville, A. R. (1966). 'Identity of the "Pink Spot" '. *Nature, Lond.* **211**, 1405

11. Berlet, H. H., Spaide, J., Kohl, H., Bull, C. and Himwich, H. E. (1965). 'Effects of Reduction of Tryptophan and Methionine Intake on Urinary Indole Compounds and Schizophrenic Behavior'. *J. nerv. ment. Dis.* **140**, 297

12. — Matsumoto, K., Pscheidt, G. R., Spaide, J., Bull, C. and Himwich, H. E. (1965). 'Biochemical Correlates of Behavior in Schizophrenic Patients'. *Archs gen. Psychiat.* **13**, 521

13. — Bull, C., Himwich, H. E., Kohl, H., Matsumoto, K., Pscheidt, G. R., Spaide, J., Tourlentes, T. T. and Valverde, J. M. (1964). 'Endogenous Metabolic Factor in Schizophrenic Behavior'. *Science* **144**, 311

14. Boards, F., Persky, H. and Hamburg, D. A. (1956). 'Psychological Stress and Endocrine Functions, Blood Levels of Adrenocortical and Thyroid Hormones in Acutely Disturbed Patients'. *Psychosom. Med.* **18**, 324

15. Boulton, A. A. and Felton, C. A. (1966). 'The "Pink Spot" and Schizophrenia'. *Nature, Lond.* **211**, 1404

16. — Pollitt, R. J. and Majer, J. R. (1967). 'Identity of Urinary "Pink Spot" in Schizophrenia and Parkinson's Disease'. *Nature, Lond.* **215**, 132

17. Bourdillon, R. E., Clarke, C. A., Ridges, A. P., Sheppard, P. M., Harper, P. and Leslie, S. A. (1965). ' "Pink Spot" in the Urine of Schizophrenics'. *Nature, Lond.* **208**, 453

18. Brune, G. G. and Himwich, H. E. (1960). 'Effects of Reserpine on Urinary Tryptamine and Indole-3-acetic Acid Excretion in Mental Deficiency, Schizophrenia and Phenylpyruvic Oligophrenia'. *Acta International Meeting for the Technical Study of Psychotropic Drugs.* Bologna, p. 1

19. —— (1961). 'Correlations between Behavior and Urinary Indole Amines During Treatment with Reserpine and Iso-carboxazid, Separately and Together'. *Neuro-psychopharmacology* **2**, 465

20. —— (1962). 'Indole Metabolites in Schizophrenic Patients'. *Archs gen. Psychiat.* **6**, 324

21. —— (1962). 'Effects of Methionine Loading on the Behavior of Schizophrenic Patients'. *J. nerv. ment. Dis.* **134**, 447

22. —— (1963). 'Biogenic Amines and Behavior in Schizo-phrenic Patients'. *Recent Adv. biol. Psychiat.* **5**, 144

23. — and Pscheidt, G. R. (1961). 'Correlations Between Behavior and Urinary Excretion of Indole Amines and Catecholamines in Schizophrenic Patients as Affected by Drugs'. *Fedn Proc. Fedn Am. Socs exp. Biol.* **20**, 889

24. — Kohl, H. H. and Himwich, H. E. (1963). 'Urinary Ex-cretion of Bufotenin-like Substance in Psychotic Patients'. *J. Neuropsychiat.* **5**, 14

25. — Pscheidt, G. R. and Himwich, H. E. (1963). 'Different Responses of Urinary Tryptamine and of Total Catecholamines During Treatment with Reserpine and Isocarboxazid in Schizo-phrenic Patients'. *Int. J. Neuropharmac.* **2**, 17

26. Bumpus, F. M. and Page, I. H. (1955). 'Serotonin and Its Methylated Derivatives in Human Urine'. *J. biol. Chem.* **212**, 111

27. Burch, P. R. J. (1964). 'Schizophrenia: Some New Aetiological Considerations'. *Br. J. Psychiat.* **110**, 818

28. Buscaino, G. A. and Stefanachi, L. (1958). 'Urinary Excretion of 5-Hydroxyindoleacetic Acid in Psychotic and Normal Subjects'. *A.M.A. Archs Neurol. Psychiat.* **80**, 78

29. Capella, P. and Horning, E. C. (1966). 'Separation and Identifica-tion of Derivatives of Biologic Amines by Gas–liquid Chromato-graphy'. *Analyt. Chem.* **38**, 316

30. Christodoulou, G. N. and Papaevangelou, G. J. (1966). 'High Protein, High Carbohydrate Diets, and Electroshock Treatment Related to 5-Hydroxyindoleacetic Acid Excretion in Schizo-phrenics and Normal Controls'. *Am. J. Psychiat.* **123**, 738

31. Cohen. S. and Ditman, K. S. (1962). 'Complications Associated With Lysergic Acid Diethylamide (LSD-25)'. *J. Am. Med. Ass.* **181**, 161

32. —— (1963). 'Prolonged Adverse Reactions to Lysergic Acid Diethylamide'. *Archs gen. Psychiat.* **8**, 475

33. Connell, P. H. (1958). *Amphetamine Psychosis.* Maudsley Mono-graph No. 5, p. 57. London: Oxford University Press

34. Creveling, C. R. and Daly, J. W. (1967). 'Identification of 3,4-Dimethoxyphenylethylamine from Schizophrenic Urine by Mass Spectrometry'. *Nature, Lond.* **216,** 190

35. Downing, D. F. (1964). 'Psychotomimetic Compounds'. *Psychopharmacological Agents,* Vol. 1, p. 555. Ed. by M. Gordon. New York: Academic Press

36. Ederle, W. (1957). 'Zur Frage der Millon-Reaktion in der Modifikation von SANO und DECKER bei der Schizophrenie'. *Nervenarzt* **28,** 131

37. Editorial (1967). 'Antibody, Antimind?' *Lancet* **1,** 828

38. Elmadjian, R., Hope J. M. and Lamson, E. T. (1957). 'Excretion of Epinephrine and Norepinephrine in Various Emotional States'. *J. clin. Endocr. Metab.* **17,** 608

39. Fabing, H. D. and Hawkins, J. R. (1956). 'Intravenous Bufotenine Injection in the Human Being'. *Science* **123,** 886

40. Faurbye, A. and Pind, K. (1968). 'Occurrence of Bufotenin in the Urine of Schizophrenic Patients and Normal Persons'. *Nature, Lond.* **220,** 489

41. Feldstein, A., Hoagland, H. and Freeman, H. (1961). 'Radioactive Serotonin in Relation to Schizophrenia'. *Archs. gen. Psychiat.* **5,** 246

42. Fischer, E. and Spatz, H. (1967). 'Determination of Bufotenin in the Urine of Schizophrenics'. *Int. J. Neuropsychiat.* **3,** 226

43. — Fernández Lagravere, T. A., Vázquez, A. J. and Di Stefano, A. O. (1961). 'A Bufotenin-like Substance in the Urine of Schizophrenics'. *J. nerv. ment. Dis.* **133,** 441

44. Friedhoff, A. J. and van Winkle, E. (1962). 'Isolation and Characterization of a Compound from the Urine of Schizophrenics'. *Nature, Lond.* **194,** 897

45. Gessner, P. K. and Page, I. H. (1962). 'Behavioral Effects of 5-Methoxy-N:N-dimethyltryptamine, Other Tryptamines, and LSD'. *Am. J. Physiol.* **203,** 167

46. Gjessing, R. (1932). 'Beiträge zur Kenntnis der Pathophysiologie des katatonen Stupors. I. Über periodisch rezidivierenden Katatonen Stupor, mit kritischem Beginn und Abschlug'. II. Über periodisch rezidivierende verlaufende katatonen Stupor mit lytischem Beginn und Abschlug'. *Arch. Psychiat.* **96,** 319, 391

47. Gross, H. and Franzen, Fr. (1964). 'Zur Bestimmung körpereigenen Amine in biologischen Substraten'. *Biochem. Z.* **340,** 403

48. Gullotta, S. (1930). 'Untersuchung Über den Harn von Amentia und Dementia praecox-Kranken'. *Biochem. Z.* **218,** 472

49. Heath, R. G. and Krupp, I. M. (1967). 'Schizophrenia as an Immunologic Disease. I. Demonstration of Antibrain Globulins by Fluorescent Antibody Techniques'. *Archs gen. Psychiat.* **16,** 1

50. Heller, B. (1966). 'Influence of Treatment with Amino Oxidase Inhibitor on the Excretion of Bufotenin and the Clinical Symptoms in Chronic Schizophrenic Patients'. *Int. J. Neuropsychiat.* **2,** 193

51. Himwich, H. E. (Ed.) (1967). *Amines and Schizophrenia,* p. 137. London: Pergamon Press

52. Hoch, P. H. (1951). 'Experimentally Produced Psychoses'. *Am. J. Psychiat.* **107,** 607

53. Horwitt, M. K., Meyer, B. J., Meyer, A. C., Harvey, C. C. and Haffron, D. (1957). 'Serum Copper and Oxidase Activity in Schizophrenic Patients'. *A.M.A. Archs Neurol. Psychiat.* **78,** 275

54. Kakimoto, Y., Sano, I., Kanazawa, A., Tsujio, T. and Kaneko, Z. (1967). 'Metabolic Effects of Methionine in Schizophrenic Patients Pretreated with a Monoamine Oxidase Inhibitor'. *Nature, Lond.* **216,** 1110

55. Kallmann, F. J. (1946). 'The Genetic Theory of Schizophrenia. An Analysis of 691 Schizophrenic Twin Index Families'. *Am. J. Psychiat.* **103,** 309

56. Kety, S. S. (1959). 'Biochemical Theories of Schizophrenia. I. Critical Review of Current Theories and of the Evidence Used to Support Them'. *Science* **129,** 1528

57. — (1961). 'Possible Relation of Central Amines to Behavior in Schizophrenic Patients'. *Fedn Proc. Fedn Am. Socs exp. Biol.* **20,** 894

58. — (1965). 'Biochemical Theories of Schizophrenia'. *Int. J. Psychiat.* **1,** 409

59. Kopin, I. J. (1959). 'Tryptophan Loading and Excretion of 5-Hydroxyindole-acetic Acid in Normal and Schizophrenic Subjects'. *Science* **129,** 835

60. Kraepelin, E. (1909–1913). *Psychiatry,* 8th edn. Leipzig

61. Leach, B. E. and Heath, R. G. (1956). 'The *In Vitro* Oxidation of Epinephrine in Plasma'. *A.M.A. Archs Neurol. Psychiat.* **76,** 444

62. McDonald, R. K. (1958). 'Ceruloplasmin and Schizophrenia'. *Chemical Concept of Psychosis,* p. 230. Ed. by M. Rinkel and H. C. B. Denber. New York: McDowell, Obolensky

63. McGeer, P. L., McNair, F. E., McGeer, E. G. and Gibson, W. C. (1957). 'Aromatic Metabolism in Schizophrenia. I. Statistical Evidence for Aromaturia'. *J. nerv. ment. Dis.* **125,** 166

64. Matsumoto, K., Berlet, H. H., Bull, C. and Himwich, H. E. (1966). 'Excretion of 17-Hydroxycorticosteroids and 17-Ketosteroids in Relation to Schizophrenic Symptoms'. *J. psychiat. Res.* **4,** 1

65. Mitsuda, H. (Ed.) (1967). 'A Clinico-genetic Study of Schizophrenia'. *Clinical Genetics in Psychiatry,* p. 49. Tokyo: Igaku Shoin

66. Nishimura, T. and Gjessing, L. R. (1965). 'Failure to Detect 3,4-Dimethoxyphenylethylamine and Bufotenine in the Urine From a Case of Periodic Catatonia'. *Nature, Lond.* **206,** 963

99

67. Osmond, H. and Smythies, J. (1952). 'Schizophrenia: A New Approach'. *J. ment. Sci.* **98,** 309

68. Park, L. C., Baldessarini, R. J. and Kety, S. S. (1965). 'Methionine Effects on Chronic Schizophrenics'. *Archs gen. Psychiat.* **12,** 346

69. Perry, T. L., Hansen, S., MacDougall, L. and Schwarz, C. J. (1966). 'Urinary Amines in Chronic Schizophrenia'. *Nature, Lond.* **212,** 146

70. Pollin, W., Cardon, P. V. and Kety, S. S. (1961). 'Effects of Amino Acid Feedings in Schizophrenic Patients Treated with Iproniazid'. *Science* **133,** 104

71. Pscheidt, G. R., Berlet, H. H., Bull, C., Spaide, J. and Himwich, H. E. (1964). 'Excretion of Catecholamines and Exacerbation of Symptoms in Schizophrenic Patients'. *J. psychiat. Res.* **2,** 163

72. Richter, D. (Ed.) (1957). *Somatic Aspects of Schizophrenia.* London: Pergamon Press

73. Rodnight, R. (1956). 'Separation and Characterization of Urinary Indoles Resembling 5-Hydroxytryptamine and Tryptamine'. *Biochem. J.* **64,** 621

74. Runge, T. M., Lara, F. Y., Thurman, N., Keyes, J. W. and Hoerster, S. H. (1966). 'Search for a Bufotenin-like Substance in the Urine of Schizophrenics'. *J. nerv. ment. Dis.* **142,** 470

75. Sano, I. (1954). Über die Kälte Millon-Reaktion beim Schizophrenen Formenkreis und den Trager derselben'. *Folia psychiat. neurol. jap.* **8,** 218

76. — and Decker, P. (1955). Über die in der kälte auftretenden Millon-Reaktion'. *Klin. Wschr.* **33,** 614

77. — and Nagasaka, G. (1956). 'Über chronische Weckaminsucht in Japan'. *Fortschr. Neurol. Psychiat.* **24,** 391

78. Scheiner, E. (1929). 'Über die Millonsche Reaktion des Harns bei Geisteskranken'. *Biochem. Z.* **204,** 361

79. Schottstaedt, W. W., Grace, W. J. and Wolff, H. G. (1956). 'Life Situations, Behavior, Attitudes, Emotions, and Renal Excretion of Fluid and Electrolytes'. *Psychosomat. Res.* **1,** 147, 292

80. Siegel, M. (1965). 'A Sensitive Method for Detection of N,N-Dimethylserotonin (Bufotenin) in Urine; Failure to Demonstrate its Presence in the Urine of Schizophrenic and Normal Subjects'. *J. psychiat. Res.* **3,** 205

81. Slater, E. (1953). 'Psychotic and Neurotic Illness in Twins'. *Medical Research Council Special Report No.* 278. London: Her Majesty's Stationery Office

82. Smythies, J. R., Bradley, R. J. and Johnston, V. S. (1967). 'The Behavioral Effects of some Derivatives of Mescaline and N,N-Dimethyltryptamine in the Rat'. *Life Sci.* **6,** 1887

83. Snyder, S. H. and Richelson, E. (1968). 'Psychedelic Drugs: Steric Factors Which Predict Psychotropic Activity'. *Proc. natn Acad. Sci.* **60,** 206

84. Sourkes, T. L. (1962). *Biochemistry of Mental Disease.* New York: Hoeber Medical Division, Harpers and Row

85. Spaide, J., Tanimukai, H., Ginther, R., Bueno, J. and Himwich, H. E. (1967). 'Schizophrenic Behavior and Urinary Tryptophan Metabolites Associated with Cysteine Given with and without a Monoamine Oxidase Inhibitor (Tranylcypromine)'. *Life Sci.* **6,** 551

86. Sprince, H., Parker, C. M., Jameson, D. and Alexander, F. (1963). 'Urinary Indoles in Schizophrenic and Psychoneurotic Patients after Administration of Tranylcypromine (Parnate) and Methionine or Tryptophan'. *J. nerv. ment. Dis.* **137,** 246

87. — — — and Josephs, J. A., Jun. (1965). 'Effect of Methionine and its Metabolites on Tryptophan Metabolism'. *Fedn Proc. Fedn. Am. Socs exp. Biol.* **24,** 169

88. Szara, S. (1956). 'Dimethyltryptamine: Its Metabolism in Man; The Relation of its Psychotic Effect to the Serotonin Metabolism'. *Experientia* **12,** 441

89. — (1967). 'Hallucinogenic Amines and Schizophrenia'. *Amines and Schizophrenia*, p. 181. Ed. by H. E. Himwich. London: Pergamon Press

90. Takesada, M., Kakimoto, Y., Sano, I. and Kaneko, Z. (1963). '3,4-Dimethoxyphenylethylamine and Other Amines in the Urine of Schizophrenic Patients'. *Nature, Lond.* **199,** 203

91. — Miyamoto, E., Kakimoto, Y., Sano, I. and Kaneko, Z. (1965). 'Phenolic and Indole Amines in the Urine of Schizophrenics'. *Nature, Lond.* **207,** 1199

92. Tanimukai, H. (1967). 'Modifications of Paper and Thin Layer Chromatographic Methods to Increase Sensitivity for Detecting N-Methylated Indoleamines in Urine'. *J. Chromatog.* **30,** 155

93. — Ginther, R., Spaide, J. and Himwich, H. E. (1967). 'Psychotomimetic Indole Compound in the Urine of Schizophrenics and Mentally Defective Patients'. *Nature, Lond.* **216,** 490

94. — — — Bueno, J. R. and Himwich, H. E. (1967). 'Occurrence of Bufotenin (5-Hydroxy-N,N-dimethyltryptamine) in Urine of Schizophrenic Patients'. *Life Sci.* **6,** 1697

95. — — — — — (1968). 'Psychotogenic N, N-Dimethylated Indole Amines and Behavior in Schizophrenic Patients'. *Recent Adv. biol. Psychiat.* **10,** 6

96. — — — — — (1969). 'Detection of Psychotomimetic N,N-Dimethylated Indoleamines in the Urine of Four Schizophrenic Patients' *Br. J. Psychiat.* In Press

97. Thudichum, J. W. E. (1884). *A Treatise on the Chemical Constitution of the Brain.* London: Bailliere, Tindall and Cox

98. Turner, W. J. and Merlis, S. (1959). 'Effect of some Indolealkylamines on Man'. *A.M.A. Archs Neurol. Psychiat.* **81,** 121

99. Ungerleider, J. T., Fisher, D. D. and Fuller, M. (1966). 'The Dangers of LSD. Analysis of Seven Months' Experience in a University Hospital's Psychiatric Service'. *J. Am. med. Ass.* **197,** 389

100. Yuwiler, A. (1965). 'Psychopathology and 5-Hydroxyindoleacetic Acid Excretion'. *J. psychiat. Res.* **3,** 125

CHAPTER 5

LIFE CHANGE, STRESS AND MENTAL DISORDER: THE ECOLOGICAL APPROACH

BRIAN COOPER

and

MICHAEL SHEPHERD

HISTORICAL AND INTRODUCTORY

The search for causes of mental disorder can be traced back at least to Graeco-Roman times. Once primitive belief in animistic magic had begun to yield to the concept of illness as a natural phenomenon, men turned for an explanation of abnormal mental states to the environment and life-experience of those afflicted. Emotional disturbances were invoked, the 'passions of sensations' of Asclepiades. Drugs and digestive upsets, as well as grief and fear, were the demonstrable causes of melancholia according to Soranus of Ephesus; mania he ascribed to over-exertion, licentiousness, alcoholism and amenorrhoea. In the sixteenth century, the Hippocratic doctrine of natural causation was reaffirmed by Johann Weyer and by Paracelsus, who considered certain mental disorders to be secondary to physical illness through the ascent to the head of fumes given off by the affected organs.

Throughout the centuries, medical opinions on this topic were derived at best from clinical impressions heavily augmented by speculation. No systematic study was undertaken of the relationship between supposed causal agents and the onset of disease. On the other hand, the writings of social historians provide a wealth of evidence for some connection between natural or man-made events and the incidence of mental disorder. The classic example is supplied by the great plague epidemics of the Middle Ages. 'The times', writes Galdston[23], 'were full of strife and sorrow, and hence of great madness. The Black Death, raging between 1347–50, had carried off, it is estimated, a third of the population of Europe, and utterly demoralized those surviving.'

The first manifestation of irrational behaviour following on this catastrophe was a mass persecution of the Jews. Already disliked

102

because of their association with money-lending, they were now accused of spreading the pestilence by poisoning water-supplies and the advance of the plague across Europe was attended by a wave of pogroms in which whole communities were burned to death.

Soon afterwards there occurred a revival of the ancient Brotherhood of Flagellants, whose members inflicted on one another ritual whipping and scourging. Their appearance in Western Europe, says Hirst[41] was 'one of the most remarkable infective psychoses in history. It spread like an epidemic. . . .' From their origin in Hungary the flagellant bands moved north and west, reaching Dresden early in 1349 and thence travelling across Germany and on to France, England, Denmark, Sweden and Poland. Although essentially a layman's cult of repentance, the movement had its darker side, for there is good evidence that besides taking an active part in the massacres of Jews, the Flagellants in some instances were directly responsible for spreading the contagion.

The bizarre outbreaks of dancing mania have been widely regarded as another sequel of the plague. In the words of Hecker[34] 'The effects of the Black Death had not yet subsided and the graves of millions of its victims were scarcely closed, when a strange delusion arose in Germany which took possession of the minds of men and . . . hurried away body and soul into the magic circle of hellish superstition.' In Italy a like condition was ascribed to the bite of the poisonous Tarantula. The origin of choreomania and tarantism can be traced back to the plague dances which were used in many areas to ward off the disease, to combat despair or to celebrate the end of an epidemic. Even stranger was the resurgence of lycanthropy, dormant since Greek times. Men were said ' . . . to run howling about graves and fields in the night, and [would] not be persuaded but that they were wolves, or some such beasts'[34]. Nor were the children exempt from the universal malaise. According to the historian Nohl[62], 'The excessive unrest which during the tribulations of plague time had taken possession of humanity is further revealed by the wanderings and pilgrimages of the children'. In the face of these compulsive migrations, parental admonitions and even physical restraint were of no avail and thousands of children vanished from their homes.

Up to the seventeenth century, repeated epidemics of plague were accompanied by outbreaks of abnormal behaviour as well attested as those which followed on the Black Death[41]. In modern Western society, however, mass catastrophes have been increasingly confined to times of war. Indeed, since systematic recording has become feasible, major conflicts have provided our main source of evidence on the pathogenic significance of acute environmental stress,

103

although local disasters such as earthquakes, volcanic eruptions, fires and floods have made their contribution.

Despite their dramatic nature, such occurrences do not figure at all prominently in the psychiatric literature. Clinical psychiatrists, working for the most part under peaceful conditions, have been concerned rather with the effects of more commonplace changes in the individual life pattern which, though not usually pathogenic, may be conducive to mental illness in susceptible persons. Hence in the textbooks of the past 200 years it is very largely such events as acute physical illness, childbirth, bereavement and abrupt social change which have been cited as the precipitants of insanity.

Modern notions of psychiatric aetiology may be said to date from the publication in 1801 of Pinel's *Traité Medico-philosophique*. It is claimed that Pinel's first question to his patients was always 'Have you recently had to suffer anger, grief or annoyance?'[24] This at least conveys the spirit of his enquiries, as the accompanying reproduction of a table from the Treatise clearly shows (Table 1).

Among the principal causes of mental infirmity Pinel counted the spasmodic passions of rage and fright, the oppressive passions of grief, hate, fear and remorse, and the presence of harmful factors in the social environment. He clearly recognized the effect of physical disturbances such as fever, head injury, childbearing and alcoholic excess and specifically mentioned the dangers of transition from an active to an inactive way of life, as at retirement. But Pinel's most outstanding contribution was his insistence, which his pupil Esquirol was to take up, on the importance of the statistical approach if questions of causation were ever finally to be resolved.

Two further advances in psychiatric thought during the nineteenth century helped to pave the way for modern research in this field. One was the development by Kraepelin and the German descriptive school of a system of classification which could serve as a basis for epidemiological research. The other, less widely recognized but of comparable importance, was the growth of the idea of multifactorial causation, first clearly enunciated by Griesinger[28]. The following passage is quoted because it is a striking century-old illustration both of the actuarial approach to causation and of the application to psychiatry of the epidemiological triad of agent, host and environment.

The causes [of insanity] comprehend, on the one hand, the external circumstances (nationality, climate, season of the year) under the influence of which insanity is generally, with more or less frequency, observed; on the other hand, they signify certain external injuries (sunstroke, wounds of the head) of which insanity is frequently a consequence; finally, they comprehend certain internal states de-

A General Table* of Cases of Insanity Cured at the Asylum de Bicêtre, in the Second Year of the Republic, by Regimen and Exercise Exclusively

Periods of admission	English calendar days inclusive	Age	Trade or profession	Cause	Species	Relapses where they occurred
November, 1790	—	45	Gardener	Disappointment in love	Periodical mania with delirium	Two relapses on seeing the beloved object
July, 1792	—	22	Mason's labourer	Excessive labour	Periodical mania with delirium	—
November, 1790	—	22	Soldier	Consequence of acute fever	Accidental dementia	—
Frimaire, year 2	Nov. 22, Dec. 21	21	Soldier	Consequence of acute fever	Accidental dementia	—
Pluviôse, year 2	Jan. 21, Feb. 19	24	Soldier	Terror	Periodical mania with delirium	Relapsed for a fortnight
Ventôse, year 1	Feb. 20, Mar. 21	30	Soldier	Excessive ambition	Periodical mania with delirium	Three relapses
Ventôse, year 1	Feb. 20, Mar. 21	24	Soldier	Excessive ambition	Periodical mania with delirium	One relapse from premature dismission
Germinal, year 1	Mar. 22, Apr. 20	36	Tailor	Loss of property	Periodical mania with delirium	—
Germinal, year 1	—	28	Waterman	Jealousy	Periodical mania with delirium	Relapsed after his dismission
Floreal, year 1	Apr. 21, May 20	36	Tailor	Distress of mind	Melancholia	—
Messidor, year 1	June 20, July 19	44	Labourer	Heat of the sun	Periodical mania with delirium	Relapsed three times before his dismission
Vendemaire, year 2	Sep. 23, Oct. 22	46	Shopkeeper	Loss of property	Melancholia	—
Vendemaire, year 2	—	64	Labourer	Distress of mind	Periodical mania with delirium	—
Messidor, year 2	—	25	Tanner	Distress of mind	Convalescent from acute mania	—
Thermidor, year 2	July 20, Aug. 18	46	Tanner	Distress of mind	Convalescent from acute mania	—
Thermidor, year 2	—	56	Hairdresser	Terror	Convalescent from acute mania	—
Thermidor, year 2	—	25	Soldier	Excessive ambition	Convalescent from acute mania	—
Thermidor, year 2	—	22	Soldier	Terror excited by the discharge of artillery	Periodical mania with delirium	—

Reproduced from Pinel (1962) by courtesy of Hafner

pendent on the organism itself (hereditary disposition, previous disease, or other general disturbance of the organic mechanism, such as disease of the lungs, the genital organs, etc.) which we know by experience have an influence on the development of insanity. In very many of these circumstances the intimate connection between them and the influences ascribed to them, the mode in which from them the mental disease is developed, is scarcely ever or not at all evident. The conclusion post hoc ergo propter hoc depends, therefore, on a simple empirical (statistical) knowledge of the fact that these particular circumstances (for example, hereditary disposition) very frequently coincide with, or precede, the commencement of insanity. In other of these so-called causes, their mode of action, the manner in which, in consequence of them, the disease is established, can be comprehended. But the province of *aetiology* in the narrow sense is only to enumerate empirically the known circumstances of causation; it belongs to *pathogeny* to explain the physiological connection between cause and effect, to show the particular mechanical act by means of which insanity is induced through a given circumstance (for example, excessive depressing emotion, heart disease, etc.), a task towards which we have hitherto done little more than prepare the way.

One could wish to see this text framed on the walls of every psychiatric department in the land. While the term aetiology has come to be used more broadly than in Griesinger's day, it is clear from the above passage that he employed the word in an essentially epidemiological sense; that is, to denote the study of statistical associations between various medical, social and environmental factors and the onset of mental disorder. Furthermore, his schema places firmly under the heading of pathogeny all those investigations of physiological and psychological mechanisms which have made up the great bulk of modern psychosomatic research. It is, indeed, a logical corollary to Griesinger's line of argument that such studies can usefully proceed only within the framework provided by epidemiological enquiry. This review emphasizes how scattered and fragmentary have been the attempts to apply these principles and what relatively small advances have been made since Griesinger's day.

The use of the epidemiological method in psychiatry has been extensively discussed[53, 73, 80] and Hare[32, 33] has demarcated the common frontier with medical ecology*. The present survey will be restricted to those studies which have considered the relationship of clearly defined environmental change to the onset of psychiatric

* In this chapter *ecology* denotes the study of the effects on health of the physical, biological and social environment and *epidemiology* the method by which such effects are measured by comparison of the rates of morbidity in defined populations.

morbidity. Such studies have the distinguishing characteristic that they are concerned with the chronological sequence of events; hence valid comparisons may be drawn not only between different populations, but also and more readily between the same population at different periods of time. Not surprisingly, a high proportion of important modern studies in this field have been done in wartime either with military personnel or civilian populations.

EFFECTS OF WAR

Combatants on Active Service

Already in World War I, a number of medical observers had come to recognize the psychogenic nature of many battle casualties[95]. In consequence, military psychiatry was awarded a much more important role in the second conflict and an extensive literature grew up on the form and treatment of the 'war neuroses'[11, 20, 25, 76, 77]. The development of 'forward psychiatry'[3] led to a steep reduction in the rates for lasting disability by dint of prompt and intensive treatment in the battle zones.

One by-product of this new emphasis on preventive psychiatry in the armed services was an appreciation of the need for statistical studies. In the words of the American official history[26]

> The application of certain principles of epidemiology was found to be useful. For example, when hospital admission rates were determined and studied, it was clear that although the psychiatric problem was Army-wide, the rates were from 5 to 10 times as high among troops engaged in actual combat as in training centres or in isolated overseas posts or elsewhere in the Army. . . . It was epidemiological studies of hospital admission rates which showed the direct role of physical danger from enemy shellfire in causing psychiatric disorders. Similarly, the steady increase in hospital admission rates with duration of exposure to enemy shellfire represented strong evidence of the role of physical exhaustion in these cases.

In *Figure 1* the point is clearly illustrated by the close correlations between battle injury and psychiatric casualty rates occurring in three army divisions during a seven-week period of active service. The relationship remained fairly constant throughout at one psychiatric admission to every four or five troops wounded in action.

While figures of this kind speak for themselves, military psychiatrists were not slow to recognize the importance of constitutional predisposition[81]. Grinker and Spiegel[29] wrote

> Repeated observation has demonstrated that the men who became psychiatric casualties can be divided into two arbitrary groups on the

basis of the intensity of external stress to which they had been subjected. In the first group the stress has been minimal, and yet has led
to severe symptoms. In the second and by far the larger group, the
stress has been severe, and has only produced marked symptoms after
a prolonged exposure. It is apparent therefore that some other factor
besides the intensity of the stress is sresponsible for the production of
symptoms.

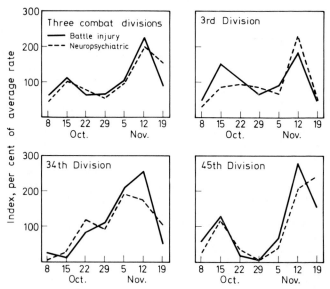

(Reproduced from Glass and Burnucci (1966) by courtesy of the Office of the Surgeon
General, Department of the Army, Washington, D.C.)

*Figure 1. Relation between trend of battle injury and neuropsychiatric
admissions, Fifth U.S. Army*

In their veiw, the first group's vulnerability was related to previous
psychiatric disturbance and personality defects.

Though the implications for personnel selection may have been
well understood, few epidemiologicol studies were conducted in this
field. The investigation of 'flying stress' in the Royal Air Force by
Reid[72] remains a model of its kind. In World War I, this condition
in aviators had been attributed to oxygen lack, noise and cold. Since,
however, clinical histories strongly suggested an acute type of
neurotic reaction[89], Reid set out to examine more systematically the
incidence in different units. He found the highest rates in Bomber
Command (U.K.), the next in Middle East Air Force, the next in

Fighter Command and the lowest in home-based training formations. The distribution of cases was thus related to the intensity of the air war, rather than to distance from home.

Further analysis showed that within Bomber Command the incidence was related to casualty rates rather than to the number of flying hours. A period of heavy casualties was accompanied by an increase of reported 'flying stress' in the same month and followed by a sharp rise in venereal disease in the following month. It could thus be inferred that danger to life was a more important factor than cumulative fatigue.

Since the peak incidence occurred early rather than late in the operational careers of men exposed to the hazards of combat flying, it seemed that individual predisposition was also of greater weight than any cumulative effect. This personal factor was highlighted by the finding that air-gunners, who had been less rigorously screened, suffered a higher incidence than pilots and navigators, despite the fact that the latter had more onerous and responsible duties.

In general, war service studies predicated an increase in nervous tension as the direct antecedent cause, but there are instances of small epidemics being triggered off by an abrupt and unexpected *relief* of tension. Murphy[61], for example, cites a Jugoslav report of an outbreak of acute psychosis among the partisans in that country immediately following on the cessation of fighting. A similar phenomenon observed by Tredgold[91] in the British Army provides a striking example of this paradoxical effect.

In August 1945, when the Japanese capitulated, preparations for the invasion of Malaya were in the final stages and Allied service units in the Far Eastern theatre had been undergoing intensive training. Tredgold, having noted several cases of acute manic excitement which developed immediately afterwards, set out to collect others and was able to trace 23, of whom he personally examined 16. A number of characteristic features indicated the essential similarity of these cases: most of the patients were officers who had been exposed to increased mental strain and responsibility in the months preceding 'V.J. Day'. All but one were under 30 and almost all had good service records. Only two had any previous psychiatric history. Eleven were known to have developed a low-grade pyrexia, but all physical investigations, including white-cell counts, blood culture and examination for malarial parasites, were negative. The patients were not confused or disorientated and in no case could a primary organic diagnosis be confirmed.

On these grounds, the author concluded that in the majority of cases the illness was psychogenic:

. . . . there were mental factors which must have played a part. There was a very sudden and acute change in the tempo of work with a sudden relief of tension. This must have affected strongly the over-conscientious responsible type of staff officer who had been employed in circumstances . . . . calculated to increase those obsessional tendencies and anxiety.

That the cluster of reported cases corresponded to a minor epidemic was confirmed by comparison of the number of patients invalided home from this war theatre during the immediate post-war period with the figures for preceding months.

Civilian Populations

The effects of war on civilian populations could seldom be so nicely gauged, largely because the environmental stresses to which they were exposed were not as a rule so clear and massive as those of combat situations. Official disquiet lest wartime conditions should give rise to any alarming increase in mental disorder was soon allayed. No such consequence was observed; indeed the statistics pointed to a decrease in the rates both for mental hospital admissions[35, 42] and for suicide. A survey of neurotic disorders undertaken for the Medical Research Council led Lewis[51] to conclude that there had been no general upward trend, although the records of one London general practice did suggest a temporary increase immediately following major air raids on the metropolis.

In view of the attendant difficulties of method, this finding must be accepted with some reserve. Nevertheless, a good deal of evidence was accruing at about that time for a positive association between large-scale air raids and the incidence of a much more reliably ascertained medical condition; namely, perforated peptic ulcer. During the first two months of the 1940 blitz, figures from 16 London hospitals showed a significant increase in the numbers of perforations[86], an association neatly demonstrated by *Figure 2*. Subsequently, the rate was shown to have fallen steeply from the end of the blitz in May 1941[83].

The difficulties of interpreting such correlations are well known. In this context, a group of Scottish workers[44] were able to show that while the incidence of perforated peptic ulcer in Glasgow likewise began to rise sharply in the autumn of 1940 and remained high until June 1941, this increase antedated the period of heavy air raids on that city, which did not begin until March 1941. They concluded, therefore, that the phenomenon was linked not with the specific stress of air raids but with more general factors such as overwork, weariness, irregular feeding habits and food shortages, noting moreover that 'during the period in question the whole country was in a state of nervous strain as a result of the war situation.' However valid this interpretation, the rapid fall after June 1941 remains something of a mystery.

Although national statistics on the whole revealed no definite psychiatric trends associated with wartime conditions, investigation of relatively small groups of civilians known to have undergone

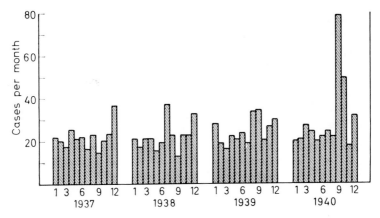

(Reproduced from Stewart and Winser (1942) by courtesy of the Editor of *Lancet*)

Figure 2. Cases of perforated peptic ulcer each month for the period 1937–40, in 16 London Hospitals

severe personal experiences showed a very high incidence of subsequent psychiatric morbidity. Thus, a follow-up study of a series of civilians who had been admitted to First Aid Posts after being buried in bombed houses[21] showed that of those who had been immured for an hour or more about two-thirds later developed neurotic symptoms and that approximately half of these were still suffering from neurotic ill-health a year later.

EFFECTS OF COMMUNITY DISASTER

Similar findings have been reported by psychiatrists who have had opportunities for observing the after-effects of personal involvement in communal disasters. A famous instance was the fire which broke out at the Cocoanut Grove night club in Boston one night in November 1942, in which nearly 500 people lost their lives. Within two hours of this event over 100 casualties were brought to the Massachussetts General Hospital, which fortunately was well equipped to deal with such an emergency because of the current state of war and the presence of a burns research unit. A week later, because one of the surviving patients developed an acute psychotic reaction, psychiatrists attached to the hospital were invited to examine all the casualties still on the wards[9]. Of 17 examined at that time, all but three were thought to show evidence of psychiatric morbidity, a finding which excluded any transient delirious reactions. The long-term effects were indicated by Adler[1], who found that of 46 victims of the fire admitted to the Boston City Hospital, 25 were still suffering from anxiety neuroses three months afterwards and 13 nine months afterwards.

Psychological reactions to the disaster were thought to be determined not only by the acute physical trauma, but also by subsequent experiences. Once the initial stages of shock and anguish had passed, many of the patients expressed strong feelings of resentment because their immediate requirements of comfort, reassurance and personal contact had not been satisfied by the hospital regime. At this stage, too, problems of rehabilitation became increasingly prominent and the psychiatrists found a strong need for co-operation with the medical social workers, a need in many instances persisting beyond the patient's discharge from hospital. The investigators concluded that

> . . . . it is desirable to have psychiatric evaluation of patients early in the course of their hospital care, continuous psychiatric attention to those patients who are in a precarious emotional state, and lastly aid in making readjustment, especially to bereavement, immediately after leaving hospital.[9]

These opinions have received support from the findings of a number of investigators. In particular, a systematic exploration of this field of enquiry was made by Tyhurst[92, 93], who studied a number of civilian disasters in Canada. His observations of the 'natural history' of psychiatric phenomena led him to postulate three overlapping phases of reaction: (1) a period of impact; (2) a period of recoil; (3) a post-traumatic period. In the first stage, lasting for a few minutes or up to an hour after the acute catastrophe, as many as a quarter of the survivors showed manifestly inappropriate responses such as states of confusion, paralysing anxiety or 'hysterical' crying and screaming which could be readily distinguished from the stunned, bewildered air of the majority. In the second, recoil stage many survivors showed florid anxiety with a strong need to ventilate their emotions and a conspicuous dependence on those who ministered to their needs: in particular, they craved to be comforted and were afraid to be left alone. This child-like state of dependence was also of short duration. Reactions in the third, post-traumatic stage were much more akin to those with which the psychiatrist is familiar under normal conditions. Depressive reactions, fatigue and loss of concentration were the common symptoms, while recurrent catastrophic dreams were frequent. Fugue states and psychotic episodes also occurred, but were relatively uncommon. The third stage was of much longer duration and in a proportion of cases the symptoms appeared to be chronic and intractable.

A number of attempts to formulate normal responses to acute stress in terms of psychological mechanisms have been made on the basis of experience with combat flying[5], severe burns[31] and major surgery[45], as well as communal disasters[93, 96]. Most workers have emphasized the importance of predisposition in determining the severer types of reaction. In this context, however, it is as well to bear in mind the heterogeneous nature of the events which have been subsumed under the term 'acute stress'. An illustration of this point is provided by Adler[2], who compared the survivors of the Cocoanut Grove fire with a control series of closed head-injury patients and concluded that two distinct forms of 'post-traumatic neurosis' were involved. The prevalence of acute anxiety and catastrophic dreaming among the disaster victims led her to believe that terrifying experiences of the kind they had undergone lead to a higher rate of neurotic reactions than is found after civilian head injuries and that the nature of the symptoms is directly influenced by the circumstances of the traumatic event.

The risk of further exposure may also be a crucial factor in determining the response to a 'near miss' situation. A study of the survivors of a marine explosion[50], for example, revealed that since most of them were virtually compelled by economic necessity to return to work on oil tankers, they felt themselves continually under the threat of another such disaster. The high prevalence of neurotic ill-health manifest at follow-up was considered by the investigators to be mainly attributable to this circumstance, rather than to any predisposing constitutional factors. They argued that the role of such factors has been over-emphasized and that there is a case for regarding post-traumatic neurosis in previously normal individuals as a distinct entity.

As a rule, the importance of predisposition can be assessed only in retrospect, since no normal population has been psychiatrically screened before the occurrence of a major disaster. One study which indirectly supplied evidence on this point was that which Rawnsley and Loudon[71] undertook for the Medical Research Council on the mental health of the Tristan da Cunha islanders evacuated to Britain when the island volcano erupted in October 1961. As it transpired, this enforced migration was followed by no major psychiatric disturbance, perhaps because of the remarkably strong social cohesion of the island people. Nevertheless, minor symptoms were commonly reported when they were examined in England and chief among these was headache which in the great majority of cases was thought to be psychogenic. During a six-month period, those individuals with the symptom of headache of no apparent cause consulted the medical officer at their camp significantly more often than a matched control group. Furthermore, the distribution of headache in 1962 was found to be closely related to that of an epidemic of gross hysteria which was known to have occurred on Tristan da Cunha in 1937. This outbreak had been fully documented by the medical members of a Norwegian scientific expedition[8] and it was known that 21 of the islanders had at that time manifested hysterical faints, fits, 'choking spells' and bouts of acute excitement. Among 19 survivors of this group, 16 had psychogenic headache after the volcanic eruption.

EFFECTS OF SOCIO-CULTURAL CHANGE

In Tristan da Cunha no loss of life occurred and the nature of the environmental stress may be said to have resided less in the acute disaster than in the consequent disruption of the islanders' normal pattern of life. From this point of view, the episode provides a simple model of the phenomenon which in one form or another has been held responsible for many increases in psychiatric morbidity; namely, rapid socio-cultural change. Such change can be extremely difficult to define and measure for the purpose of ecological research. It may be sudden or relatively insidious in onset, of permanent or only transient effect, gladly accepted or reluctantly endured, common to a whole population or restricted to special groups. It is thus understandable that studies in this field have for the most part yielded incomplete, unreliable and often contradictory information.

In a few instances it has proved possible to make use of national statistics to establish ecological correlates of the incidence of psychiatric disorder. The suicide rate during the inter-war years, for example, was shown in the United States to be inversely correlated with a business index reflecting the state of the market[16] and in Great Britain to be positively related to unemployment figures[88]. More commonly, however, such relationships can be demonstrated only with the aid of special surveys of those subgroups of the population most directly at risk. Studies of this kind have been comprehensively reviewed by Murphy[61], who gives as the principal factors, besides war and the transition from peace to war, emigration, internal migration, and the rapid acculturation process which is found where people in primitive cultures are brought into contact with modern Western society. Perhaps the most forcible conclusion to emerge from Murphy's very careful and detailed survey is the extreme difficulty of forming any conclusions in an area where there are so many uncontrolled variables to be considered.

Emigration provides the paradigm of social change. Earlier findings suggested that the rates of mental illness among immigrant groups were greatly in excess of those in the indigenous populations. As more sophisticated studies were undertaken and it became possible to control for such related variables as age, social class, employment level and ethnic status, the observed differences diminished until it can be said that 'Today the relationship has become quite doubtful, and its meaning equally so.'[61] Confusion has been heightened by reports from some countries that immigrant groups actually have lower psychiatric rates than the native populations[59, 87]. The problem is complex, involving such factors as the reasons leading to migration, the selection procedures enforced by the host country and the kind of adaptation required of immigrant groups. More rigorous screening, for example, may serve to modify the high rate of immigration of unstable individuals such as Odegaard[63] showed to have occurred among the Norwegian community in Minnesota.

The highest rates of mental disorder have been found in those immigrant groups such as refugees and displaced persons whose migration could scarcely be classed as voluntary[18, 67]. In this context it is virtually impossible to differentiate between what Murphy[60] has described as the four interlocking factors of loss of homeland, experience of persecution, cultural difficulties of readjustment and social isolation. Moreover, it has been shown that even when emigration occurs under strong political pressures, as for example following the Hungarian uprising of 1956, there is still a selective tendency for unstable, pre-psychotic individuals to join the exodus[57].

While large-scale movements of population, wars and mass catastrophes have provided the 'experiments of opportunity' by which the epidemiologist can hope to study the effects of environmental stress in pure culture, the bulk of the evidence under peaceful conditions has to be collected by means of numerous painstaking studies of the reactions associated with commonplace events and circumstances. Many of these are more or less randomly distributed throughout the general population, being linked only with epochs of the normal life cycle. University examinations[56, 75], engagement[12], change of house[30], interpersonal conflicts at work[82] and bereavement[65] are among the life stresses which have been held responsible for the advent of psychiatric illness in susceptible persons. Better accredited, however, are the consequences for mental health of those biological events marked by changes of the *milieu interne*—in particular, childbirth, trauma and illness.

EFFECTS OF BIOLOGICAL CHANGE: CHILDBIRTH, TRAUMA AND ILLNESS

Childbirth is a life-event with physiological, psychological and socio-cultural aspects which render it in many ways an ideal subject for studies of stress. Furthermore, it constitutes a readily identifiable point-event of a kind which lends itself to epidemiological research. It is, nonetheless, remarkable how few surveys have been undertaken in this field. The most authoritative is that of Paffenbarger[64], who reviewed the medical records of all women aged 15–44 years who were in-patients of any psychiatric hospital in Hamilton County, Ohio, from 1940 to 1958. Events of pregnancy, labour and the puerperium were compiled from the local maternity hospital records and comparative data obtained from the records of the maternity patients of the same ethnic status delivered in the same obstetric unit immediately before and after each psychiatric patient. *Figure 3* clearly illustrates the temporal relationship of parturition to the onset of mental illness in the index group.

Comparison with the control group of mentally normal subjects showed that postpartum illness was associated with certain obstetric and perinatal abnormalities, as well as with a previous history of psychiatric disturbance which suggested the importance of predisposing factors. This finding conforms with the conclusion drawn by Seager[78] from his own controlled study that the puerperium acts as a non-specific stress which may precipitate mental illness in susceptible women.

Major physical trauma supplies another type of event which can be precisely defined in time. In particular, the medico-legal implications of head injury have been sufficiently important to warrant several systematic attempts to evaluate the part which it may play in the development of psychiatric disability. A study by Dencker[13] is of some interest as an illustration of the overlapping interests of epidemiology and genetics. The author set out to assess the psychiatric sequelae of closed head-injury by follow-up of a large twin series. Since a complete index of all twins born in the south of Sweden was available, it was possible to identify all those born after 1880 among a total of some 15,000 persons treated for closed head-injury in the hospitals of two counties of Scandinavia. Of 128 living twin pairs who were traced, 37 were monozygotic and 91 dizygotic. The results indicated that most of the psychiatric morbidity and

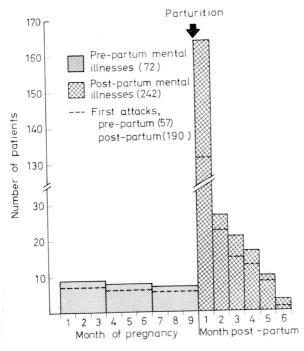

(Reproduced from Paffenbarger (1964) by courtesy of the Editor of the *British Journal of Preventive and Social Medicine*)

Figure 3. Onset of parapartum mental illnesses among hospitalized patients in Hamilton County, Ohio, 1940–58. First attacks represent women without previous mental illness

character abnormalities found among the propositi had antedated their head injuries and could be termed constitutional. Complaints such as irritability, fatigue and anxiety were not found significantly more often among the propositi than among the probands, while the small differences in cognitive ability were not regarded as clinically significant. The monozygotic twins showed a higher concordance than the dizygotic in respect of headache, vertigo, impairment of memory, sensitivity to noise and reduction of alcohol tolerance. In general, the findings underlined the importance of constitutional factors.

Major surgical procedures constitute a form of physical trauma which lends itself to research. Analysis of large case-series have revealed that severe psychiatric reactions occur after a wide variety of surgical procedures at an average rate of about 1 in 1,500[47, 52]. The existence of a separate clinical entity of 'postoperative psychosis' has been postulated[85], but the evidence so far adduced seems rather tenuous.

Certain operations have long been thought to carry a special risk of psychiatric complications: cataract extraction, for example, has been regarded throughout this century as a precipitating cause of acute psychosis[47, 55]. Gynaecological operations, and in particular hysterectomy, have also been reported to have a high incidence of psychiatric sequelae[54, 85]. More recently, a number of conflicting reports have appeared on the effects of open heart surgery[10, 17, 48], perhaps because, as Knox[48] suggested, the selective criteria for this type of procedure vary widely between different hospitals.

While clinical studies of this kind provide valuable inferential evidence, there is a dearth of controlled investigations. The lead in this direction given by Lindemann[54] has recently been followed by Barker[4], who examined the incidence of psychiatric referral among a large sample of women who had undergone hysterectomy four to five years previously. He found a rate three times that for women of comparable age in the general population and more than twice that for a control group of women who had had cholecystectomy.

A number of workers have explored the relationship in distribution of psychiatric illness and systemic disease in populations[6, 14, 15, 74]. These enquiries have for the most part been confined to establishing associations either at a given point in time or over the life span. There has been an almost complete lack of studies relating the onset in time of different forms of morbidity. Kellner[46], however, was able to take advantage of his general practice medical records for this purpose. For two years he kept a special record of all consultations by a patient population of 1,600. Each attendance with overt emotional disturbance or 'functional' symptoms (i.e. those with no known organic pathology) was labelled 'neurotic ill-health', while 'physical illness' was defined as any organic conditions or surgical procedure which confined a previously healthy person to bed for at least three weeks or necessitated a stay in hospital of at least one week. 'Convalescence' he defined as the period of four weeks following discharge from hospital or from the time of becoming ambulant. Using these operational definitions, Kellner established that of 60 patients who had 'physical illness' during a two-year period, 12 had developed 'neurotic ill-health' during the illness or in 'convalescence'. This total compared with 120 episodes in the remainder of the patient population and represented a significant excess. Bearing in mind the possible fallacies, Kellner considered the findings so positive as to suggest strongly the likelihood of a real temporal clustering of physical and neurotic illness.

EFFECTS OF LIFE CHANGE
LONGITUDINAL STUDIES

An essentially similar technique has been employed to examine the temporal clustering of all types of illness episode. A series of studies initiated by the late Harold Wolff at Cornell University[37, 38, 39, 40] explored the morbidity experience of several groups including female telephone operators, skilled workmen, college graduates and two immigrant samples. The main focus of these investigations was the distribution of illness episodes over a long period of time and for this purpose medical histories extending for up to 20 years were obtained. Psychiatric disorders were included together with organic disease and accidents. It soon became apparent that characteristic patterns of low and high illness experience could be delineated, individuals tending to have a relatively constant average over the years. Nevertheless, there were periods in the individual life histories when marked increases had occurred in the numbers of illness episodes: a phenomenon which at once raised the question as to whether or not any association could be discerned with changes of life pattern. More detailed histories were taken from subsamples of the groups concerned, with a view to examining for such associations. In one study the social and cultural background of 68 Hungarian refugees was explored and the resulting data submitted to three independent assessors who rated the subject's own perceptions of their experiences year by year on a 5-point scale ranging from 'very satisfactory' to 'highly unsatisfactory'. An average of 20 years for each subject was rated in this way and the scores proved highly reliable. When the data were compared with the subject's medical records over the same period it was found that 'highly unsatisfactory' years were mostly those in which illness clusters had occurred.

These studies of the Cornell Human Ecology Program carried an intrinsic weakness in that they relied on retrospective collection of data. Moreover, insofar as the individual perception of life difficulties was highly subjective, it could not be assumed to be independent of the informant's current state of mental and physical health. These difficulties have been largely surmounted by another group of American workers using refinements of the same method. Holmes and Rahe and their co-workers[69, 70] devised a rating scale for severity of illness based on the risk of serious disability and the threat to life. More important was their attempt to quantify changes in the life pattern. To this end they scored a series of 41 types of life-change according to their estimate of the extent of the change and the amount of adjustment required of the individual. The scale employed ranged from major events such as the death of a spouse (100 Life Change Units, or L.C.U.) down to minor occurrences such as a spell of leave for a serviceman (13 L.C.U.).

> In this fashion, a person's yearly amount of life-changes can be numerically represented by the total of that year's L.C.U. This method attempts to examine every area of significant life-change regardless of whether the change is considered to be desirable, undesirable, volitional or not under the person's direct control.[9]

In an intensive study of a random sample of 50 U.S. Navy and Marine Corps personnel discharged on psychiatric grounds, it was found that years of greater than average life-change had uniformly preceded illnesses or illness clusters. Furthermore, severe illnesses and clusters of illnesses were preceded by L.C.U. significantly higher than those preceding minor illness. Two instances of death and one of near-death were also preceded by clusters of high life-change magnitude.

This technique represents a clear advance in research method, avoiding in large measure the pitfalls of subjective reporting which trapped many earlier workers. There remain, however, serious limitations to its application. Only under special conditions, such as obtain in the regular armed forces, is it possible as a rule to secure reliable and comprehensive medical records for representative samples over a period of years. The retrospective charting of all categories of 'life-change' must also be regarded as an unreliable procedure under ordinary conditions, when it is subject to errors of omission, distortion and falsification. Finally, the method as described would be difficult to apply to any one diagnostic entity.

EVENTS PRECEDING THE ONSET OF PSYCHIATRIC ILLNESS

Two recent studies by another group of American research workers attempted to apply the study of life events specifically to current psychiatric illness. In the more recently reported study[58] they describe a comparison of 100 psychiatric in-patient admissions with the same number of matched controls drawn from the general wards of the same hospital. The events checked comprised the birth, death and illness of family members; educational history and school performance; military service; marital history; occupational and financial record of patient and spouse; changes of residence; changes in household; changes in close personal relationships and interpersonal conflicts in the home, at work or at school. The chief finding was the striking similarity between index and control groups in respect of the incidence of such identifiable life-stresses. This fact led the authors to conclude that while psychosocial stress might well be implicated in the genesis of illness, it did not appear to lead to psychiatric illness rather than to other forms of morbidity.

In their earlier study[43], the same group studied a sample of 40 hospital in-patients suffering from relatively severe affective illness (34 with depression and six with manic states). Among these patients the onset of illness had been fairly clear-cut, so that it was possible to rate this approximate point in time to the occurrence of identified life-events. Here again the findings were compared with those for a control group matched in respect of age, sex, race, religion, marital status, education, social class and income level. The findings showed significant differences between index and control groups only in respect of more frequent change of residence and a higher incidence of interpersonal conflict for the index patients during the year prior to admission, when their illnesses were already becoming florid. In only ten of the 40 psychiatric patients had the onset of affective disorder followed within six months of objective life stress and among this group no definite temporal association could be demonstrated between such life stresses and earlier episodes of psychiatric illness. In short, the data appeared to favour the view that the temporal relationship between affective illness and life events is purely random.

A very different result was obtained by two British workers studying the onset of acute schizophrenia[7], who introduced two further refinements into their research design. First, they accepted for inclusion in their sample only those schizophrenic patients admitted to two London mental hospitals with a first illness or clearly defined relapse of acute onset, such that the appearance of grossly abnormal behaviour could be reliably dated. Secondly, to reduce the possibility of memory errors they charted the occurrence of life events for the preceding three months only. The basis of comparison which they employed was also different from that of the American team, healthy factory workers being sampled for a control group, instead of hospital patients with physical ailments.

Whether because of the use of a healthy control group, or because of the more reliable and comprehensive recording of recent events, or indeed because of the different diagnostic category under scrutiny, the findings of this latter study were strikingly positive, showing a highly significant excess of life events among the index group during the period of three weeks preceding the onset of acute schizophrenia (*Figure 4*).

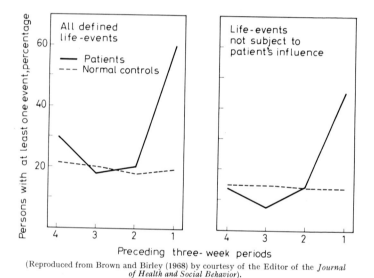

(Reproduced from Brown and Birley (1968) by courtesy of the Editor of the *Journal of Health and Social Behavior*).

Figure 4. Experience of life-events during four consecutive three-week periods. (a) 50 patients immediately prior to onset of schizophrenic illness; (b) 325 normal controls immediately prior to interview

DISCUSSION

In psychiatry, much confusion has resulted from the lack of any clear definition of the term 'stress'. The ambiguities surrounding this word spring in part from its uncertain etymology[66]. In this connection, Vickers[94] has pointed out the need to distinguish between three sets of variables: the environmental situation, the physiological and psychological changes which it engenders in the individual, and the behaviour consequent upon those changes. These factors he suggested should be designated respectively 'stress-situation', 'stress-change' and 'stress-behaviour': a recommendation which, if adopted, might achieve a useful clarification.

If Vickers' formulation be compared with that made by Griesinger 90 years earlier (*see* p. 104), it will be seen that they correspond neatly. In the German's view, aetiology proper comprised only studies of the associations between 'stress-situation 'and 'stress-behaviour'; that is to say, those which nowadays would be termed ecological or epidemiological. Studies concerned with 'stress-change', or the nature of the physiological and psychological mechanisms which result in morbid phenomena, were subsumed by him under the separate heading of pathogeny.

The pathogenic concept of stress has dominated this field of research for a number of decades, during which time most clinical and experimental investigators have been preoccupied with the intervening variable of 'stress-change'. As Leigh[49] has commented, the whole history of psychosomatic medicine, under the influence first of psychoanalytic doctrine and more recently of psychophysiological theory, has centred round the notion of stress-change within the individual. That this should have been the case is readily understandable in historical terms, for it is clear from the writings of pioneer workers like Selye[79] that their twin sources of inspiration were Freud and W. B. Cannon. Nevertheless, in the long run, this preoccupation with mechanisms has proved detrimental to clinical science, for many attractive lines of enquiry have yielded disappointing results and the assumptions on which they were based have not always been confirmed by experimental investigation.

In this situation, a strong case can be made for a more intensive and systematic application of the epidemiological method than has yet been attempted. Only by means of epidemiological studies which fully establish the relationship between 'stress-situations' and 'stress-behaviour' can a firm aetiological basis be secured for future research.

To discern a need for the ecological approach is not to exaggerate its achievements to date. Although this review has been confined to studies dealing with events, crises and life-change on the one hand and the onset of mental disorder on the other, it has served to highlight problems of method and definition which have greatly impeded all environmental research in psychiatry. With hindsight it is clear that little progress could be made until the stage had been set by the development of research techniques in other disciplines and particularly in the social sciences. A sophisticated ecological design may call for the use of sampling procedures, standardized measuring instruments, controlled matching and other refinements which are only now gaining acceptance among medically trained investigators. To add to these difficulties, there has been a lack of any generally agreed diagnostic classification and the psychiatric nomenclature is still bedevilled by question-begging terms such as 'reactive psychosis' and 'pyschogenic psychosis'[19].

The problems of case-identification, classification and measurement with which the epidemiologist has to contend in all fields of medicine are especially troublesome in psychiatry because of the paucity of suitable laboratory tests and biological indices. Where measuring procedures are simple, the effects of stress-situations on exposed populations may be expressed in terms of related physiological variables, as in Graham's study of blood pressure changes among combat troops[27]. No doubt modern technology will further extend the range of physiological and biochemical investigations which can be conducted on large population samples, but commonsense decrees that the place of intricate and expensive tests in epidemiology will always be limited. Ethical considerations also demand some restraint on the procedures to which individuals in stress-situations may be subjected, as at least one study of the parents of dying children makes clear[22].

The inability to examine observed reactions to environmental change in terms of the mediating adaptive changes within the organism may prove a serious handicap where the significance of certain types of stimulus are not fully understood. Psycho-analytic teaching, for example, emphasizes the profound symbolic meaning for the individual of many events and experiences which to the observer may appear too trivial to merit attention. It does not need a psycho-analyst to point out that certain universal experiences such as puberty, marriage, child-bearing, change of domicile and of employment are not uniformly perceived and do not carry universal significance. Some ecologists—for example, Hinkle[36]—have argued strongly that the investigator cannot afford to ignore the patient's account of what specific events mean to him. In applying epidemiological techniques, however, it is essential at the present stage of knowledge to treat certain classes of environmental change as standard units which can be objectively and reliably measured.

The dangers of over-simplification are also inherent in the need to treat stress-situations as point-events. In the real world, environmental stress is almost always of a complex nature. Thus, the experience of pregnancy may be traumatic in a variety of ways: through the initial shock of recognition, the effect on future plans and expectations, the ensuing changes in personal relationships, the various related social problems such as inadequate housing and loss of earnings, the woman's increasing fatigue and physical discomfort, her fear of impending labour and the unconscious meaning which pregnancy and childbirth may hold for her. The emergence of psychiatric symptoms may be conditional on the interaction of several or all of these factors.

Finally, the scope and limitations of the epidemiological method must be borne in mind. Being by definition concerned with associations, it cannot be used to elucidate cause-and-effect relationships. While, therefore, ecological studies can be regarded as essential for further advance, they can never stand alone. Rather, serious research programmes must in the future move towards a more logical integration and differentiation of clinical, epidemiological and laboratory methods. Fifty years ago, Goldberger and his co-workers by their patient uncovering of the aetiology and pathogeny of pellagra provided a model for such a programme in psychiatry[90]. The example remains unique to the present day, but the climate is changing and there are some grounds for hoping that collaborative studies of this kind are destined to become the rule rather than the exception.

REFERENCES

1. Adler, A. (1943). 'Neuropsychiatric Complications in Victims of Boston's Cocoanut Grove Disaster'. *J. Am. med. Ass.* **123,** 1098
2. —— (1945). 'Two Different Types of Post-traumatic Neuroses'. *Am. J. Psychiat.* **102,** 237
3. Ahrenfeldt, R. H. (1958). *Psychiatry in the British Army in the Second World War.* London: Routledge and Kegan Paul
4. Barker, M. G. (1968). 'Psychiatric Illness after Hysterectomy'. *Br. med. J.* **1,** 91
5. Bond, D. (1953). 'The Common Psychological Defenses to Stressful Situations and the Patterns of Breakdown When They Fail'. *Symposium on Stress,* p. 142. National Research Council and Walter Reed Army Medical Centre. Washington D.C.
6. Brown, A. C. (1965). 'The General Morbidity of Neurotic Patients'. *Unpublished M.D. thesis.* University of Cambridge
7. Brown, G. W. and Birley, J. L. (1968). 'Social Change and the Onset of Schizophrenia'. *J. Hlth soc. Behav.* **9,** 203
8. Christophersen, E. (Ed.) (1946). *Results of the Norwegian Scientific Expedition to Tristan da Cunha, 1937–8.* Oslo: Norske Videnskaps Akademi
9. Cobb, S. and Lindemann, E. (1943). 'Neuropsychiatric Observations'. In *Management of the Cocoanut Grove Burns at the Massachussetts General Hospital. Ann. Surg.* **117.** Special Suppl.

10. Cohen, S. I. (1964). 'Neurological and Psychiatric Aspects of Open Heart Surgery'. *Thorax* **19**, 575

11. Craigie, H. B. (1942). 'Physical Treatment of Acute War Neurosis'. *Br. med. J.* **2**, 675

12. Davies, D. L. (1956). 'Psychiatric Illness in Those Engaged to be Married'. *Br. J. prev. soc. Med.* **10**, 123

13. Dencker, S. J. (1958). 'A Follow-up Study of 128 Closed Head Injuries in Twins using Co-twins as Controls'. *Acta psychiat. neurol. scand.* Suppl. 123

14. Doust, J. W. Lovett (1952). 'Psychiatric Aspects of Somatic Immunity: Differential Incidence of Physical Disease in the Histories of Psychiatric Patients'. *Br. J. soc. Med.* **6**, 49

15. Downes, J. and Simon, K. (1954). 'Characteristics of Psychoneurotic Patients and Their Families as Revealed in a General Morbidity Study'. *Milbank meml Fund q. Bull.* **32**, 42

16. Dublin, L. I. and Bunzel, B. (1933). ' "To Be or Not To Be"—A Study of Suicide'. New York: Harrison Smith and Robert Haas

17. Egerton, N. and Kay, J. H. (1964). 'Psychological Disturbances Associated with Open Heart Surgery'. *Br. J. Psychiat.* **110**, 433

18. Eitinger, L. (1959). 'The Incidence of Mental Disease Among Refugees in Norway'. *J. ment. Sci.* **105**, 326

19. Faergeman, P. M. (1963). 'Psychogenic Psychoses: A Description and Follow-up of Psychoses Following Psychological Stress'. London: Butterworths

20. Fairbairn, W. R. D. (1943). 'The War Neuroses: Their Nature and Significance'. *Br. med. J.* **1**, 183

21. Fraser, R., Leslie, I. M. and Phelps, D. (1943). 'Psychiatric Effects of Severe Personal Experiences During Bombing'. *Proc. R. Soc. Med.* **36**, 119

22. Friedman, S. B., Mason, J. W. and Hamburg, D. A. (1963). 'Urinary 17-Hydroxycorticosteroid Levels in Parents of Children with Neoplastic Disease: A Study of Chronic Psychological Stress'. *Psychosom. Med.* **25**, 364

23. Galdston, I. (1965). 'Community Psychiatry: Its Social and Historic Derivations'. *Can. psychiat. Ass. J.* **10**, 461

24. Georget, E. J. (1820). *De la Folie.* Paris

25. Gillespie, R. D. (1945). 'War Neuroses after Psychological Trauma'. *Br. med. J.* **1**, 653

26. Glass, A. J. and Bernucci, R. J. (Eds) (1966). *Neuropsychiatry in World War II.* Office of the Surgeon General, Department of the Army. Washington D.C.

27. Graham, J. D. P. (1945). 'High Blood Pressure after Battle'. *Lancet* **1**, 239

28. Greisinger, W. (1867). 'Mental Pathology and Therapeutics'. Translated by C. L. Robertson and J. Rutherford. London: New Sydenham Society

29. Grinker, R. R. and Spiegel, J. P. (1945). *Men under Stress*. London: Churchill
30. Hall, P. (1964). 'Moving House in the Aetiology of Psychiatric Symptoms'. *Proc. R. Soc. Med.* **57,** 83
31. Hamburg, D. A., Hamburg, B. and Degoza, S. (1953). 'Adaptive Problems and Mechanisms in Severely Burned Patients'. *Psychiatry* **16,** 1
32. Hare, E. H. (1952). 'The Ecology of Mental Disease'. *J. ment. Sci.* **98,** 579
33. —— (1967). 'The Epidemiology of Schizophrenia. In *Recent Developments in Schizophrenia: A Symposium*. Ed. by A. Coppen and A. Walk. London: Royal Medico-Psychological Association
34. Hecker, J. F. C. (1840). *The Epidemics of the Middle Ages*. (Translated by B. G. Babington). London: Sydenham Society
35. Hemphill, R. E. (1941). 'Importance of the First Year in War in Mental Disorder'. *Bristol med. chir. J.* **85,** 11
36. Hinkle, L. E. (1957). 'Health and the Social Environment: Experimental Investigations'. In *Explorations in Social Psychiatry*. Ed. by A. H. Leighton, J. A. Clausen and R. N. Wilson). London: Tavistock Publications
37. —— Plummer, N. (1952). 'Life Stress and Industrial Absenteeism: The Concentration of Illness and Absenteeism in One Segment of a Working Population'. *Ind. Med. Surg.* **21,** 363
38. —— and Wolff, H. G. (1957). 'The Nature of Man's Adaptation to his Total Environment and the Relation of this to Illness'. *A.M.A. Archs internal Med.* **99,** 442
39. —— Pinsky, R. H., Bross, I. D. J. and Plummer, N. (1956). 'The Distribution of Sickness Disability in a Homogeneous Group of Healthy, Adult Men'. *Am. J. Hyg.* **64,** 220
40. —— Redmont, R., Plummer, N. and Wolff, H. G. (1960). 'An Examination of the Relation Between Symptoms, Disability and Serious Illness in Two Homogeneous Groups of Men and Women'. *Am. J. publ. Hlth* **50,** 1327
41. Hirst, L. F. (1953). *The Conquest of Plague*. London: Oxford University Press
42. Hopkins, F. (1943). 'Decrease in Admissions to Mental Observation Wards During War'. *Br. med. J.* **1,** 358
43. Hudgens, R. W., Morrison, J. R. and Barchha, R. G. (1967). 'Life Events and Onset of Primary Affective Disorders'. *Archs gen. Psychiat.* **16,** 134
44. Illingworth, C. F. W., Scott, L. D. W. and Jamieson, R. A. (1944). 'Acute Perforated Peptic Ulcer: Frequency and Incidence in West of Scotland'. *Br. med. J.* **2,** 617
45. Janis, I. L. (1958). 'Psychological Stress: Psychoanalytic and Behavioural Studies of Surgical Patients'. New York: John Wiley
46. Kellner, R. (1966). 'Psychiatric Ill-health Following Physical Illness'. *Br. J. Psychiat.* **112,** 71

47. Knox, S. J. (1961). 'Severe Psychiatric Disturbances in the Post-operative Period—A Five Year Survey of Belfast Hospitals'. *J. ment. Sci.* **107**, 1078

48. — (1963). 'Psychiatric Aspects of Mitral Valvotomy'. *Br. J. Psychiat.* **109**, 656

49. Leigh, D. (1968). 'The Form Complete: The Present State of Psychosomatic Medicine'. *Proc. R. Soc. Med.* **61**, 375

50. Leopold, R. L. and Dillon, H. (1963). 'Psycho-anatomy of a Disaster: A Long-term Study of Post-traumatic Neuroses in Survivors of a Marine Explosion'. *Am. J. Psychiat.* **119**, 913

51. Lewis, A. J. (1942). 'Incidence of Neurosis in England Under War Conditions'. *Lancet* **2**, 175

52. — (1955). 'The Relation Between Operative Risk and the Patients' General Condition'. *Report of the Sixteenth Congres International de Chirurgie.* Copenhagen

53. Lin, T-Y and Standley, C. C. (1962). 'The Scope of Epidemiology in Psychiatry'. *Public Health Papers No. 16.* Geneva: W. H. O.

54. Lindemann, E. (1941). 'Observations on Psychiatric Sequelae to Surgical Operations in Women'. *Am. J. Psychiat.* **98**, 132

55. Linn, L., Kahn, R. L., Coles, R., Cohen, J., Marshall, D. and Weinstein, E. A. (1953). 'Patterns of Behaviour Disturbance Following Cataract Extraction'. *Am. J. Psychiat.* **110**, 281

56. Mechanic, D. (1962). *Students under Stress. A Study in the Social Psychology of Adaptation.* Glencoe, Ill.: Free Press

57. Mezey, A. G. (1960). 'Personal Background, Emigration and Mental Disorder in Hungarian Refugees'. *J. ment. Sci.* **106**, 618

58. Morrison, J. R., Hudgens, R. W. and Barchha, R. G. (1968). 'Life Events and Psychiatric Illness: A Study of 100 Patients and 100 Controls'. *Br. J. Psychiat.* **114**, 423

59. Murphy, H. B. M. (1955). *Culture, Society and Mental Disorder in in South East Asia.* Unpublished MS

60. — (Ed.) (1955). *Flight and Resettlement.* Paris: Unesco

61. — (1961). 'Social Change and Mental Health'. *Milbank meml Fund q. Bull.* **39**, 385

62. Nohl, J. (1961). 'The Black Death: A Chronicle of the Plague'. Translated by C. H. Clarke. London: Allen & Unwin

63. Ødegaard, Ø. (1932). 'Emigration and Insanity'. *Acta psychiat. neurol. scand.* Suppl. 4

64. Paffenbarger, R. S. Jun. (1964). 'Epidemiological Aspects of Parapartum Mental Illness'. *Br. J. prev. soc. Med.* **18**, 189

65. Parkes, C. M. (1964). 'Recent Bereavement as a Cause of Mental Illness. *Br. J. Psychiat.* **110**, 198

66. Pearson, H. E. S. and Joseph, J. (1963). 'Stress and Occlusive Coronary-artery Disease'. *Lancet* **1**, 415

67. Pfister-Ammende, M. (1955). 'The Symptomatology, Treatment and Prognosis in Mentally Ill Refugees and Repatriates in Switzerland'. In *Flight and Resettlement.* Ed. by H. B. M. Murphy. Paris: Unesco

68. Pinel, P. (1962). 'A Treatise on Insanity'. *History of Medicine Series No. 14.* (Translated by D. D. Davis). New York Academy of Medicine. New York: Hafner

69. Rahe, R. H., McKean, J. D. and Arthur, R. J. (1967). 'A Longitudinal Study of Life Change and Illness-patterns'. *J. Psychosom. Res.* **10,** 355

70. — Meyer, M., Smith, M., Kjaer, G. and Holmes, T. H. (1964). 'Social Stress and Illness Onset'. *J. Psychosom. Res.* **8,** 35

71. Rawnsley, K. and Loudon, J. B. (1964). 'Epidemiology of Mental Disorder in a Closed Community'. *Br. J. Psychiat.* **110,** 830

72. Reid, D. D. (1948). 'Sickness and Stress in Operational Flying'. *Br. J. soc .Med.* **2,** 123

73. — (1960). 'Epidemiological Methods in the Study of Mental Disorders'. *Public Health Papers No. 2.* Geneva: W.H.O.

74. Roessler, R. and Greenfield, N. S. (1961). 'Incidence of Somatic Disease in Psychiatric Patients'. *Psychosom. Med.* **23,** 413

75. Rook, Sir Alan (1959). 'Student Suicides'. *Br. med. J.* **1,** 599

76. Sargant, W. and Slater, E. (1940). 'Acute War Neuroses'. *Lancet* **2,** 1

77. — and Shorvon, H. J. (1945). 'Acute War Neurosis: Special Reference to Pavlov's Experimental Observations and the Mechanism of Abreaction'. *Archs Neurcl. Psychiat., Chicago,* **54,** 231

78. Seager, C. P. (1960). 'A Controlled Study of Post-partum Mental Illness'. *J. ment. Sci.* **106,** 214

79. Selye, H. (1956). *The Stress of Life.* New York: Longmans, Green

80. Shepherd, M. and Cooper, B. (1964). 'Epidemiology and Mental Disorder: A Review'. *J. Neurol. Neurosurg. Psychiat.* **27,** 277

81. Slater, E. (1943). 'The Neurotic Constitution: A Statistical Study of 2000 Neurotic Soldiers'. *J. Neurol. Neurosurg. Psychiat.* **6,** 1

82. Smith, J. A. (1956). 'Occupational Stress and Emotional Illness'. *J. Am. med. Ass.* **161,** 1038

83. Spicer, C. C., Stewart, D. N. and Winser, D. M. de R. (1944). 'Perforated Peptic Ulcer During the Period of Heavy Air-raids'. *Lancet* **1,** 14

84. Stengel, E. (1964). *Suicide and Attempted Suicide.* Harmondsworth, Middlesex: Penguin

85. — Zeitlyn, B. B. and Rayner, E. H. (1958). 'Post-operative Psychoses'. *J. ment. Sci.* **104,** 389

86. Stewart, D. N. and Winser, D. M. de R. (1942). 'Incidence of Perforated Peptic Ulcer: Effect of Heavy Air Raids'. *Lancet* **1,** 259

87. Sunier, A. (1956). *Mental Illness and Psychiatric Care in Israel.* Mimeograph. Amsterdam

88. Swinscow, D. (1951). 'Some Suicide Statistics'. *Br. med. J.* **1,** 1417

89. Symonds, C. P. (1943). 'The Human Response to Flying Stress'. *Br. med. J.* **2,** 703, 740

90. Terris, M. (Ed.) (1964). *Goldberger on Pellagra.* Baton Rouge: Louisiana State University Press

91. Tredgold, R. F. (1947). 'Manic States in the Far East'. *Br. med. J.* **2,** 522

92. Tyhurst, J. S. (1951). 'Individual Reactions to Community Disaster: The Natural History of Psychiatric Phenomena'. *Am. J. Psychiat.* **107,** 764

93. —— (1958). 'The Role of Transition States—Including Disasters —In Mental Illness'. In *Symposium on Preventive and Social Psychiatry.* Walter Reed Army Institute, Washington, D.C.

94. Vickers, Sir Geoffrey (1958). 'Congress on Stress and Mental Illness'. *Lancet* **1,** 205

95. Wittkower, E. and Spillane, J. P. (1940). 'A Survey of the Literature of Neuroses in War'. In *The Neuroses in War.* Ed. by E. Miller. London: Macmillan

96. Wolfenstein, M. (1957). *Disaster.* Glencoe, Ill.: Free Press

CHAPTER 6

ANOREXIA NERVOSA: ITS IDENTITY AS AN ILLNESS AND ITS TREATMENT

G. F. M. RUSSELL

INTRODUCTION

Anorexia nervosa is an illness which excites considerable interest from physicians and psychiatrists alike, with the result that an extensive literature has accumulated. This review will select only those contributions which appear to the author to have advanced the subject. Inevitably there is a danger of failing to do justice to a considerable number of carefully made observations. In the interest of brevity, references will be largely confined to those articles published during the last 15 years or so and which have broken fresh ground. It is necessary first to sum up some of the important points that have been stressed prior to the period covered by this review.

(1) A clear distinction between the clinical features of anorexia nervosa and those resulting from total loss of function of the anterior pituitary gland followed the publication by Sheehan and Summers[108]. They demonstrated that disease confined to the pituitary gland did not give rise to a loss of body weight and as a result of this work the ghost of Simmond's cachexia was finally laid. It was thus possible for Michael and Gibbons[82] to state categorically that the problem of distinguishing between the two diagnoses was a mythical one.

(2) The view that anorexia nervosa has a psychogenic basis has steadily gained ground from the time that the illness was ascribed to a 'morbid mental state'[48] with a resulting loss of appetite. The formulation[120] that the refusal of food signifies a defence against unconscious fantasies of oral conception, is probably the psychodynamic model which aroused the greatest interest.

(3) Increasingly, patients with anorexia nervosa have been referred to psychiatrists for treatment. Williams[130], however, has given a sharp reminder that their lives may be in danger from malnutrition and its consequences and he has stressed the need for 'somatic' methods of treatment.

(4) Although several series of patients had been reported in the literature previously, it was the follow-up study[60] that provided

the most systematic detailed information regarding the psychiatric features, natural course and outcome of this illness. Their findings led Kay and Leigh to conclude that anorexia nervosa does not consist of a distinct 'clinical entity' but of a variety of psychiatric disorders. On the whole they formed an optimistic view of the natural course of the illness.

Most of the views summarized above need qualification today and it is proposed to discuss recent advances supporting the argument for recognizing the identity of anorexia nervosa. They will be examined under the following headings: the diagnostic criteria of the illness, its natural course and the elucidation of its causation. These advances are the outcome of research in clinical psychiatry, applied psychology, endocrinology and nutritional physiology, and their consideration will be followed by an appraisal of the hypothalamic model. Finally, the treatment of anorexia nervosa will be discussed.

IDENTITY OF ANOREXIA NERVOSA

To discuss the identity of anorexia nervosa might appear an idle scholarly exercise were it not for the danger that to dismiss it as a mere symptom of a variety of psychiatric illnesses[73] might result in a loss of interest and a stifling of research. In a similar discussion on the nosological status of hysteria, Sir Aubrey Lewis[70] has underlined the confusion that has arisen from the verbal quibbles surrounding terms such as 'illness,' 'syndrome' and 'clinical entity'. In any such argument, it is crucial to be explicit about the definition of these terms. Several authors who have rejected the view that anorexia nervosa is a 'clinical entity' have failed to define what they mean by this term[11, 60]. They merely indicated that their patients varied greatly in their premorbid personalities or differed in some of the psychopathological features. The same can be said of any psychiatric illness of uncertain causation, including schizophrenic and manic-depressive psychoses. In contrast, Scadding[106] has given a lucid account of how the criteria used in the diagnosis of various physical diseases may evolve as more becomes known about them. For example, a disease may first become identified by observing that it presents a number of clinical features which are usually associated with each other; this is the clinical-descriptive or 'Hippocratic' procedure of diagnosis. Subsequently the clinical-descriptive approach may become supplemented or modified by the acquisition of data gleaned from more precise fields of enquiry such as morbid anatomy, applied physiology, biochemistry, cytogenetics, etc. Eventually, the identification of noxious agents, deficiency states, disordered body chemistry or genetic abnormalities may lead to elucidation of the aetiology of the disease.

Our present state of knowledge does not yet permit us to state categorically that anorexia nervosa is a distinct illness, but in order to attempt to establish its identity, three sets of operational criteria will be used: (1) the constancy of association of the various clinical features; (2) the similarity in the course and outcome of the illness and more especially whether the illness 'breeds true', that is, remains fundamentally the same in those patients who suffer later relapses or who reach chronicity; (3) the elucidation of a clear-cut aetiology; causes may be multiple and may consist of psychogenic and/or physiogenic factors. Ultimately this last criterion is the only satisfactory one, but we seem far from satisfying it with the majority of psychiatric disorders.

DIAGNOSTIC CRITERIA

The view is gaining ground that anorexia nervosa has a 'consistent nucleus'[115]. The following clinical features should be elicited before accepting the diagnosis.

(1) The patient's behaviour leads to a marked loss of body weight* and malnutrition. The abnormal behaviour consists of a studied and purposive avoidance of foods considered to be of a 'fattening nature', usually carbohydrate-containing foods such as sugar, bread and cereals, potatoes, pastries and confectionary. Often, but not invariably, the patient resorts to additional devices which ensure a loss of weight: self-induced vomiting or purgation, or excessive exercise. Occasionally a patient may indulge in bouts of overeating but these are usually compensated for by subsequent vomiting or prolonged starvation which effectively counteract the transient increase in the caloric intake.

(2) There is an endocrine disorder which manifests itself clinically by cessation of menstruation in those patients who are most commonly afflicted by the illness—adolescent girls or women during the reproductive period of life. The amenorrhoea is an early symptom and may precede the onset of weight loss; it is often very persistent and may last for several years.

In male subjects the equivalent symptom is a loss of sexual interest and lack of potency, but in adolescent boys it may be difficult to elicit these symptoms. In them, it is desirable to establish by means

---

* A weight loss of 25 lb or more has been stipulated[11] but this figure obviously should be modified according to the patient's weight before the onset of the illness and the body build.

133

of hormone assays evidence for the hormonal disturbance which will be discussed later.

In children before puberty, it is not yet possible to demonstrate an endocrine disorder characteristic of anorexia nervosa. The diagnosis can still be made tentatively by relying on other criteria, (1) and (3), but there may remain room for uncertainty. Tolstrup[116], however, has stated that anorexia nervosa in these young patients resembles closely the illness that occurs after puberty.

(3) There are aspects of the psychopathology which are characteristic of anorexia nervosa, irrespective of the patient's sex. They are essentially manifestations of a morbid fear of becoming fat, which may be fully expressed by the patient or may be more explicit in her behaviour[16, 17]. To safeguard herself against what the patient often calls 'losing control'—meaning not being able to stop eating—she strives to remain abnormally thin. She defends her attitude by asserting that to be thin is for her right and desirable, and she often appears to be absolutely convinced of the justification of her ideas. She loses all judgement as to her requirements for food and may protest that she is eating satisfactorily; she often over-estimates her body weight and sets herself a precise weight, above which she dare not rise.

There are, in addition, greatly varying psychopathological manifestations, especially depressive symptoms, but also obsessional, hysterical or phobic symptoms. Even some of the commoner features rightly stressed, such as the 'perceptual and conceptual disturbances'[16] and the 'asceticism at puberty'[115], are not as characteristic of anorexia nervosa as the fear of fatness. It is also true that the patient's premorbid personality is extremely variable, but these divergences are not necessarily in conflict with the uniformity of the syndrome. Neither does one need to claim that there should be a specific psychogenesis in order to delineate anorexia nervosa; at the present time this is still not possible. In short, anorexia nervosa is an illness or syndrome with a constellation of symptoms and signs which should permit a reliable diagnosis to be made. One may confidently state at least that the term 'anorexia nervosa' conveys far more to a professional colleague than say 'obsessional neurosis with a feeding disorder'.

Conclusion

Recently, interest has been shown in the question of the reliability of psychiatric diagnoses[3, 109]. It is likely that with the use of clear-cut criteria for diagnosis, such as those enumerated above, the degree of agreement in identifying patients with anorexia nervosa is likely to be at least as good as with patients suffering from other recognized psychiatric disorders. Admittedly, this opinion should be put to the test by using standardized diagnostic techniques in the ways suggested in the Lancet article[3].

COURSE OF ANOREXIA NERVOSA

Sir Aubrey Lewis[70] has pointed out that, if knowledge about an illness is limited, a requirement for its identification as a 'clinical entity' is that it breeds true: if patients relapse or their illness runs a chronic course, there should be no fundamental change in its salient clinical features. A far less reliable method for establishing the identity of an illness is to ascertain whether there is some uniformity in its course. For example, when discussing the diagnosis of schizophrenia, Fish[41] pointed out the limitations of restricting it to illnesses which leave permanent defects of personality. He also noted, however, that the criterion of incurability led to the isolation of leukaemia and addisonian anaemia. The method of isolating illnesses on the basis of their course, in the hands of Kraepelin, laid the early foundations of the classification of psychiatric disorders.

Data are now available on the natural course and outcome of anorexia nervosa as a result of well conducted follow-up studies extending over several years. It must first be conceded that the prognosis of patients with this illness is variable: a proportion recover completely after two, three or more years; a sizeable proportion remain permanently unwell. The relative numbers belonging to each category again vary according to the author, most probably as a result of factors related to the selection of the patients and the criteria accepted by the investigators. Whereas Beck and Brøchner-Mortensen[7] reported a recovery or improvement in four-fifths of their 20 patients, Meyer[81] found that only seven out of his 20 patients had recovered. Kay and Shcapira[61] described an outcome lying in between these two extremes. They further pointed out that many patients are left with residual disabilities, an observation also made by Cremerius[19] who personally followed up in detail over 15 to 18 years a series of 11 patients. Warren[123] emphasized the gravity of anorexia nervosa occurring in 20 very young girls, including eight who were prepubertal at the time of onset.

If the course of anorexia nervosa is variable, however, the present evidence supports the view that the illness 'breeds true'. Kay has summarized two studies, the first conducted at the Maudsley

Hospital in London[60] and the second in Newcastle[61]: 60 per cent of his patients continued to show disturbances of appetite of some degree or kind, 50 per cent remained underweight or had marked fluctuations in weight, menstruation remained irregular or absent in 60 per cent of the female patients. The psychiatric assessment of the patients at follow-up showed that 28 per cent were preoccupied with problems connected with food, 33 per cent had a variety of neurotic symptoms, another 33 per cent were better adjusted, but even they had a number of deficiencies in the social or sexual sphere. Kay and Schapira concluded: 'Generally speaking, the basic form of the psychiatric disturbances associated with anorexia nervosa remains constant, and new developments seldom arise.' Similarly, Cremerius emphasized the persistence of abnormal attitudes to food and amenorrhoea in 5 of his 11 patients; 5 others had improved markedly but remained rather eccentric, and 3 of them he described as having character neuroses*. Most sizeable studies include an occasional patient who later develops schizophrenia[19, 61, 123], but few authors take the view that this is anything but a chance findnig. In his study, Warren emphasized his observation that many of his 11 girls who had recovered from the feeding and menstrual disorders continued to show neurotic or personality disturbances of different degree, thus questioning the significance or the basic nature of anorexia nervosa. Nevertheless, even among these 11 patients 5 continued to 'watch their figures and tended to avoid carbohydrates such as bread and potatoes, but probably not more so tha ' many normal young women'. The normality of such behaviour is obviously difficult to assess and is at least questionabţe. Preliminary findings of a prognostic study conducted on patients treated in the Metabolic Unit of the Maudsley Hospital confirm the view of Kay and Schapira that abnormal attitudes to body weight and eating persist for very long, even in patients whose illness follows a relatively favourable course[84].

Conclusion

The evidence is still incomplete but, as far as it goes, it lends weight to the thesis that anorexia nervosa does not as a rule evolve into a different kind of psychiatric disorder and has, therefore, an identity of its own. There may persist a variety of neurotic symptoms or evidence of social or sexual maladjustment, but many of these features are often present at the onset of the anorexia nervosa, though overshadowed by the more dramatic feeding disturbance.

* Only 1 was said to have recovered.

ELUCIDATION OF THE AETIOLOGY OF ANOREXIA NERVOSA

Psychogenesis

From the earliest descriptions of anorexia nervosa, it has been accepted without question that the illness is at least partly of psychogenic causation, but the early psychodynamic speculations have given way to more cautious formulations based on sounder clinical observations. For example, the rather sweeping generalization of Waller, Kaufman and Deutsch[120] that anorexia nervosa is a defence against unconscious fantasies of oral insemination has been questioned. Instead, recent studies have stressed the significance of feeding and nutrition in early infancy and the importance of the influences, including biological influences, that overwhelm the patient at the time of puberty. Moreover, there is greater awareness that descriptions of psychodynamic mechanisms are not synonymous with aetiological explanation[115].

The penetrating studies of Bruch[16, 17] have already been mentioned. Bruch relates the patient's fear of fatness to a failure to perceive bodily sensations appropriately, including the awareness of her own body image. For example, she may not accept that she is too thin, even when she has become emaciated, and appears surprised to learn that her weight is as low as it actually is. She acquires an abnormal concept of ideal bodily proportions and may protest with anguish when she sees herself becoming 'fat' (meaning somewhat less scraggy when treatment is put into effect). Bruch also attaches some importance to her observation that in adolescent girls there is often an inability to achieve self-expression and independence from the parents. This is accompanied by a sense of ineffectiveness and the patient feels that she cannot act as she wants but only in response to external demands. There is some experimental evidence that supports Bruch's observations: Griffiths[45] showed that patients with anorexia nervosa judged their weight to be more or less than 'normal' in a way similar to a control group of normally nourished neurotic patients: the thin patients thus tended not to view their own weights as too low. Moreover, the patients with anorexia nervosa considered being fat as much more unpleasant than did the control groups of neurotic patients and normal student nurses.

Psychodynamic formulations purporting to explain the evolution of anorexia nervosa may not be accepted universally, but still deserve careful evaluation. The interested reader should refer to Thomä's work[115] in which he makes a spirited defence of the role of psycho-dynamic factors, but is careful not to ascribe automatically causal significance to them. He also demurs from characterizing the family environment as pathogenic. He prefers to emphasize the abnormal psychic development of the patient and stresses that only seldom can a psychological trauma be elicited before the onset of the illness. Thomä describes the following psychodynamic processes: a defence mechanism not directed against external danger but against the developmental process of puberty itself; a regression so that the patient abandons the genital-sexual stage of development and sexual impulses vanish from consciousness; 'fixation at an oral level' so that thought is dominated by food and hunger; striving towards an ascetic ideal and an asexual life. There would appear to result a perpetual struggle to escape from guilt and anxiety; abstinence from food may serve as self-punishment; they may also seek to protect and feed other members of their families or other patients.

The importance of the efflorescence of puberty has also been emphasized by Crisp[21, 24] who views the effects of starvation and the resulting malnutrition as leading to a reduction in sexual drive and thus to a secondary reinforcement of the self-starvation. Novlyan-skaya[86] describes anorexia nervosa as a prolonged abnormal reaction to puberty. Meyer[81] refers to Pubertäts magersucht, the term 'mager-sucht' (seeking after thinness) being a German equivalent to anorexia nervosa and describing more aptly the principal psycho-pathology of the illness.

The interaction between the patients' mental state and their food intake has been measured in a systematic way in a small number of patients[94]. After treatment had resulted in a partial or total restora-tion of their nutrition, they were permitted to select their own diet while under observation in a metabolic ward. From daily records by the nursing staff on a Phipps behaviour chart, it was possible to assess fluctuations in symptoms such as anxiety, depression and irritability, and correlate them with the intake of food. The daily calorie consumption was measured by burning samples of the diet in a bomb calorimeter. Three out of four patients showed that, on the days when they chose of their own volition to eat more food, they ex-perienced more distress, as shown by highly significant correlations. The obvious conclusion was that, in those patients whose abnormal attitudes towards food and body image persist, relief from their more distressing symptoms is achieved by eating less. In them, relapse and weight loss would appear to be inevitable, thus empha-sizing the importance of trying to modify the 'morbid mental state' which Gull recognized as being the core of the problem.

Conclusion

The importance of the psychological disorder in anorexia nervosa cannot be doubted, but a specific psychogenesis remains elusive.

Familial and Developmental Factors

Kay, Schapira and Brandon[62] have questioned the validity of the shorthand intuitive descriptions of family situations, such as the robust nagging mother and the passive father, assumed to predispose to anorexia nervosa. They point out the importance of allowing for a two-way interaction between the child and the family and ask the pertinent question 'how does a "normal" mother behave when her daughter is intent on self-starvation?' These authors described a number of features found more frequently among the anorexia nervosa patients and their families than among control groups of neurotic patients and nursing students. They were the occurrence of abnormal marriages in the parents (mainly periods of separation), birth complications (e.g. forceps deliveries), infant feeding difficulties, and environmental difficulties such as overcrowding and economic hardship. They also found that patients with anorexia nervosa were often only children, but Kay (Personal communication, 1969) has expressed reservations about this observation which has not been confirmed by others. Kay, Schapira and Brandon confirmed an earlier finding[20] that these patients were often overweight in childhood. Crisp thought that even their birth weight was relatively high and that their early good nutrition might have contributed to an early puberty and hence to an early confrontation with sexual and emotional conflicts.

Conclusion

The identification of pathogenic family situations will have to await stringent studies similar to that of Kay and his colleagues.

The Endocrine Disorder in Anorexia Nervosa

Reference has already been made to the work of Sheehan and Summers[108] which cleared up the confusion that surrounded the mythical problem of distinguishing between anorexia nervosa and the effects of a destructive disease of the anterior pituitary gland. Bliss and Migeon[10] assessed the function of the adrenal cortex and the thyroid—two of the target glands of the anterior pituitary—and showed conclusively that there was no diminution in their activity. Indeed, more recent work[77] revealed that in anorexia nervosa the anterior pituitary can maintain elevated plasma levels of growth hormone and cortisol (the latter presumably through the agency of

ACTH). In some patients the plasma levels of these hormones can be raised further by administering insulin[68]. The earlier view that the malnutrition of anorexia nervosa gives rise to a secondary global failure of anterior pituitary function[131] can, therefore, be rejected.

Whereas it can be concluded that many of the actions of the anterior pituitary gland are preserved in anorexia nervosa, there is now a growing body of evidence that one of the functions mediated by the anterior pituitary is impaired, namely the release of gonadotrophins which act on the gonads and regulate sexual and reproductive activity. Moreover, this isolated endocrine failure may be of a specific nature, though more work is needed before this can be established. The interaction between the nutritional and the endocrine disorders in anorexia nervosa is complex, but the malnutrition is only partly the cause of the gonadal failure.

The evidence in the female patient with anorexia nervosa for these statements is as follows. For a long time clinicians have observed that the cessation of menstruation may be the earliest manifestation of the illness and antedates weight loss or even eating disturbances in at least a quarter of patients[7, 60]. Recent laboratory investigations have confirmed that there is a failure in the output of gonadotrophins and oestrogens in patients before they receive treatment. A number of earlier studies reported widely differing findings in their hormonal assays[35, 40, 55, 90] but they will not be reviewed as they failed to express their results in terms of a reference standard and were thus unreliable. A marked reduction in the urinary output of human pituitary gonadotrophins was found in 18 out of 19 patients admitted to the Maudsley Hospital[8, 100, 102]; the method of assay was the mouse uterus test[74] and the first international reference preparation of human menopausal gonadotrophin was used as a standard. In these studies, three oestrogen fractions were also measured by the method of Brown[14] and Brown, Bulbrook and Greenwood[15]—oestriol, oestrone and oestradiol. All three fractions were much reduced, but the reduction of oestriol (normally the largest fraction) was even greater than that of the other two oestrogens.

By refeeding the patients and inducing a considerable restoration of the lost body weight, and at the same time continuing the hormonal assays, it was possible to assess whether the malnutrition had been responsible for the diminished output of gonadotrophins and oestrogens. To some extent it had, for refeeding led to increased excretion of these hormones in the urine, but recovery was not complete. The gonadotrophin levels did not return to normal and, more important, there was no cyclical variation in the output of the hormones such as would herald a resumption of normal menstrual cycles with ovulation. This incomplete recovery persisted for several months in those patients who underwent prolonged studies, in spite of the very considerable gains in body weight. In one of the studies, factors affecting the reappearance of gonadotrophins in the urine on refeeding were examined further[100]. Weight gain was indeed one of the necessary factors, but not the only one: in fact the variation in response between different patients depended more on the duration of their illness: paradoxically, patients with a longer illness showed an earlier and brisker excretion of gonadotrophins than those who had been ill for shorter periods. It appears, therefore, that as at the onset of the illness, there can be a dissociation between the feeding and the endocrine disorders: the patient may have become chronically undernourished, yet hormonal function may be restored more readily than in a patient with a shorter illness.

The method used in the above studies for the gonadotrophin assays were non-specific and did not distinguish between follicle-stimulating hormone and luteinizing hormone. In view of the function of luteinizing hormone in causing ovulation and inducing the menstrual cycles, it is possible that this is the hormone which is selectively deficient in anorexia nervosa. Further work using immunological methods of assay would elucidate this question.

In male patients with anorexia nervosa there is probably a hormonal disorder analogous to that present in the female. Ismail and Harkness[57, 58] reported low testosterone outputs in the urine of two male patients in whom a diagnosis of anorexia nervosa had been made at the Maudsley Hospital, using the criteria of the characteristic feeding and psychiatric disorders. More recent work at the Maudsley has shown that male patients also have very low urinary levels of gonadotrophins and gonadal (testosterone) hormones[6]. The analogy cannot be pursued any further for the time being because it has not yet been possible to study the effects of refeeding in a sufficiently large series of male patients. It is fair to say, however, that the available information to date supports the view that the endocrine disorder in anorexia nervosa is of a similar kind in the male as in the female. Hormonal assays should, therefore, permit a more certain diagnosis to be made in male patients.

The isolated failure of the release of gonadotrophins from the anterior pituitary in patients with anorexia nervosa almost certainly reflects a disturbance at the level of the hypothalamus. Harris, Reed and Fawcett[51] have reviewed the evidence that the hypothalamus controls the anterior pituitary gland by means of releasing factors which in their turn regulate the secretion of a number of hormones, including follicle-stimulating and luteinizing hormones.

Thus, it can be concluded that in anorexia nervosa there is a disturbance of neural function, the end-stage of which is an isolated hypothalamo-pituitary failure which manifests itself clinically in the female by amenorrhoea. It would, moreover, be too facile to dismiss this endocrine disorder as being of 'psychogenic origin'. As already pointed out, a clear-cut psychogenesis is elusive; moreover, little is known of the physiological mechanisms of amenorrhoea which clearly follows emotional disturbances[42]. It must also be pointed out that whereas amenorrhoea is an invariable manifestation of anorexia nervosa in female patients of the appropriate age, it is much less common in other forms of mental illness, even in the psychoses[44].

The relationship between the secondary gonadal failure in anorexia nervosa and abnormal sexual attitudes and frigidity should also be considered. These psychological changes are usually interpreted as a form of regression away from the developmental processes of puberty and assumed to be of psychogenic origin; but it is pertinent to ask whether the gonadal failure itself (with the deficient secretion of oestrogens or testosterone) might not contribute to the loss of sexual interest. This may not seem likely in the female in view of the evidence that castration or the menopause have little effect on sexuality and only loss of adreno-cortical function has a profound depressing effect on libido[124]. On the other hand, these observations are mainly pertinent to the mature adult woman; the situation might be different when gonadal failure occurs soon after the onset of puberty. In the case of the male, however, it is more likely that reduction of testosterone activity leads to the loss of libido and potency which have been recorded[67]. These questions are still *sub judice*. Recent experimental work on the role of the central nervous system in determining the timing of puberty and consequent patterns of behaviour may be highly relevant. This function of the nervous system is determined at an early stage of its development: neonatally in the rat[4], and during intra-uterine life in the guinea pig[89]. Such an early organization of the nervous system has been shown to be susceptible to interference by a number of intra-uterine factors[37]. The integration of the efflorescence of puberty and the laying down of sexual behaviour and psychological attitudes is obviously a complex and uncharted field: one can only speculate about its importance in human illness, but it is conceivable that it has some bearing on the genesis of anorexia nervosa.

Conclusion

The finding of a relatively distinct and isolated endocrine disorder in anorexia nervosa supports the view that it has an identity of its own.

The Nutritional Disorder in Anorexia Nervosa

Malnutrition is probably responsible for most of the physical complications of anorexia nervosa, with the exception of the amenorrhoea, and may contribute to the mental ill-health. Fatalities are usually the result of the malnutrition, except in the case of patients who commit suicide. It is, therefore, important for doctors, including psychiatrists, to be aware of the nutritional deficiencies that arise so that they can be corrected and serious complications avoided. There is also a theoretical reason for wanting to investigate the nutritional disorder in anorexia nervosa: only by doing so can the pathogenesis of the various clinical manifestations be understood. Whereas it is reasonable to expect that many of the physical complications are secondary to the malnutrition, it is desirable to establish this beyond doubt. It has already been pointed out that such investigations led to the conclusion that the endocrine disorder in anorexia nervosa is not simply the result of weight loss, but is a primary feature of the illness. In spite of these arguments in favour of nutritional studies, there have been comparatively few until recently and there was little more than the observation that specific vitamin deficiencies are rare in anorexia nervosa[11].

The loss of weight is mainly due to the purposive reduction of food intake, but may be accelerated by self-induced vomiting and/or purgation which are particularly pernicious in leading to metabolic complications. In reducing the amount of food eaten, the patients selectively avoid carbohydrate-containing foods: the foods chosen are relatively rich in protein or even in fats. As a result, the contribution made by protein foods to the total calorie intake is relatively high: 18 per cent on the average, compared with 10 to 12 per cent in normal subjects, though the *absolute* intake of protein is still low[94].

Body Composition—Loss of weight represents a loss of body tissue which varies in its composition according to the patient's age and sex, the original state of his nutrition and the kind of starvation that he is enduring. Studies of body composition have been carried out in male concentration camp victims[127, 128] and in starved male human volunteers[63, 64] but similar investigations in anorexia nervosa, or even in females, are very sparse. Ljunggren, Ikkos and Luft[71] did, however, carry out such a study, relying on body dilution techniques. They found that in their patients with anorexia nervosa the greater part of the lost tissue consisted of solid matter (68 per cent) and the water content was only 32 per cent. Russell and Mezey[96] used nitrogen balances and indirect calorimetry as described by Passmore, Strong and Ritchie[88], and found an even greater proportion of solids in the tissue laid down during refeeding, most of this tissue consisting of fat (77 per cent fat, 7 per cent protein and 16 per cent water). The high rate of fat deposition was confirmed by measurement of skin-fold thickness at different sites and by determinations of respiratory quotients. These findings contrasted with previous studies in other kinds of malnutrition, but they were attributed to the sex difference rather than the nature of the malnutrition in anorexia nervosa. This conclusion was confirmed by nitrogen balance studies in male patients with anorexia nervosa: they retained greater amounts of nitrogen during refeeding, thus falling into line with previous studies done on male patients suffering from other kinds of malnutrition[94]. Further work on protein metabolism in female patients with anorexia nervosa confirms that they show little in the way of protein in-sufficiency: plasma amino acid levels were found to be normal in contrast with the abnormalities reported in states of protein in-sufficiency such as kwashiorkor[54]. Only when a measurement of plasma albumen turn-over was carried out by injecting intra-venously labelled iodinated albumen (^{131}I), was it possible to demonstrate a protective mechanism which reduced the breakdown of albumen, presumably in order to conserve body protein[94]. Kassenaar, Graeff and Kouwenhoven[59] showed that there was no impairment of protein synthesis during the refeeding of patients with anorexia nervosa, as assessed by studies using ^{15}N-labelled glycine.

Another feature of malnutrition which may be looked on as a protective device is a reduction in the body's metabolic rate. This was also found in anorexia nervosa when the calorie expenditure was expressed in terms of the body's total consumption of oxygen[96] or even when expressed in terms of oxygen uptake per kilogram body weight[72]. Traditionally, the basal metabolic rate (B.M.R.) is calculated by dividing the basal oxygen consumption by the body surface area and expressing it as a percentage of normal. In wasted patients the estimation of surface area by the Dubois formula is unreliable and falsely high, so that the B.M.R. result obtained is often even lower than the true reduction in metabolic rate.

Electrolyte Disturbances and Renal Function—In many patients with anorexia nervosa there is a depletion of body potassium[39]. In patients who do not vomit or purge themselves, the serum potassium levels usually remain normal, but the depletion of potassium can be shown by comparing potassium and nitrogen balances during refeeding[92]. In other patients, the serum levels of sodium and especially of potassium may be reduced, and there may be an accompanying hypochloraemic alkalosis. This is most likely to happen when there are multiple sources of potassium loss from the body, combined with the poor food intake. Additional factors may contribute to the hypokalaemia: Truninger-Rathe and Spühler[117] reported a high urinary aldosterone excretion in a patient with anorexia nervosa who took purgatives. Wolff and colleagues[132] found evidence of secondary hyperaldosteronism and raised renin levels in their nine patients. Renal biopsies revealed hyperplasia and increased granularity of the juxtaglomerular cells, features commonly associated with increased quantities of renin in the plasma. Secondary hyperaldosteronism is thought to lead to an increase in alimentary and urinary losses of potassium[34]. Whatever the mechanisms, hypokalaemia is a complication which should be recognized: it may lead to tetany, E.C.G. abnormalities, muscle weakness or paralysis, and death[129]. Chronic hypokalaemia may also give rise to renal tubular vacuolation and a reduced renal function.

Quite apart from the renal complications of hypokalaemia, the malnutrition of anorexia nervosa may cause a failure of urinary dilution in patients whose illness has been of long duration—three years or longer[99]. The mechanism of this impairment of diuresis is uncertain. It could not be attributed to adrenocortical insufficiency nor to excessive antidiuretic hormone secretion. The defect was found to be usually associated with a diminished glomerular filtration rate, but this is probably only a contributory factor. Confirmation of this finding came from a further enquiry by Dare[32] who measured the glomerular filtration rate by the clearance of ^{57}CO cyanocobalamin. Wolff and colleagues[132] suggested that raised renal or plasma angiotensin levels might be another factor. Whatever the cause, the impaired diuresis is eventually reversible by refeeding the patients, thus proving that it is secondary to the nutritional disturbance.

In patients who are vigorously treated by feeding them with a high calorie and protein diet, there is a limit to their ability to clear nitrogenous products with the result that high blood urea levels may be recorded (up to 80–100 mg per cent), in the absence of dehydration. This is probably partly the result of the renal disturbances in anorexia nervosa.

Other Complications of Malnutrition in Anorexia Nervosa—A dry skin and an excessive growth of dry brittle hair over the nape of the neck, the cheeks, the forearms and the thighs (lanugo hair) is found in anorexia nervosa as well as in other kinds of malnutrition. These changes have been attributed to a follicular keratosis[76].

The hands and feet are often cold and blue, and there is an accompanying delay in peripheral vasodilatation such as should normally occur when the patient is placed in a warm room. This phenomenon is at least partly due to the malnutrition and reflects a disturbance in the regulation of body temperature. It may lead to hypothermia which can be fatal. Patients with severe inanition should have their rectal temperature recorded with a low-reading thermometer and chlorpromazine should not be prescribed without caution.

Peripheral oedema may develop, especially when a severely malnourished patient is treated by rapid refeeding. Dietary factors are important—high intakes of salt, water and carbohydrate increase the tendency to water retention. Electrolyte disturbances may also be contributory, as may postural factors such as the patient standing immobile for long periods, but, as in other forms of famine oedema, the exact mechanism is unknown. The oedema is not necessarily due to hypoproteinaemia; in fact plasma protein levels are usually normal in anorexia nervosa[13]. The oedema reflects the relative preservation of the extracellular fluid space, together with a diminution in the elasticity of the skin now too large to sheathe the wasted body structure[33, 75].

Hypercholesterolaemia has for long been known to occur in anorexia nervosa[87] and hypothyroidism is no longer considered to be the cause. Klinefelter[65] found raised levels of cholesterol only in younger patients, and found no correlation between these levels and the duration of the illness or the type of food consumed. Blendis and Crisp[9] attributed the raised serum cholesterol at least in part to the patient's feeding pattern of intermittent overeating, whether or not it was associated with vomiting; when they were treated by refeeding, their serum cholesterol levels tended to fall.

Carotenaemia leading to a yellow pigmentation of the skin, and especially of the palms and soles, has been described in anorexia nervosa[28]. Its presence can be confirmed by measuring the level of carotene in the serum. A high ingestion of carotene-containing foods such as carrots and spinach seems to be the cause[26]. It is unlikely that any symptoms of anorexia nervosa are due to carotenaemia.

A moderate normochromic, normocytic anaemia often arises during the refeeding of patients, the haemoglobin levels falling to 10 to 11 g per cent, usually as a result of haemodilution[101]. This anaemia corrects itself within a few weeks without any specific treatment. Occasionally there occurs a more severe anaemia with haemoglobin levels around 6 to 7 g per cent. This is due to a temporary hypoplasia of the bone marrow akin to that described in kwashiorkor[122]; in time, and with continued feeding, a spontaneous regeneration of the red cells takes place. In yet another small group of patients, there develops an iron deficiency anaemia shown by hypochromic red cells

146

and a low level of serum iron. Only in these patients is the administration of iron salts necessary and beneficial.

Conclusions

Most of the nutritional disturbances that have been described are secondary features of the illness. The study of the malnutrition of anorexia nervosa has hitherto been neglected. Further study is essential not only because these complications may be dangerous to physical health and need treatment in their own right, but because the malnutrition may contribute to the psychological symptoms.

The Feeding Disorder in Anorexia Nervosa and the Hypothalamic Model

The importance of the psychogenesis of anorexia nervosa cannot be doubted, but it is evident that there may well be multiple factors contributing to the illness, including primary abnormalities of body chemistry and physiology. In a search for fundamental causes of this illness, it may be useful to examine as a theoretical model the group of disturbances which arise in various species of animal as a result of experimental lesions of the hypothalamus. The resemblance between this model and the clinical features of anorexia nervosa has already been noted[1, 93, 121]. For example, experimental hypothalamic lesions in rats have led to food and water refusal[2], disturbances of water balance[83] and of oestrus, ovulation and mating behaviour[107]. The analogy with the symptoms of anorexia nervosa, including amenorrhoea, is admittedly rather crude. Yet the hypothesis that a disturbance of neural function—possibly at the level of the hypothalamus—may be partly responsible for anorexia nervosa points to useful avenues of enquiry.

The disturbance of water metabolism in anorexia nervosa is almost certainly secondary to the malnutrition[99] and need not be discussed further. A strong case for a disorder of neural function leading to amenorrhoea has already been made, but this feature of the illness is overshadowed by the feeding disorder. Is there any evidence to support the view that there may be a failure of the mechanisms normally regulating food intake? It will immediately be objected that the feeding disorder of anorexia nervosa is a purposive refusal of food, and indeed several authors have pointed out that often there is no true loss of appetite, so that the term 'anorexia' is a misnomer[11, 81]. This is certainly correct, though a definite proportion of patients consistently maintain that they sense no hunger and have lost all interest in food[111]. Even if food refusal rather than true anorexia is the rule, this is not out of keeping with a disorder of the food-regulatory mechanisms: such a disorder might conceivably lead to abnormal attitudes to eating, including even 'rationalizations' expressed as fears concerning body weight.

It is, therefore, reasonable to search for sigrs of disturbed food intake regulation. Again, this presents many difficulties. Grossman[46] has pointed out that multiple mechanisms operate in the control of hunger, appetite and food intake. More is known about the function of the central nervous mechanisms—the lateral 'feeding centres' and the ventromedial 'satiety areas'. In animals, destruction of the lateral areas leads to food and water refusal[2, 114]. Destruction of the ventro-medial areas (or irritation of the lateral areas) gives rise to over-eating and diminished activity, both of which lead to obesity[53, 83, 91]. There remains, however, much uncertainty as to the peripheral mechanisms which monitor information about the need for food, and pass it on to the central nervous areas. Thus, it is difficult to search for disturbances of these mechanisms in anorexia nervosa. Neverthe-less, such enquiries have been undertaken, modelled on the different theories of the peripheral control of feeding.

(1) Cannon and Washburn[18] ascribed considerable importance to the activity of the stomach in giving rise to sensations of hunger. The truth is not so simple, as is evident from the fact that patients who have had much of their stomach removed surgically are still capable of regulating their food intake. Nevertheless, it is thought that the quality of the sensations of hunger in such patients is altered and that they no longer feel hunger pangs[47]. Silverstone and Russell[111] looked for abnormal or diminished gastric motility in anorexia nervosa patients, but did not find any. A few patients did, however, tend to deny feeling hunger in the presence of vigorous gastric contractions, thus adding some support to Bruch's[17] view that there is a perceptual disturbance for bodily sensations in anorexia nervosa.

(2) Glucose metabolism, and especially the surmised differences in arteriovenous glucose levels within the hypothalamic feeding area is considered by Mayer[79, 80] to be most important in regulating food intake. Mayer's theory, when applied to patients with anorexia nervosa, failed, however, to yield any information which might have indicated an anomaly in the utilization of glucose and thus explain the loss of appetite or the food refusal[97]. These patients did show transient 'diabetic' changes in their glucose tolerance test (increased blood levels of glucose and greater capillary–venous glucose differ-ences), but they proved to be readily reversible by refeeding on an adequate diet for a few days.

(3) The third peripheral mechanism considered important in the

normal regulation of food intake is the heat produced by food during its assimilation (its specific dynamic action), which acts on the central nervous system, possibly on the feeding areas of the hypothalamus[12]: this additional heat would lead to an inhibition of food intake. Looked at this way, an animal would eat in order to keep warm. Applying this theory to the clinical situation of anorexia nervosa, the feeding disorder might be due to an increased sensitivity of the heat-responsive areas of the central nervous system. In cats and dogs the preoptic region of the hypothalamus has been shown to be sensitive to local temperature changes[50, 85]. In order to measure the regulation of temperature in patients with anorexia nervosa, Wakeling[119] compared their responses to a heat load with those of normal controls. He did this by immersing one of the subject's arms in hot water and measuring over a period of time the resulting rise in central (oral) temperature and peripheral temperature (in the finger of the opposite hand). Normally, there is only a slight increase in the central temperature $(0·2°C)$ before the occurrence of a brisk rise in the peripheral temperature. The patients, on the other hand, were relatively unresponsive: they started with a lower basal central temperature, but it increased to a significantly higher level before the onset of a rise in peripheral temperature which was delayed and slow. Thus the heat regulatory mechanism in response to a heat load is relatively insensitive in anorexia nervosa and the adjustments which normally dissipate the heat are sluggish and inefficient. In order to test if these abnormalities are secondary to the malnutrition, Wakeling retested the patients after they had been treated and had gained weight. There was indeed some recovery: the sensitivity of the central mechanisms returned to normal and there was no increased rise in oral temperature after a heat load, but the peripheral responses (presumably due to vasodilatation in the limbs) still remained somewhat sluggish. Wakeling was cautious to point out that his patients had not fully regained their lost weight, so that he was uncertain if the disturbance that persisted could be considered as primary. It is evidently desirable to extend this work in order to ascertain if patients with anorexia nervosa have a primary impairment of another hypothalamic function—temperature regulation—which may be closely linked with the control of the intake of food.

If physiological studies have not yet revealed definite abnormalities of the mechanisms controlling food intake, is there any more direct clinical or pathological evidence of a central nervous disorder? There is no doubt that disease of the hypothalamus can lead to emaciation. Bauer[5], in a review of 60 patients with hypothalamic disease collected from the literature, reported that 11 had become emaciated: in most of them a tumour had been revealed at autopsy. In recent years, there have been several descriptions of young children with tumours of the base of the brain—often invading the hypothalamus—which have caused marasmus[36, 126]; however, none of these patients presented a clinical picture resembling anorexia nervosa. There have, in fact, been very few pathological studies of patients dying from anorexia nervosa and most of them were concerned principally with the state of the endocrine glands rather than the brain[103, 110, 131]. White and Hain[125] described a cystic lesion of the third ventricle in a patient who had had profound anorexia and weight loss, but she was aged 62 and was quite unlike a patient with anorexia nervosa; similarly the young child reported by Udvarhelyi, Adamkiewicz and Cooke[118] as having anorexia nervosa caused by a tumour of the fourth ventricle was quite atypical of this illness. Martin[78] did, however, succeed in carrying out pathological examinations of two patients who had suffered from chronic anorexia nervosa. He found widespread cortical loss of nerve cells and gliosis and attributed these to long-standing malnutrition.

Cerebral structure and function have also been examined in living patients. Heidrich and Schmidt-Matthias[52] found by air-encephalography a moderate dilatation of the lateral ventricles and widening of the subarachnoid spaces in three patients, one of whom had a dilated third ventricle. They too consider these changes to be secondary to the malnutrition. Eitinger[38] has also described a chronic atrophic cerebral process as a result of malnutrition in concentration camp victims and he compares them with anorexia nervosa patients. Finally, there have been a number of electroencephalographic studies. Crisp, Fenton and Scotton[27] found generalized abnormalities consisting of excess theta activity and unstable responses to hyperventilation; these abnormalities were attributed to the malnutrition and electrolyte disturbances. In a minority of patients, who gave a history of epileptic attacks, there were discharges of fast spikes and waves. Goor[43] interpreted the EEG abnormalities he found as indicative of 'diencephalic disturbance', and Sing and colleagues[113] also purported to provide EEG evidence of abnormal hypothalamic activity in one patient. These latter reports appear less convincing than the study of Crisp and his colleagues.

Conclusion

The best evidence in favour of a primary disorder of neural function in anorexia nervosa is provided by the endocrine studies, but a search for further hypothalamic disturbances should be pursued and should include studies of feeding and temperature control.

TREATMENT OF ANOREXIA NERVOSA

Whereas the general management of patients with anorexia nervosa can be very effective, at least during its early stages, it must be conceded that no specific treatment has yet been devised. Pronouncements on the efficacy of the treatment have expressed sentiments varying from supreme optimism[56] to reasoned caution[81]. Williams[130] reported a high mortality rate (10 out of 53 patients). It is obvious that therapeutic success can only be gauged by controlled studies taking into account the variable course of the illness and the overriding importance of processes of selection. Beck and Brøchner-Mortensen[7] were certainly correct when they pointed out that the outcome in patients treated in general hospitals is, as a rule, more favourable than in those referred to psychiatrists working in mental hospitals. Evidently the latter patients show a more florid psychopathology which makes for a more severe and entrenched illness. It is useless, therefore, to compare methods of treatment carried out in different centres by different practitioners.

The treatment of patients with anorexia nervosa can be subdivided into two phases:

(1) The initial treatment aimed at saving life, restoring nutrition and relieving the acute psychiatric disturbance.

(2) The long-term treatment where the aims should be the consolidation of the patient's improvement, and the prevention of relapses which are only too common.

During the first phase, treatment is relatively simple and successful results are easily obtained so long as a few elementary principles are adhered to. It is easy to induce a very considerable weight gain in wasted patients. The long-term treatment is much more difficult and the outcome is often unpredictable. Therapeutic efficacy should, therefore, be assessed more by these long-term results, but there have been no such controlled studies so far.

EARLY PHASES OF TREATMENT

If the illness has resulted in considerable weight loss, admission to a suitably staffed hospital ward is usually necessary—out-patient treatment is seldom successful. Patients often view admission to hospital as a threat and are reluctant to be separated from their families. They can usually be persuaded to accept admission if the co-operation of the family is enlisted. On rare occasions, there is no alternative to compulsory treatment under the Mental Health Act, 1959.

151

Nursing and Dietary Treatment

The most important factor in the early treatment of anorexia nervosa is the placing of the patient in surroundings favourable to breaking the entrenched habits which have led to the loss of weight. It is imperative to detect and correct the complications of malnutrition, and to restore normal nutrition. Gull[49] described the requisite 'moral conditions' as follows: 'The patients should be fed at regular intervals, and surrounded by persons who would have more control over them, relations and friends being generally the worst attendants.' Ryle[104] and Hurst[56] reiterated these principles and simply laid down that the patient should not be left at mealtimes until the whole meal has been consumed. They did not believe that expert psychotherapy was required. French psychiatrists recommend the 'cure d'isolement', thus emphasizing the importance of separating the patient from her family. In essence, treatment should be delegated to specially trained nursing staff who are conversant with the behaviour patterns and psychological problems of these patients[98]. The nurses should anticipate that the patient may evade finishing her meal, dispose of her food secretly, induce vomiting after meals, take strong purgatives or exercise vigorously. Firm rules and careful observation usually discourage such deceptions. By remaining close at hand at mealtimes and by an artful combination of cajolery and gentle bullying, a skilful nurse can persuade practically any patient to finish the food placed before her. Reassurance is often needed that the patient's appearance will improve after gaining weight and that the nurse will not allow her to overeat or become too fat; but she must avoid being trapped into promises of keeping the patient's body weight at an abnormally low level. Vomiting also often responds to nursing measures: the patient is forbidden access to the toilet and is asked to use a bedpan, she is carefully observed after meals and is told to lie down for a while any time she feels nauseated. At first, many restrictions on the patient's activities must be imposed; later 'rewards' can be given by gradually removing these restrictions as she accepts food more readily and gains weight.

Dietary treatment takes second place to the nursing care and a normal mixed diet is often best. For the first six or eight weeks, however, a liquid diet may have advantages when given as an addition or as an alternative to normal food[98]. For example, a 2,388 calorie diet is provided by mixing the following in 2,000 lm water: Complan* (300 g), lactose or glucose (113 g), Prosparol† (113 g) and Nescafé‡

* Glaxo Ltd.   † Duncan Flockhart Co. Ltd.   ‡Nestlé & Co. Ltd.

152

(30 g) for flavouring. Lactose is usually preferred to glucose because it tastes less sweet, but has the disadvantage of causing diarrhoea in some patients who have a reduced tolerance to disaccharides. The caloric value of the diet is increased each week until 3,000 to 5,000 calories are consumed daily. On this regime, it is not difficult to induce a weight gain of up to 28 lb (12·7 kg) in eight weeks.

As well as restoring nutrition, these general nursing and dietary measures frequently bring about an amelioration in the patient's attitudes to eating and a reduction in the psychiatric disturbance. In others, however, the abnormal attitudes persist and relapse is likely. In a small minority, there is a sharp worsening of the psychiatric disorder, but the subsequent course is often favourable[95].

The nutritional complications—hypokalaemia, hypoglycaemia or hypothermia—may need the appropriate specific treatment when they arise. Except in rare intractable cases, however, the general measures suffice: serum potassium levels rapidly return to normal once the vomiting and purgation are controlled, and body temperature rises after a satisfactory calorie intake has been assured.

Drugs and Physical Treatment

By administering large doses of chlorpromazine (rising to over 1000 mg daily) in combination with modified insulin therapy, Dally and Sargant[30] were able to induce rapid weight gain in their patients. Sim[112] rightly questions if this success is due to the drugs or to the general measures they adopted, including bed rest. In any case, this heroic treatment is not without risk. Hypoglycaemic coma may ensue from insulin to which patients with anorexia nervosa may be sensitive[68]; chlorpromazine may lead to hypothermia. In a later publication, Dally and Sargant[31] said that the insulin can be omitted from the treatment. They also endeavoured to assess the long-term results of their treatment. Although they claimed its superiority over other methods of treatment (bed rest and high calorie diets) the differences were not very marked when reassessed after a follow-up of three to five years. The value of the chlorpromazine appears to be in allaying fear and diminishing resistance to eating[29].

Tube-feeding is generally condemned[29] and is usually unnecessary[98]. Laboucarié and Barrès[66] advocated electroconvulsive therapy for patients with anorexia nervosa to reduce anxiety and resistance, and as a prelude to psychotherapy, but few psychiatrists would accept such a recommendation. Electroconvulsive therapy is probably only of very limited value in patients showing a severe degree of depression persisting in spite of general measures. Even then, antidepressant drugs should first be given a trial.

Behaviour Therapy

Leitenberg, Agras and Thomson[69] have reported a satisfactory gain in weight in two patients treated by 'selective positive reinforcement'. This treatment included having a male psychology student sitting with the patient at supper and engaging her in 'non-contingent, pleasant conversation'. In addition, the patient was praised when she ate more; restrictions had been imposed soon after admission, but they were replaced by rewards of pleasurable activities in return for gaining weight. Such behaviour therapy is evidently almost identical with the general nursing care already described; it does not, therefore, merit any claim to specificity.

LONG-TERM TREATMENT

It has already been stressed that even after an impressive amelioration of the nutritional and mental state of the patient, relapse is only too common. Moreover, in spite of the patient remaining relatively well, amenorrhoea may persist and there may be a faulty or eccentric social and sexual adjustment. The long-term treatment is, therefore, of paramount importance, but is unfortunately often ineffective.

Psychotherapy

In theory at least, psychotherapy should provide the patient with anorexia nervosa with the best chance of lasting recovery. Thomä[115] has presented a detailed and objective account of psychotherapy, given according to psychoanalytic precepts, to patients treated in the psychiatric hospital of Heidelberg University. Out of 30 patients with anorexia nervosa, 19 received psychotherapy varying in duration from 28 to 440 hours; the majority of the remaining patients refused psychotherapy. Thomä's criteria of the patient's progress were clinical and not merely psychoanalytic; they included changes in body weight as well as in the mental state. It is again necessary to distinguish between short-term and long-term results of treatment.

Thomä concluded that in eight of his patients the considerable improvement or cure that took place could only have been obtained with psychotherapy. He appears cautious in the appraisal of his results and attributes a success to psychotherapy, not only when there is a clinical improvement, but when he can discern the mode of action of the treatment. Accordingly, he sometimes considered improvement to have been spontaneous, even though psychotherapy had been given. Nevertheless, the study is not entirely conclusive and illustrates the enormous difficulties that are encountered in assessing as complex a procedure as psychotherapy. The groups of patients were largely self-selected according to whether or not they accepted psychotherapy: it might be expected that the more co-operative patients would show a more favourable outcome. Moreover, the results seem to bear little relation to the duration of psychotherapy which, as already pointed out, varied a great deal. Eight of the 19 patients given psychotherapy showed an initial improvement as compared to only two out of ten patients who improved spontaneously. It has been emphasized that short-term favourable results are obtained relatively easily with general therapeutic measures. When Thomä's assessment of his patients at follow-up is examined, 4 of the 8 responders to psychotherapy were found to have recovered, 2 still had chronic symptoms and 2 'bleak prospects'. The remaining 11 showed no improvement, or one which could not be attributed to psychotherapy. Even if it is considered that eight out of 17 patients showed a marked response to psychotherapy as opposed to the spontaneous recovery of two out of ten patients not given psychotherapy, the difference is not statistically significant. It may be objected, however, that it is not entirely fair to rebuff Thomä's claims by means of a simple calculation which does not do credit to his painstaking work. Thomä made a number of additional observations: psychotherapy is more difficult in young adolescent patients who showed less favourable results; he did not encounter any serious suicidal attempts nor any psychotic episodes among his patients.

The long-term results of Crisp[23] should also be mentioned. He reported a favourable outcome in nine out of 21 patients who had received psychotherapy as well as chlorpromazine. The average duration of the follow-up was 18 months.

Leucotomy

Sargant[105] reported satisfactory long-term results after modified leucotomy (limited anterior cuts) in patients with anorexia nervosa and Dally[29] agreed that this treatment can be very effective in the more obsessional patients; but the operation may be followed by compulsive overeating and determined or successful suicidal attempts[24]. In any case, the outcome of a modified leucotomy seems largely unpredictable and this treatment should, therefore, be undertaken very seldom and only as a last resort.

General Measures

In the absence of any specific and enduring treatment for anorexia nervosa, the best plan is to continue over as long a period of time as is necessary the out-patient supervision and support of the patient. General guidance and supportive psychotherapy should be directed at improving interpersonal relationships and the adjustment at home and at work. The patient should be gently encouraged to mix socially with members of both sexes. Drug treatment and dietary measures are seldom effective with out-patients. At the present stage of knowledge there seems little advantage in administering hormones with the aim of inducing menstruation. A significant proportion of the patients will need readmission to hospital on one or several occasions to restore body weight and relieve the psychological symptoms. In time, the majority will recover or achieve a *modus vivendi*, but this may take anything from two to five years or longer after the onset of the illness.

Conclusions

Skilled nursing and dietary treatment are extremely effective during the early phases of treatment. The long-term treatment is more problematical: general supportive measures should be taken to prevent relapses and psychotherapy may be rewarding in selected patients.

SUMMARY

Identity of Anorexia Nervosa

Evidence has been put forward which supports the view that anorexia nervosa deserves a firm place in classifications of psychiatric illness. Certainly, anorexia nervosa compares favourably for this claim with other mental illnesses which have gained wider acceptance in current systems of classification.

(a) Anorexia nervosa can be readily identified by its chief clinical features—behaviour leading to a considerable weight loss, an endocrine disorder and a psychopathology characterized by a morbid fear of fatness. The endocrine disorder manifests itself by amenorrhoea in postpubertal girls in whom the illness is commonest.

(b) The course of the illness is variable. Many patients make a complete or almost complete recovery, but this may take several years. In others, the illness becomes chronic, but it seldom undergoes any fundamental change.

(c) No clear-cut causes for anorexia nervosa have yet emerged, but data are being accumulated from more precise fields of enquiry— applied psychology, family studies, endocrinology, and nutritional physiology and chemistry:

(i) The endocrine abnormality is primary and is not simply explicable as a result of the malnutrition; it leads to a failure in the release of gonadotrophins from the anterior pituitary and hence of hormones from the gonads (oestrogens or testosterone).

(ii) The characteristics of the nutritional disorder have been described; their study is important in view of their contribution to the morbidity and mortality of this illness.

(iii) Consideration has been given to the experimental hypothalamic preparations which bear some resemblance to the clinical features of anorexia nervosa. So far, only the endocrine disorder lends support to this experimental model, but further searches for disturbances of the feeding and temperature-regulating mechanisms in anorexia nervosa are indicated.

Treatment

The treatment of patients with anorexia nervosa is rewarding and effective, but it must be conceded that no specific treatment has yet emerged. The principle of sound nursing and dietary treatment that was enunciated by Gull, Ryle and Hurst still remains the essential basis of treatment. The greatest need is for a form of treatment that accelerates recovery and prevents relapses. For the chronic patient, repeated admissions to hospitals may be required, together with general supportive measures and possibly psychotherapy.

REFERENCES

1. Anand, B. K. (1961). 'Nervous Regulation of Food Intake'. *Physiol. Rev.* **41,** 677
2. — and Brobeck, J. R. (1951). 'Localization of a "Feeding Center" in the Hypothalamus of the Rat'. *Proc. Soc. exp. Biol. Med.* **77,** 323
3. Annotation (1969). 'Analysis of Psychiatric Diagnosis'. *Lancet* **1,** 35
4. Barraclough, C. A. (1961). 'Production of Anovulatory Sterile Rats by Single Injections of Testosterone Propionate'. *Endocrinology* **68,** 62
5. Bauer, H. G. (1954). 'Endocrine and Other Clinical Manifestations of Hypothalamic Disease. A Survey of 60 Cases, with Autopsies'. *J. clin. Endocr. Metab.* **14,** 13
6. Beardwood, C. J., Beumont, P. J. V., Owens, C. and Russell, G. F. M. (1969). 'Gonadotrophin and Testosterone Excretion in Male Patients with Anorexia Nervosa'. In preparation
7. Beck, J. C. and Brøchner-Mortensen, K. (1954). 'Observations on the Prognosis in Anorexia Nervosa'. *Acta med. scand.* **149,** 409

8. Bell, E. T., Harkness, R. A., Loraine, J. A. and Russell, G. F. M. (1966). 'Hormone Assay Studies in Patients with Anorexia Nervosa'. *Acta endocr., Copenh.* **51,** 140

9. Blendis, L. M. and Crisp, A. H. (1968). 'Serum Cholesterol Levels in Anorexia Nervosa'. *Postgrad. med. J.* **44,** 327

10. Bliss, E. L. and Migeon, C. J. (1957). 'Endocrinology of Anorexia Nervosa'. *J. clin. Endocr. Metab.* **17,** 766

11. — and Branch, C. H. H. (1960). 'Anorexia Nervosa: Its History, Psychology and Biology'. *Psychosom. Med. Monogr. Suppl.* 1939

12. Brobeck, J. R. (1960). 'Food and Temperature'. *Recent Prog. Horm. Res.* **16,** 439

13. Brothwood, J. (1964). 'The Plasma Proteins in Anorexia Nervosa'. *Dissertation of the Academic Diploma in Psychological Medicine.* University of London

14. Brown, J. B. (1955). 'A Chemical Method for the Determination of Oestriol, Oestrone and Oestradiol in the Human Urine'. *Biochem. J.* **60,** 185

15. — Bulbrook, R. D. and Greenwood, F. C. (1957). 'An Evaluation of a Chemical Method for the Estimation of Oestriol, Oestrone and Oestradiol-17β'. *J. Endocr.* **16,** 41

16. Bruch, H. (1962). 'Perceptual and Conceptual Disturbances in Anorexia Nervosa'. *Psychosom. Med.* **24,** 187

17. — (1965). 'Anorexia Nervosa and its Differential Diagnosis'. *J. nerv. ment. Dis.* **141,** 555

18. Cannon, W. B. and Washburn, A. L. (1911–1912). 'An Explanation of Hunger'. *Am. J. Physiol.* **29,** 441

19. Cremerius, J. (1965). 'Zur Prognose der Anorexia Nervosa'. *Arch. Psychiat. u.z.ges. Neurol.* **207,** 378

20. Crisp, A. H. (1965). 'Some Aspects of the Evolution, Presentation and Follow-up of Anorexia Nervosa'. *Proc. R. Soc. Med.* **58,** 814

21. — (1965). 'Clinical and Therapeutic Aspects of Anorexia Nervosa—A Study of 30 Cases'. *J. psychosom. Res.* **9,** 67

22. — (1965). 'A Treatment Regime for Anorexia Nervosa'. *Br. J. Psychiat.* **112,** 505

23. — (1966). 'A Treatment Regime for Anorexia Nervosa'. *Br. J. Psychiat.* **112,** 505

24. — (1967). 'The Possible Significance of Some Behavioural Correlates of Weight and Carbohydrate Intake'. *J. psychosom. Res.* **11,** 117

25. — (1967). 'Anorexia Nervosa'. *Hosp. Med.* **1,** 713

26. — and Stonehill, E. (1967). 'Hypercarotenaemia as a Symptom of Weight Phobia'. *Postgrad. med. J.* **43,** 721

27. — Fenton, G. W. and Scotton, L. (1968). 'A Controlled Study of the EEG in Anorexia Nervosa'. *Br. J. Psychiat.* **114,** 1149

28. Dally, P. J. (1959). 'Carotenaemia Occurring in a Case of Anorexia Nervosa'. *Br. med. J.* **1,** 1333

29. — (1967). 'Anorexia Nervosa—Long-term Follow-up and Effects of Treatment'. *J. psychosom. Res.* **11,** 151

30. — and Sargant, W. (1960). 'A New Treatment of Anorexia Nervosa'. *Br. med. J.* **1,** 1770

31. — — (1966). 'Treatment and Outcome of Anorexia Nervosa'. *Br. med. J.* **2,** 793

32. Dare, C. (1967). 'Glomerular Filtration Rate in Anorexia Nervosa'. *Dissertation for the Academic Diploma in Psychological Medicine.* University of London

33. Davidson, S. and Passmore, R. (1966). *Human Nutrition and Dietetics*, 3rd Ed., p. 356. Edinburgh, London: Livingstone

34. Dawborn, J. K. and Ross, E. J. (1967). 'The Effect of Prolonged Administration of Aldosterone on Sodium and Potassium Turnover in the Rabbit'. *Clin. Sci.* **32,** 559

35. Decourt, J., Jayle, M. F., Lavergne, G. H. and Michard, J. P. (1950). 'L'amenorrhée des Anorexies Mentales; Notions Cliniques; Étude Biologique and Biochimique'. *Ann. Endocr., Paris* **11,** 571

36. Diamond, E. F. and Averick, N. (1966). 'Marasmus and the Diencephalic Syndrome'. *Archs Neurol., Chicago* **14,** 270

37. Donovan, B. T. and Van der Werff ten Bosch, J. J. (1965). 'Physiology of Puberty'. *Monographs of the Physiology Society, p. 163.* London: Edward Arnold

38. Eitinger, L. (1965). 'Der Parallelismus Zwischen dem KZ-Syndrom und der Chronischen Anorexia Nervosa'. In *Anorexia Nervosa*, p. 118. Stuttgart: Thieme Verlag

39. Elkington, J. R. and Huth, E. J. (1959). 'Body Fluid Abnormalities in Anorexia Nervosa and Undernutrition'. *Metabolism* **8,** 376

40. Emanuel, R. W. (1956). 'Endocrine Activity in Anorexia Nervosa'. *J. clin. Endocr. Metab.* **16,** 801

41. Fish, F. J. (1962). In *Schizophrenia*, p. 3. Bristol: John Wright

42. Gibbons, J. L. (1961). 'Psychological Factors in Ovarian and Uterine Dysfunction'. In *Modern Trends in Endocrinology—2.* Ed. by H. Gardiner-Hill. London: Butterworths

43. Goor, C. (1954). 'EEG in Anorexia Nervosa'. *Electroenceph. clin. Neurophysiol.* **6,** 349

44. Gregory, B. A. J. C. (1957). 'The Menstrual Cycle and its Disorders in Psychiatric Patients, II'. *J. psychosom. Res.* **2,** 199

45. Griffiths, R. D. P. (1967). 'An Investigation of Hypotheses Derived from the Clinical Observation of Anorexia Nervosa'. *Dissertation of the Master of Philosophy Degree in Abnormal Psychology.* University of London

46. Grossman, M. I. (1955). 'Integration of Current Views on the Regulation of Hunger and Appetite'. *Ann. N.Y. Acad. Sci.* **63,** 76

47. — and Stein, I. F. (1948). 'Vagotomy and the Hunger-producing Action of Insulin in Man'. *J. appl. Physiol.* **1,** 263

48. Gull, W. W. (1868). 'The Address in Medicine'. *Lancet* **2,** 171

49. — (1874). 'Anorexia Nervosa (Apepsia Hysterica, Anorexia Hysterica)'. *Trans. clin. Soc. Lond.* **7**, 22

50. Hardy, J. D., Hellon, R. F. and Sutherland, K. (1964). 'Temperature-sensitive Neurones in the Dog's Hypothalamus'. *J. Physiol.* **175**, 242

51. Harris, G. W., Reed, M. and Fawcett, C. P. (1966). 'Hypothalamic Releasing Factors and the Control of Anterior Pituitary Function'. *Br. med. Bull.* **22**, 266

52. Heidrich, R. and Schmidt-Matthias, H. (1961). 'Encephalographische Befunde bei Anorexia Nervosa'. *Arch. Psychiat. NervKrankh.* **202**, 183

53. Hetherington, A. W. and Ranson, S. W. (1940). 'Adiposity in the Rat'. *Anat. Rec.* **78**, 149

54. Holt, L. E., Snyderman, S. E., Norton, P. M. and Roitman, E. (1963). 'The Plasma Aminogram in Kwashiorkor'. *Lancet* **2**, 1343

55. Hubble, D. (1952). 'The Course of Anterior Hypopituitarism'. *Lancet* **1**, 1123

56. Hurst, A. (1939). 'Discussion on Anorexia Nervosa'. *Proc. R. Soc. Med.* **32**, 744

57. Ismail, A. A. A. and Harkness, R. A. (1966). 'Factors Associated with Alterations in Urinary Testosterone Levels'. *J. Endocr.* **35**

58. — — (1967). 'Urinary Testosterone Excretion in Men in Normal and Pathological Conditions'. *Acta Endocr., Copenh.* **56**, 469

59. Kassenaar, A., Graeff, J. de and Kouwenhoven, A. T. (1960). '15N-glycine Studies of Protein Synthesis During Refeeding in Anorexia Nervosa'. *Metabolism* **9**, 831

60. Kay, D. W. K. and Leigh, D. (1954). 'The Natural History, Treatment and Prognosis of Anorexia Nervosa, Based on a Study of 38 Patients'. *J. ment. Sci.* **100**, 411

61. — and Schapira, K. (1965). 'Prognosis in Anorexia Nervosa'. In *Anorexia Nervosa*, p. 113. Stuttgart: Thieme Verlag

62. — — and Brandon, S. (1967). 'Early Factors in Anorexia Nervosa Compared With Non-anorexic Groups'. *J. psychosom. Res.* **11**, 133

63. Keys, A and Brozek, J. (1953). 'Body Fat in Adult Man'. *Physiol. Rev.* **33**, 245

64. — — Henschel, A., Mickelsen, O. and Taylor, H. L. (1950). In *The Biology of Human Starvation*. Minneapolis: The University of Minnesota Press

65. Klinefelter, H. F. (1965). 'Hypercholesterolaemia in Anorexia Nervosa'. *J. clin. Endocr. Metab.* **25**, 1520

66. Laboucarié, J. and Barrès, P. (1954). 'Les Aspects Cliniques, Pathogéniques et Therapeutiques de l'Anorexie Mentale (d'après 50 Observations)'. *L'Evolut. Psychiat.* **1**, 119

67. Ladewig, D. (1968). 'Die Anorexia Nervosa des Mannes'. *Schweizer Arch. Neurol. Neurochir. Psychiat.* **101**, 383

68. Landon, J., Greenwood, F. C., Stamp, T. C. B. and Wynn, V. (1966). 'The Plasma Sugar, Free Fatty Acid, Cortisol and Growth Hormone Response to Insulin and the Comparison of this Procedure with Other Tests of Pituitary and Adrenal Function. II. In Patients with Hypothalamic or Pituitary Dysfunction or Anorexia Nervosa'. *J. clin. Invest.* **45,** 437

69. Leitenberg, H., Agras, W. S. and Thomson, L. E. (1968). 'A Sequential Analysis of the Effect of Selective Positive Reinforcement in Modifying Anorexia Nervosa'. *Behav. Res. Therapy* **6,** 211

70. Lewis, A. J. (1966). 'Survivance de l'Hystérie'. *L'Evolut. Psychiat.* **2,** 159

71. Ljunggren, H., Ikkos, D. and Luft, R. (1957). 'Studies on Body Composition'. *Acta Endocr. Copenh.* **25,** 187, 199, 209

72. — — — (1961). 'Basal Metabolism in Women with Obesity and Anorexia Nervosa'. *Br. J. Nutr.* **15,** 21

73. Loo, P. and Duflot, J.-P. (1958). 'L'anorexie Mentale'. *Annls méd.-psychol.* **116,** 734

74. Loraine, J. A. and Brown, J. B. (1959). 'A Method for the Quantitative Determination of Gonadotrophins in the Urine of Non-pregnant Human Subjects'. *J. Endocr.* **18,** 77

75. McCance, R. A. (1951). In *Studies of Undernutrition, Wuppertal, 1946–9.* Medical Research Council Special Report Series, No. 275, Chap. 2, p. 21. London: Her Majesty's Stationery Office

76. — and Barrett, A. M. (1951). In *Studies of Undernutrition, Wuppertal, 1946–9.* Medical Research Council Special Report Series, No. 275, Chap. 3, p. 83. London: Her Majesty's Stationery Office

77. Marks, V. and Howorth, N. (1965). 'Plasma Growth-hormone Levels in Chronic Starvation in Man'. *Nature, Lond.* **208,** 687

78. Martin, F. (1955). 'Pathologie des Aspects Nevrologiques et Psychiatriques dans quelques Manifestations Carentielles avec Troubles Digestifs et Neuro-endocriniens. II. Etudes des Alterations du Systeme Nerveux Central dans Deux Cas d'anorexie Survenue Chez la Jeune Fille (Dite Anorexie Mentale)'. *Helv. med. Acta* **22,** 522

79. Mayer, J. (1953). 'Glucostatic Mechanism of Regulation of Food Intake'. *New Engl. J. Med.* **249,** 13

80. — (1964). 'Regulation of Food Intake'. In *Nutrition,* Vol. 1. Ed. by G. H. Beaton and E. W. McHenry. New York, London: Academic Press

81. Meyer, J.-E. (1961). 'Das Syndrom der Anorexia Nervosa: Katamnestische Untersuchungen'. *Arch. Psychiat. u.z. ges. Neurol.* **202,** 31

82. Michael, R. P. and Gibbons, J. L. (1963). 'Interrelationships Between the Endocrine System and Neuropsychiatry'. *Int. Rev. Neurobiol.* **5,** 243

83. Miller, N. E., Bailey, C. J. and Stevenson, J. A. F. (1950). 'Decreased "Hunger" but Increased Food Intake Resulting from Hypothalamic Lesions'. *Science* **112**, 256

84. Morgan, H. G. and Russell, G. F. M. (1969). 'A Prognostic Study of Anorexia Nervosa'. In preparation.

85. Nakayama, T., Hammel, H. T., Hardy, J. D. and Eisenman, J. S. (1963). 'Thermal Stimulation of Electrical Activity of Single Units of the Preoptic Region'. *Am. J. Physiol.* **204**, 1122

86. Novlyanskaya, K. A. (1958). 'One of the Forms of Prolonged Pathological Reactions in Puberty (Anorexia Nervosa in Adolescents)'. *Zh. Nevropat., Psikhiat.* **58**, 861

87. Parienté, M. and Trillat, E. (1955). 'Troubles des conduites alimentaires. II. Les conduites nevrotiques de restriction alimentaire chez l'adolescent et l'adulte'. *Encyclopédie Médico-chirurgicale*, 37105, C^{10}, p. 2. Paris

88. Passmore, R., Strong, J. A. and Ritchie, F. J. (1958). 'The Chemical Composition of the Tissue Lost by Obese Patients on a Reducing Regimen'. *Br. J. Nutr.* **12**, 113

89. Phoenix, C. H., Goy, R. W., Gerall, A. A. and Young, W. C. (1959). 'Organizing Action of Prenatally Administered Testosterone Propionate on the Tissues Mediating Mating Behaviour in the Female Guinea-pig'. *Endocrinology* **65**, 369

90. Rakoff, A. E. (1962). 'Polycystic Disease of the Ovaries: Its Relationship to the Stein-Leventhal Syndrome and Other Endocrine Dysfunctions'. *J. Germantown Hosp.* **3**, 25

91. Reynolds, R. W. (1965). 'An Irritative Hypothesis Concerning the Hypothalamic Regulation of Food Intake'. *Psychol. Rev.* **72**, 105

92. Russell, G. F. M. (1964). 'Psychological Factors in the Control of Food Intake'. In *Diet and Bodily Constitution*, p. 69. Ciba Foundation Study Group No. 17. London: Churchill

93. — (1965). 'Metabolic Aspects of Anorexia Nervosa'. *Proc. R. Soc. Med.* **58**, 811

94. — (1967). 'The Nutritional Disorder in Anorexia Nervosa'. *J. psychosom. Res.* **11**, 141

95. — (1969). 'Metabolic, Endocrine and Psychiatric Aspects of Anorexia Nervosa'. In *The Scientific Basis of Medicine. Annual Reviews*, Chap. 14. London: Athlone Press

96. — and Mezey, A. G. (1962). 'An Analysis of Weight Gain in Patients with Anorexia Nervosa Treated with High Calorie Diets'. *Clin. Sci.* **23**, 449

97. — and Bruce, J. T. (1964). 'Capillary-venous Glucose Differences in Patients with Disorders of Appetite'. *Clin. Sci.* **26**, 157

98. — and Gillies, C. (1964). 'Anorexia Nervosa. Investigation and Care of Patients in a Psychiatric Metabolic Ward'. *Nurs. Times* July 3, 1964

99. — and Bruce, J. T. (1966). 'Impaired Water Diuresis in Patients with Anorexia Nervosa'. *Am. J. Med.* **40**, 38

100.   —   and Beardwood, C. J. (1968). 'The Feeding Disorders, with Particular Reference to Anorexia Nervosa and its Associated Gonadotrophin Changes'. In *Endocrinology* and *Human Behaviour*, p. 310. Ed. by R. P. Michael. London: Oxford University Press

101.   —   and Willcox, D. R. C. (1969). 'Anaemia in Anorexia Nervosa'. In preparation

102.   —   Loraine, J. A., Bell, E. T. and Harkness, R. A. (1965). 'Gonadotrophin and Oestrogen Excretion in Patients with Anorexia Nervosa'. *J. psychosom. Res.* **9,** 79

103.   Russfield, A. B. and Sommers, S. C. (1963). 'Malnutrition and Tropic Hormone Storage in Hypophysis'. *A.M.A. Archs Path.* **75,** 564

104.   Ryle, J. A. (1936). 'Anorexia Nervosa'. *Lancet* **2,** 893

105.   Sargant, W. (1951). 'Leucotomy in Psychosomatic Disorders'. *Lancet* **2,** 87

106.   Scadding, J. G. (1967). 'Diagnosis: The Clinician and the Computer'. *Lancet* **2,** 877

107.   Schreiber, V. (1963). *The Hypothalamo-hypophyseal System.* Prague: Czechoslovak Academy of Sciences

108.   Sheehan, H. L. and Summers, V. K. (1949). 'The Syndrome of Hypopituitarism'. *Q. J. Med.* **42,** 319

109.   Shepherd, M., Brooke, E. M., Cooper, J. E. and Lin, T. (1968). 'An Experimental Approach to Psychiatric Diagnosis'. *Acta psychiat. scand.* **44,** *Suppl* 201

110.   Siebenmann, R. E. (1955). 'Fur Pathologischen Anatomie der Anorexia Nervosa'. *Schweiz. med. Wschr.* **85,** 530

111.   Silverstone, J. T. and Russell, G. F. M. (1967). 'Gastric "Hunger" Contractions in Anorexia Nervosa'. *Br. J. Psychiat.* **113,** 257

112.   Sim, M. (1963). 'Treatment of Anorexia Nervosa'. In *Guide to Psychiatry*, 1st edn. Edinburgh: Livingstone

113.   Sing, B., Anand, B. K., Malhotra, C. L. and Dua, S. (1958). 'Stress as an Aetiological Factor in the Causation of Anorexia Nervosa'. *Neurology, Madras* **6,** 50

114.   Teitelbaum, P. and Epstein, A. N. (1962). 'The Lateral Hypothalamic Syndrome: Recovery of Feeding and Drinking after Lateral Hypothalamic Lesions'. *Psychol. Rev.* **69,** 74

115.   Thomä, H. (1967). *Anorexia Nervosa.* Translated by G. Brydone. New York: International Universities Press

116.   Tolstrup, K. (1965). 'Die Charakteristika der Jüngeren Fälle von Anorexia Nervosa'. In *Anorexia Nervosa: Symposium am 24, 25 April, 1965 in Göttingen.* Ed. by J.-E. Meyer and H. Feldman. Stuttgart: Thieme Verlag

117.   Truninger-Rathe, I. and Spühler, O. (1960). 'Secondary Hyperaldosteronism with Cyclic Oedema as a Sequel to the Chronic Use of Laxatives in a Case of Anorexia Nervosa'. *Schweiz. med. Wschr.* **90,** 1061

118. Udvarhelyi, G. B., Adamkiewicz, J. T. and Cooke, P. E. (1966). ' "Anorexia Nervosa" Caused by a Fourth Ventricle Tumour'. *Neurology, Minneap.* **16,** 565

119. Wakeling, A. (1968). 'Regulation of Body Temperature in Patients with Anorexia Nervosa'. *Dissertation for the Academic Diploma in Psychological Medicine.* University of London

120. Waller, J. V., Kaufman, M. R. and Deutsch, F. (1940). 'Anorexia Nervosa. A Psychosomatic Entity'. *Psychosom. Med.* **2,** 3

121. Walsh, E. G. (1957). *Physiology of the Nervous System,* p. 453. London: Longmans, Green

122. Walt, F. Taylor, J. E. D., Magill, F. B. and Nestadt, A. (1962). 'Erythroid Hypoplasia in Kwashiorkor'. *Br. med. J.* **1,** 73

123. Warren, W. (1968). 'A Study of Anorexia Nervosa in Young Girls'. *J. Child Psychol. Psychiat.* **9,** 27

124. Waxenberg, S. E., Drellich, M. G. and Sutherland, A. M. (1959). 'The Role of Hormones in Human Behaviour. 1. Changes in Female Sexuality After Adrenalectomy'. *J. clin. Endocr.* **19,** 193

125. White, L. E. and Hain, R. F. (1959). 'Anorexia in Association with Destructive Lesions of the Hypothalamus'. *Archs Path.* **68,** 275

126. White, P. T. and Ross, A. T. (1963). 'Inanition Syndrome in Infants with Anterior Hypothalamic Neoplasms'. *Neurology, Minneap.* **13,** 974

127. Widdowson, E. M. (1951). In *Studies of Undernutrition, Wuppertal, 1946–9.* Medical Research Council Special Report Series, No. 275, Chap. 27, p. 313. London: Her Majesty's Stationery Office

128. — and Thrussell, L. A. (1951). In *Studies of Undernutrition, Wuppertal, 1946–9.* Medical Research Council Special Report Series, No. 275, Chap. 26, p. 296. London: Her Majesty's Stationery Office

129. Wigley, R. D. (1960). 'Potassium Deficiency in Anorexia Nervosa, With Reference to Renal Tubular Vacuolation'. *Br. med. J.* **2,** 110

130. Williams, E. (1958). 'Anorexia Nervosa: A Somatic Disorder'. *Br. med. J.* **2,** 190

131. Wilson, R. R. (1954). 'A Case of Anorexia Nervosa with Necropsy Findings and a Discussion of Secondary Hypopituitarism'. *J. clin. Path.* **7,** 131

132. Wolff, H. P., Vecsei, P., Krück, F., Roscher, S., Brown, J. J., Düsterdieck, G. O., Lever, A. F. and Robertson, J. I. S. (1968). 'Psychiatric Disturbance Leading to Potassium Depletion, Sodium Depletion, Raised Plasma-renin Concentration, and Secondary Hyperaldosteronism'. *Lancet* **1,** 257

CHAPTER 7

DIAGNOSIS OF THE REACTIVE DEPRESSIVE ILLNESSES

MARTIN ROTH and T. A. KERR

INTRODUCTION

The predisposition to depressive reactions is to some extent universal in the human race. Bereavement, failure, serious physical disease and humiliation are prone to evoke a melancholy mood of variable intensity and duration in all subjects and, while emotions of anxiety and aggression are readily recognizable over a wide range of animal species, the depressive state is probably peculiar to *homo sapiens*. The deliberate suicidal acts, in which severe and sustained depressions often culminate, are certainly so. Forms of depression that impose qualitative departures from ordinary behaviour, such as the melancholias with delusions of guilt and poverty, have probably always been recognized as illnesses. However, it is the increased number of patients seeking treatment for depressions with a kinship to normal reactions of grief and dejection, rather than the more specific disturbance of manic-depressive illness, that has made the subject such a challenging one for contemporary psychiatric practice.

Depression may form part of the response to the normal adversities and buffetings of life, it may be a symptom of a wide range of psychiatric disorders, both of the organic and the functional variety, or it may refer to one of a number of illnesses designated as 'depressive'. Most of the contemporary controversies about the classification of depression have focused upon this last group. This has served to cut the problem down to manageable proportions but has tended to separate, in a somewhat arbitrary manner, certain groups of disorders in which depression is a leading feature from others in which it is perhaps less prominent but which, nonetheless, commonly create difficulties in diagnosis. Thus a great deal of effort has been invested in an attempt to draw lines of demarcation between endogenous depression on the one hand and neurotic or reactive depression on the other. Anxiety neuroses have been largely omitted from consideration in these studies although they are very germane to the problem of classification of depression. Again, differentiations from the depressions associated with prominent paranoid symptoms and from depressions in a setting of cerebral disease have received little attention, although these are important matters not only in a practical sense but from a theoretical point of view. It is commonplace to insist that no clear lines of demarcation can be drawn between normal reactions to misfortune and depressions studied in the psychiatric clinic, although very little is known of the natural history of these normal reactions or about their response to the antidepressive remedies that are now so widely used in all forms of depressive illness. Although this chapter will be devoted largely to the neurotic depressions, any attempts to delineate them will of necessity entail some consideration of related issues.

The depressive illnesses are those in which sadness of mood is the primary and leading feature. Here we meet a semantic difficulty in that, although sadness may be directly complained of it has, in some cases, to be inferred from facial expression, general retardation or morbid ideas. In others depression may even be denied and apathy, inertia or a sense of exhaustion may be complained of instead, in the absence of any physical illness that would explain them. In other subjects, barrenness of ideas and inspiration, or a general malaise closely similar in character to that often found in association with debilitating physical illnesses are described. This last similarity is of more than diagnostic interest. The association between physical illness and psychiatric disorder which has been demonstrated in recent years in a number of enquiries[43, 45, 90] has not only served to define one factor in the causation of depressive illnesses but has also lent a new interest to some of the older biological speculations about depression which sought to answer such questions as 'Why is the capacity for response comprising sadness, retardation, resignation, despair, feelings of inferiority or worthlessness, or self-reproach ubiquitous in the human race?' Is it some contingent defect that springs from the complexity of the cerebral and mental equipment of man? Has it been positively selected in the course of evolution for its survival value to the individual or group? If depressive states are variants of the norm, does normal variation account for all the phenomena seen by the psychiatrist or are there pathological variants also? Are depressive states really ubiquitous or are there cultures immune from recognizable depressive states? If the first, we could take it that biological consideration can never bc excuded. What significance is to be attached to the partial or complete simulation of some forms of depression by a number of forms of cerebral disease or specific modes of functional disturbance of the brain produced by agents such as reserpine? Is the capacity for a depressive response neurochemically preformed in the brain, and if so, how are we to bring evidence pointing in this direction into meaningful association with the apparently reactive or socially determined character of some depressions? Finally, if depressive states are even partly determined by genetical factors, and few workers would be prepared to deny them any contribution, how are we to reconcile the very high frequency of depressive states with the disadvantages of increased mortality and possible lowered fertility[82] they impose? These general considerations arise in connection with several subjects discussed in this chapter.

The problems of classification have always been regarded as of basic importance to the advance of knowledge in psychiatry. The contemporary debate about the nature of the relationship between different forms of depressive illness might appear as no more than a fashionable, fortuitous revival of the vigorous and, at times, acrimonious discussions that were in progress some 40 years ago between figures such as Mapother[68] and Lewis[63] who, under the influence of Meyerian psychobiology, favoured unitary concepts, and Gillespie[29] and others who adhered to the Kraepelinian distinction between manic-depressive and psychogenic forms of depression. However, the situation has changed in some respects since then and the advances that have taken place have created a more favourable climate for the resolution of certain problems. Thus the validity of any classification of affective disorder can now be examined in the light of the response to treatment of entities postulated or denied.

Several metabolic changes have been described in association with depressive illness and in relation to pharmacological treatments given to relieve it. Two of the substances that have provided foci of interest are norepinephrine and 5-hydroxytryptamine which are found in substantial quantities in the diencephalon and are suspected of playing an important part in mood regulation. Both monoamines have been studied in depressed patients during illness and recovery, before and after treatment, and attempts have been made to influence their metabolism directly by the administration of drugs or of amino acids such as tryptophan[11]. Conflicting findings may have arisen in part from the failure to define precisely the patient population investigated and biochemical studies would probably benefit if more effort was devoted to ensure that clearly defined homogeneous populations were being investigated and compared with one another. The feedback from such investigations could be expected in turn to sharpen the tools for testing hypotheses about classification and ultimately for defining aetiological and pathogenic factors.

One significant methodological advance in recent years has been the introduction of rating scales for the phenomena of depression[5, 31]. Another is the important evidence which has shown that the structured clinical interview can be converted into a reliable method of examining psychiatric patients[113]. In most areas of clinical research and for studies of the problems of depression in particular, the interview must for the present remain the most important tool of investigation with the formal rating scale as a useful adjunct.

Another development of the past few decades has been in the statistical and computing techniques for investigating problems in classification and diagnosis. The modern electronic computer can undertake what would 25 years ago have been the impossible task of computing the correlations between the large number of clinical features recorded by the psychiatrist. The pattern of inter-correlations can also be readily examined and clusters of co-varying features sought with the aid of multivariate techniques such as principal component analysis and numerical taxonomy.

CULTURAL AND EPIDEMIOLOGICAL ASPECTS

The view that endogenous forms of depression with prominent guilt and retardation are rare in primitive cultures has gained wide acceptance since the observations recorded by Kraepelin[54] in Indonesia more than 60 years ago. In the years that have intervened many observations have been placed on record testifying to the low incidence and short-lived character of depressive disorders and the rarity of self-reproachful and self-punitive ideas in primitive cultures and in the lower socio-economic segments of the population in advanced societies. Many of the studies have come from Africa[9, 20]. Lambo[56], reporting from Nigeria, claimed that endogenous depression was confined to westernized segments of the population, while Stainbrook[106] found self-punitive ideas only among well-to-do patients in Brazil. In an able review of this whole subject, which includes the report of a case material studied in Hong Kong, Yap[115] concludes that when allowances have been made for age and sex differences, the reported cultural variations are most satisfactorily explained as the result of differences in emphasis and degree rather than as qualitative divergences in types of illness. Among primitive people depression is more likely to acquire a strong somatic and hypochondriacal colouring arising from the physical framework in which their ideas of disease are set. The frequency of confusional symptoms in the acute stage tends further to disguise the nature of the underlying affective disorder. Yap accepts that in Protestant cultures depressive self-reproach may be intensified in a pathoplastic manner as in the case of the puritanical Hutterite sect whose depressions tend to be marked by profound guilt feelings. However, he concludes that the cross-sectional picture, the 'bipolar' character of the illness in 29 per cent of cases and the long-term outcome of affective disorder among Chinese patients are essentially similar to those described in Euro-American groups. Aetiological theories of depressive disorder have therefore to make due allowance for the fact that it cuts across cultural boundaries.

Estimates based on population studies in developed countries have varied widely, probably on account of differences in the operational definition of depressive states that was used. Among the highest estimates recorded for manic-depressive disorders defined in strict terms have been those from Scandinavian countries. In Iceland, Helgason[32] found that the life expectancy for manic-depressive psychosis, estimated for a manifestation period of 15–74 years, was 1·80 to 2·18 per cent in men and 2·46 to 3·23 per cent in women. This estimate was similar to that found on the island of Bornholm[23]. In their important study in south-west Sweden, Essen-Möller and Hagnell[18] found a cumulative expectancy for depressive illness of 18 per cent for females and nine per cent for males; the risk for depressive psychosis for both sexes was one per cent. It was observed that only a minority of depressive cases had consulted a psychiatrist and that there was a steep decline in the number who had done so after the age of 40.

Silverman[100] carried out a comprehensive review of the epidemiological observations made on depressive illness and concluded that the prevalence rate for depressive psychosis was almost one per 1,000 and for depressive neurosis two to three per 1,000. In the light of recent careful studies of family practice in Great Britain the figure for the latter is almost certainly an under-estimate. Thus Shepherd and colleagues[98] found a total prevalence rate of 140 per 1,000 for all types of psychiatric disorder combined, in a representative sample derived from 46 general practices in Greater London; over 60 per cent of those patients given a formal psychiatric diagnosis by the family doctors were classified as neurotic. The period prevalence rate per annum for affective psychosis was estimated at 2·4 per 1,000. In another family study Crombie[13] estimated that the period prevalence rate for neurotic depression was ten per annum per 1,000 population, the incidence rising steadily with age. Watts[112] estimated that of every 1,000 patients in general practice 12 might be expected to present as new cases of depressive illness each year.

It is also of interest that, while the first admission rates for schizophrenia remained virtually constant from 1952 to 1960[84], those for affective disorders showed a striking increase over the same period, the admission rates in England and Wales increasing for both sexes by about 75 per cent[83].

PROBLEMS OF CLASSIFICATION

The establishment of a classification of affective disorders commanding wide agreement remains one of the most pressing needs in psychiatry. The partial failure to achieve this continues to impede investigations into causation along genetic, biochemical and psychological lines alike and enhances the difficulty of evaluating the efficacy of different methods of treatment. Three main areas of controversy have emerged: the nature of the relationship between the clinical variants of depressive illness, the relationship of depressive illness to anxiety states and the nosological status of 'schizo-affective' disorders.

There is now general agreement that there is little justification for regarding involutional melancholia as an entity sharply distinct from endogenous depression[37, 46, 109, 111], however, the debate continues as to whether there are qualitative differences between different forms of depression or whether the differences between the main groups denoted by the terms reactive and endogenous are of a quantitative nature. Hobson[35], Astrup, Fossum and Holmboe[3], Kiloh and Garside[50] and Carney, Roth and Garside[8] have favoured a dichotomy while Mapother[68], Lewis[63], Garmany[27] and Kendell[46] believe that depressive illnesses should be regarded as a continuum with classical neurotic depression at one pole and classical endogenous depression at the other and the majority of patients lying between. The importance of trying to reconcile this division of opinion emerges clearly from an enquiry into the reliability of psychiatric diagnosis made on 91 first admissions to a mental hospital by ten experienced psychiatrists[93]. It was shown that, if disagreement had been resolved in the areas of psychoneurosis-affective disorder and psychoneurosis-personality disorder, the overall reliability of diagnosis would have been raised from 57 per cent to 83 per cent.

Recent attempts have been made to resolve the controversy by subjecting the data obtained from depressed patients to complex statistical analysis. These studies will be discussed in some detail because of the way in which they have helped to define the problems at issue and the evidence needed to resolve them. In a prospective study of 143 patients, Kiloh and Garside[50] found that, of the two factors isolated with a simple summation factor analysis, the bipolar factor (which corresponded closely to the distinction between endogenous and reactive depression) accounted for more of the total variance than the general factor. This finding provided suggestive, though not conclusive, evidence against the concept of a single continuum of depressive disorders. It was further supported by the observation that outcome (four weeks and six months after treatment began) was significantly better in the endogenous group. However, evidence in favour of a dichotomy requires that the frequency of patients' factor scores, or scores derived from a discriminant function analysis, departs significantly from unimodality. In the investigation by Carney, Roth and Garside[8], a multiple regression analysis was carried out in those patients in whom the diagnosis could be made with confidence. The distribution of the summated symptom scores of the total population of patients proved to be clearly bimodal. The validity of the distinction between the two groups was confirmed by follow-up studies which showed that they differed sharply in outcome at three and six months after treatment with E.C.T., although a better prediction of outcome could be made directly from the features than from diagnosis. Mendels[70, 71, 72] also found that although the symptoms of reactive and endogenous forms of depression overlapped considerably, the two syndromes differed markedly in their response to E.C.T. In this study weighted scores allocated to clinical features were also found to be better predictors of outcome than diagnosis. The features which were associated with a good response to E.C.T. three months after treatment were family history of depression, early morning wakening, retardation and delusions, while neurotic traits, inadequate premorbid personality, precipitating factors and emotional lability were associated with a poor outcome.

Sandifer, Wilson and Green[94] demonstrated a bimodal distribution of symptom scores using a simple summation of items chosen for their discriminating value. On the other hand, neither of the components extracted from an analysis of 40 features in 100 private outpatients[67] differentiated the features generally associated with endogenous and neurotic depression. Rosenthal and Gudeman[86, 87] studied 100 depressed women and extracted a first factor corresponding to the endogenous constellation of complaints and a second factor corresponding to the 'self-pitying' cluster of features, but did not find that the patients were divided into distinct groups on the basis of their factor scores. Yet it was shown that patients who differed in their mean scores on the endogenous depressive factor differed also to a significant degree in respect of independently derived ratings of premorbid personality, personal history and the presence of an apparent precipitant for the illness. Carney, Roth and Garside's 143 patients were drawn largely from a local psychiatric hospital, and each patient had been judged by the psychiatrist in charge to require electroconvulsive treatment. Discrepancies between their findings and those of other enquiries may partly reflect differences in the composition of the various patient populations (*see* p. 192).

Kendell's Study

The study by Kendell[46, 47] was in a number of respects similar to that by Carney, Roth and Garside, but his findings disagreed with those recorded by these authors. On plotting the diagnostic index scores of his patients Kendell found that, although most of the low scores were obtained by neurotic patients and most of the high scores by psychotic patients, the majority obtained intermediate scores and the distribution of the scores of the total patient group was unimodal.

The interpretation of the findings in Kendell's important study raises a number of methodological problems. Principal component analysis, numerical taxonomy and other cluster analytic techniques are powerful tools, but their application to problems of classification and diagnosis is still in the developmental state. Their most fruitful uses at the present time would appear to lie in the investigation of specific hypotheses. Kendell's study consists of an attempt to submit the hypothesis advanced in the papers of Kiloh and Garside and of Carney, Roth and Garside to systematic investigation. However, the findings are relevant for these hypotheses only in so far as the patients studied and the clinical features selected can be judged to be comparable and the statistical analyses similar.

The first point concerns the list of items selected for enquiry. Even if the question of similarity of definition is ignored, the 35 features chosen by Carney, Roth and Garside, on the basis of previous observations, as specifically relevant for a study of affective disorder, do not appear to be comparable with the 60 items selected by Kendell from a large number routinely scored for general clinical purposes. Moreover, observations recorded by a number of psychiatrists in the course of ordinary clinical practice cannot be readily compared with the findings in a planned enquiry into the classification of depressive disorders in which every patient has been studied by the same psychiatrists. The larger number of clinical items used in the Kendell study might at first sight appear to carry advantages. However, even in the field of liver disease where sharp differentiations can be made with the aid of relatively hard clinical and laboratory data, the inclusion of features which did not contribute to differential diagnosis has been found to obscure existing differences and to prevent the separation of a clinical material into its constituent groups[22]. Not only does the Maudsley Item Sheet used by Kendell contain an excess of 'noise' in this sense, but its low level of reliability[30] can be expected to potentiate the tendency for such 'noise' to obscure under a blanket of smooth continuity any separate modes that might have been apparent in a distribution derived from specific clinical items.

In the study by Carney, Roth and Garside the features identified by the multiple regression analysis as having the highest discriminating value were early morning awakening, retardation, nihilistic delusions, somatic delusions, paranoid delusions, ideas of guilt, pyknic body build, weight loss, qualitative difference in affect from ordinary mood change, diurnal variation in mood, good premorbid personality, inadequate psychological reason for perpetuation of symptoms, a history of previous episodes of depression (corresponding to the endogenous pattern of Rosenthal and Gudeman) and anxiety, tendency to blame others, self-pity, hypochondriacal features and hysterical personality traits (corresponding to the 'self-pitying' pattern). Some of these items do not figure in Kendell's analysis: early morning awakening, pyknic physique, quality of the depressed mood, diurnal variation of mood, and ideas of guilt. The items used in the canonical variate analysis included seven features of premorbid personality and five types of precipitating cause in place of one each of these variables in the Carney scale of 35 items; 28 of the 35 features referred to the current illness in contrast to 25 items (differing in several particulars) out of a total of 42 in the Kendell scale.

It is claimed that the distribution of diagnostic index scores derived from discriminant function analysis was unimodal and thus differed from the result reported by Carney, Roth and Garside. However, the weights for the diagnostic index scores were derived from critical ratios and the procedure was not, strictly speaking, a discriminant function analysis; the techniques could not have yielded the optimal or independent discriminating value of each feature as the intercorrelations between features are not taken into account in the technique employed.

Kendell[45] compares the distribution of Newcastle diagnostic scores in 130 Maudsley patients, rated on the Newcastle scale by Hemsi, Kendell and McClure[33], with the distribution which Carney, Roth and Garside arrived at on the same scale in 129 of their patients (*Figure 1*). The description of the Maudsley distribution as 'unimodal' is open to question particularly as only a small proportion of the cases fall into the part of the distribution that contains the majority of the Newcastle endogenous depressions. This is all the more surprising in that a high proportion (56 per cent) of the original material had received a diagnosis of psychotic depression although

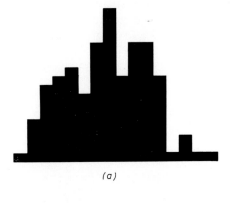

(a)

Figure 1. Comparison of the distributions of the diagnostic index scores in (a) 130 Maudsley patients and (b) 129 Newcastle patients rated on the Newcastle scale

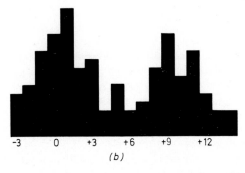

(b)

the basis on which patients were assigned to this or to the neurotic category of illness is not entirely clear.

Kendell ascribes the presence of bimodality in the Newcastle studies to a halo effect, the dichotomous distribution being in other words an artifact of prior clinical conviction. This point has some force, but bias may equally operate in a reverse direction to obscure discontinuities in the clinical material that could have been discerned by other workers.

The descriptions of the 'endogenous' and 'neurotic' types of illness that emerge from the accounts of those, on the one hand, who regard them as the opposite ends of a continuous distribution and those, on the other, who consider them to be distinct entities with some overlap are very similar. A choice between the two theories should be possible in the light of further systematic observation.

It is of interest in this context that the single factor of Kendell's fourth order analysis 'embodying the most important vector in the whole of the original matrix' was bipolar.

> It has positive loadings on retardation, abnormal rate and quantity of speech, short duration before admission, perplexity, delusions of guilt and persecution and ideas of reference; and negative loadings on previous subjective tension and hysterical symptoms, childhood neurotic traits, previous anxiety, obsessional symptoms and mood variations and precipitating psychological causes, marital and social[47].

The distribution of patients' factor scores on the bipolar factor would have been of interest, but it is not given.

UNITY AND DIVERSITY WITHIN THE DEPRESSIVE DISORDERS

An important question, about which there is little information at the present time, is the extent to which patterns of illness remain consistent over long periods. In other words, what is the degree of concordance between the clinical profile of patients in relapse and the pattern of illness they presented at the initial examination? That a limited crossover occurs is suggested by clinical observation and this was confirmed in a recent follow-up study of affective disorders[92], but more observations are needed on the long-term fate of those suffering from affective disorders.

That there is unity as well as diversity within the depressive group of disorders is not in question. The fact that antidepressive remedies such as tricyclic compounds and electroconvulsive therapy are in some degree effective in both groups of conditions testifies to the physiopathological factors they must have in common. At present enquiry in relation to the aetiology of depressive disorders requires that account is taken of these common threads. However, the more favourable response of the endogenous forms of depression, which are on the whole of greater severity, has now been clearly demonstrated in a number of studies. The fact that the less severe or neurotic forms of illness have a worse outcome presents a paradox for any theory which postulates a single continuum for all forms of depressive illness. The attempts that have been made to resolve this paradox in terms of the personality patterns associated with the disorders at the extremes of the distribution merely restate the problem in other terms.

175

Moreover, although it is possible from a phenomenological point of view to conceive of the endogenous forms of depression as being extreme variants of the norm, it is much more difficult to do this in the case of manic-depressive psychosis, particularly as the manic and depressive mood changes may be quite inappropriate to the situations in which they have arisen.

The hypothesis that the different forms of depressive illness defined by clinical observation belong to the extremes of a normal distribution and that in the range between them, which contains most of the cases, the varieties of depression merge insensibly with one another is essentially a null hypothesis. It is difficult to substantiate hypotheses of this nature, particularly where the measures employed are, as in the case of clinical observation in psychiatry, of relatively low reliability.

THE BEARING OF SOME OTHER VARIABLES ON THE RELATION BETWEEN NEUROTIC AND ENDOGENOUS DEPRESSION

The distinction between neurotic and endogenous depression is supported by a number of lines of evidence including genetical studies, physiological responses, investigations in body build as well as response to treatment. Much of the evidence until 1963 was summarized by Kiloh and Garside[50] and will not be reviewed again here. Although a number of these enquiries are consistent with a distinction between the two groups, little of it offers more than suggestive evidence in relation to the main questions at issue. However, a few of the findings are difficult to reconcile with a unitary concept of depression.

Heredity

Genetical studies[43, 101, 108] have shown close agreement in recording a morbid risk of about 12–15 per cent among the first degree relatives of manic-depressive subjects. On the other hand, in Kay's investigation of unselected depressions developing in old age the risk among first degree relatives was $3 \cdot 5 – 5 \cdot 7 \pm 1 \cdot 4$ per cent. Kallmann's twin investigation[41] showed a concordance rate of 96 per cent in 23 monozygous twin pairs and 26 per cent in dizygous twin pairs. A number of investigations appear to be in agreement that manic-depressive disorder is transmitted by a major autosomal dominant gene with a penetrance of approximately 1 in 4[102, 108].

More recently, Perris[76] has adduced impressive evidence in support of the suggestion[62] that bipolar psychoses (cycles of mania and depression) constitute a clinical entity within the body of the manic-depressive psychoses. Perris compared 138 patients with bipolar psychosis with 139 patients with unipolar psychosis. His criterion in selecting the latter was a history of at least three discrete depressive episodes. The expectation of bipolar psychosis was increased to 16·1 per cent in the relatives of bipolar patients but there was no increase in the expectation of unipolar psychosis. Conversely, the expectation of unipolar psychosis among the relatives of unipolar patients was raised to five per cent while there was no increase in the expectation of bipolar psychosis. The bipolar and unipolar groups also differed from one another in respect of physiological and psychophysiological tests. The results suggest that the two conditions are genetically independent, that they breed true and that a major gene is responsible for the bipolar psychoses. Perris also observed that unipolar mania was similar to bipolar psychosis in respect of family history.

The genetical evidence for the independence of bipolar psychoses appears compelling and accords with much existing knowledge about this form of illness. However, most of the evidence favours a substantial overlap with unipolar psychoses and Winokur and Clayton[114] suggest that, although manic-depressive illness is genetically distinct, it is manifest in attacks of mania in only half the cases. If this is accepted, the problem at issue appears to be not so much whether any clear distinction can be drawn between endogenous and neurotic forms of depression, but precisely where one or more lines of demarcation between various forms of depression should be drawn. In other words, are the depressions that occur in the families of bipolar cases identical with other 'endogenous' depressions or are the latter a clinically distinct group?

There is a wide measure of agreement with the theory[103] advanced on the strength of clinical genetical studies that (as distinct from the situation in manic-depressive psychosis) the hereditary constitution of neurotic patients is determined by a large number of genes each with a small effect, producing a quantitatively graded predisposition to neurotic disorders in the population at large. From the study by Shields and Slater[99] on same-sexed twins in which a complete lack of concordance for a diagnosis of neurotic depression was found, it would appear that it is the constitutional predisposition for depression and not the actual illness that is partly inherited.

Physiological Tests

Some of the simpler physiological tests have yielded results that have best stood the test of time so far as the distinction between neurotic and endogenous forms of depression is concerned. Strongin and Hinsie[110] measured the amount of parotid secretion in cases with

177

affective disorder. The rate of secretion in a group of endogenous depressives was well below that in a group of mixed cases of psychiatric disorder including neurotic depressions. Busfield and Wechsler[6] confirmed these findings and showed also that mild and severe depressions could not be distinguished from one another, suggesting that the endogenous cases were qualitatively rather than quantitatively apart from the reactive. In addition, Palmai and Blackwell[74] demonstrated a clear-cut reduction in salivary flow and reversal of the normal diurnal rhythm in 20 female in-patients with early morning awakening and a diurnal variation in mood in whom treatment with E.C.T. restored flow and rhythm to normal. In a later study, Palmai and colleagues[75] found a normal diurnal rhythm of salivary secretion in depressed patients without diurnal variation in mood and noted that it served to differentiate them physiologically as well as clinically from those with diurnal variation in mood.

Response to Treatment

Differences in response to treatment of the two groups with E.C.T.[8] and antidepressive drugs[51, 52, 66] have been amply reviewed and this ground will not be covered again here, except to reiterate that, if reactive and endogenous depressions are the milder and more severe forms of the same illness, it is difficult to explain the fact that the latter respond more favourably to these treatments.

Biochemical Changes

As far as the biochemistry of depression is concerned, four groups of observations are being pursued at the present time. The view that some, possibly all, depressions are associated with an absolute or relative deficiency of catecholamines, particularly norepinephrine, at important receptor sites in the brain and that elation may be associated with an excess of these amines is supported by a certain amount of evidence which has been reviewed by Schildkraut[96]. The possibility that indoleamine rather than catecholamine metabolism is disturbed has been actively investigated in recent years. Tryptophan given in large quantities by mouth is said to be an effective agent in depressive illness[12] although, as it forms tryptamine and is also the precursor of 5-HTP and 5-HT, its precise mode of action is uncertain; it is suggested that the preponderant effect may be to elevate tryptamine which can pass the blood barrier[15]. This view is contraverted by the absence of tryptamine in the brain of animals in ordinary circumstances or after administration of tryptophan unless the latter is combined with an MAO inhibitor. The finding that the concentration of 5-hydroxyindole acetic acid is reduced by half in the

C.S.F. of depressed patients[2, 14] also favours the role of 5-hydroxy-tryptamine in the brain metabolism of depressive illness. The other lines of observation which continue to be further pursued are the demonstration by Coppen and Shaw[10] of a very considerable increase in residual sodium during the depressive illness and a return to normal after recovery, and the finding by Gibbons[28] of an increased rate of secretion of cortisol in severe depressions of endogenous type. With the exception of the last group of observations, which suggested that raised plasma cortisol was a feature of endogenous rather than neurotic depressions, there is very little evidence to indicate whether clinical types of depression differ biochemically in respect of any of the groups of substances of which the metabolism is considered to be specifically disturbed in depressive states. It would appear desirable in future enquiries undertaken in human subjects to attempt both clinical classification and a quantified description derived from one or more of the validated diagnostic indices.

OTHER PROBLEMS IN THE CLASSIFICATION OF DEPRESSIVE DISORDERS

In the long drawnout controversy about the classification of affective disorders the prominence given to endogenous and reactive depressions has perhaps tended to obscure certain issues of equal importance.

The terms 'endogenous' and 'reactive' or 'neurotic' are imprecise and unsatisfactory although no one has been able to suggest better alternatives. Those who accept a qualitative distinction recognize that stressful circumstances not infrequently play some part in the precipitation and to some extent even in the causation of 'endogenous' depressions. 'Reactive' depressions often exhibit a momentum of their own and do not always respond promptly to favourable changes in circumstance. Moreover, although the two groups of conditions differ in outcome, a number of antidepressant treatments are to some extent effective in both and point to common factors as well as differences between them.

The controversy is centred on what is merely one of the main lines of demarcation. There is reason to believe that neither of the main groups of disorders can be taken as homogeneous; further differentiations may become possible in the light of future enquiries. For example, the states of depression, lethargy and inertia, following debilitating acute physical illnesses such as influenza and viral hepatitis, are broadly 'reactive' or 'neurotic' in character and so are a high proportion of the depressive states closely associated with physical illness in middle and late life[44, 45]. Although no strict comparison between the clinical features of such disorders and those of the general run of reactive depressions has been undertaken, there are reasons to believe that they may have distinctive features[48]. Further, the depressive states of young people that form the setting for impulsive 'hypereridic' suicidal attempts have broadly 'reactive' characteristics. Yet they are abrupt in onset, short lived and their termination is also sudden, the affect often being purged by the suicidal attempt. Some depressions of endogenous type undoubtedly arise after overwhelming stress which may be followed by a stuperose or inaccessible state. Many of the psychoses that have been allocated to the borderlands of schizophrenia such as the schizo-affective disorders, the 'emotion' psychoses and the strongly familial psychoses described by Leonard are also considered by some workers to be florid versions of endogenous depression.

The relationship between anxiety states and depressive disorders is also a subject of considerable practical and theoretical importance. In addition, problems of classification arise in connection with the depressive symptoms found in association with obsessional, phobic, hypochondriacal, hysterical and paranoid states, indeed in the whole area of neurotic disorders. In some of these conditions the depression is secondary to the main disability and thus an epi-phenomenon; in others the whole illness can be regarded as depressive.

Each of these problems will be considered in the sections that follow.

The Anxiety States and Depressions

Anxiety is an emotion akin to fear that arises in a state of anticipation of ordeals that are yet to come. Depression of mood is a state that follows upon bereavement, loss, defeat or humiliation. One is a state of helplessness and the other of hopelessness. Anticipation of and projection of ourselves into the future are characteristic of anxiety. The thought of the depressed subject is directed on the other hand to deprivations and disappointments in the past. The distinction was clearly made by Darwin:

> After the mind has suffered from a paroxysm of grief and the cause still continues, we fall into a state of low spirits or are utterly dejected. Prolonged pain generally leads to the same state of mind. If we expect to suffer, we are anxious, if we have no hope of relief we despair.

The differentiation of anxiety states from depression rests at the present time on far more uncertain and less generally accepted criteria than the separation of the different forms of depressive illness. Hence, if depressive illnesses are held to form a continuum, the possibility of defining any lines of demarcation within the affective disorders, or indeed neurotic illnesses as a whole, must be regarded as remote. A colouring of anxiety is frequently found in neurotic or reactive depression and may become the most prominent feature of the illness. The circumstances in which breakdown occurs and the earliest symptoms to appear assist in diagnosis, but provide no very sound basis for it. Difficulties of a similar nature arise in association with anxiety states. Here the depressive features may be in the foreground, particularly in middle and late life. This is one of the reasons why the 'agoraphobic' states of late onset are so often treated as depressive illnesses in clinical practice. Further difficulties are created by the fact that anxiety states would be expected to follow some appropriate stress. However, in a minority of cases they come out of a clear sky or follow some trivial setback. It is the seemingly endogenous quality of some forms of anxiety state that has led some workers to the concept of 'vital' anxiety[65, 97].

Here again a clear demarcation line has been suggested by some authors, while unitary views have been advanced by others. In 1926, Mapother[68] stated that the anxiety states were to be regarded as a sub-division of the manic-depressive group. Lewis[64] elaborated this unitary concept further and classified affective disorders into three main groups with major and minor variants: agitated depression and anxiety states, melancholia and neurasthenic or mild depression, manic excitement and hypomania. On the other hand, Garmany[26, 27] stated that anxiety states could be distinguished from depression in terms of the predominant symptomatology and Stenback[107] suggested that the differential diagnosis mainly depended upon the presence of 'the depressive affect (mental pain and apathy) *in the initial phase* of the psychic disturbance'. Hordern and colleagues[38] found that the first factor extracted from a factor analysis performed on the ratings of 137 patients was an anxiety-agitation factor with high saturations of somatic anxiety, psychic anxiety and agitation. Hordern pointed out that, in the absence of depression, it was not possible to label the factor 'agitated depression'. Furthermore, clinical observation suggests that the responses of anxiety and depression to treatment differ. The symptoms of patients with anxiety neurosis are frequently aggravated by tricyclic compounds and even more so when electroconvulsive therapy is administered. However, the situation is complicated by the fact that among the affective disorders in which successes are claimed with the monoamine oxidase inhibitor group of antidepressive drugs there is a group of patients regarded as 'atypical' depressions by some workers[95] and as anxiety neuroses by others[53].

In a recent enquiry, an attempt was made to sharpen discrimination between broad diagnostic groups by carrying out a systematic comparison of 145 patients tentatively allocated on the basis of the predominant mood change to the categories of anxiety state or depressive illness[89, 91]. A structured interview containing a battery of 348 items relating to a wide range of clinical features associated with anxiety and depression and containing details of the family history and background, early development, subsequent adjustment and premorbid personality was employed. A considerable overlap in symptomatology was found. A variable 'reactive' depression (in a minority of cases with suicidal ideas), as also tension, restlessness and irritability were relatively common in both groups. However, the groups differed in respect of a large number of clinical, biographical and personality indices. The patients with anxiety neurosis proved to be a constitutionally more unstable group than those with depressive illness. This was reflected in the higher incidence in the anxiety states of a family history of neurosis or personality disorder, a poor relationship with the parents and neurotic childhood traits. These patients had also fared worse at school, achieved a poorer social adjustment and showed more personality traits of anxiety, immaturity, dependence, anergia and hysterical features. Sexual maladjustment, particularly frigidity in the women, was commoner among the anxiety states. They had also experienced more frequent and severe psychological and physical stress prior to illness, the onset was more abrupt and the first breakdown had occurred at an earlier age.

The illness of patients with anxiety states was more commonly associated with severe and sustained tension and anxiety symptoms, panic attacks, situational and other phobias, depersonalization, derealization, 'temporal lobe' features, attacks of unconsciousness, aggravated frigidity and a colouring of both hysterical and obsessional features. Severe depression, diurnal variation, early awakening, suicidal tendencies, retardation, delusions and an unresponsive and unvarying affective disturbance were significantly commoner in the depressive states. The findings indicate that, in seeking to differentiate between anxiety states and depressive disorders, account has to be taken of a wide range of clinical features in addition to the predominant affective disturbance. A recently completed follow-up study carried out on these patients four years after discharge from hospital has shown that depressive illnesses carry a significantly better prognosis[92].

182

There are two further lines of evidence which bear upon the relationship between anxiety states and depressive illnesses. The first is the result of a discriminant function analysis of those of Roth and Gurney's cases in whom a diagnosis of anxiety or depressive state could be confidently made. The ten best discriminating clinical features were used to calculate summated diagnostic scores for these patients. The distribution of these summated scores was bimodal, anxiety states and depressions falling into distinct modes with a small overlap. A differentiation that is as sharp as this is unexpected but it is supported by further independent evidence. Genetical enquiries[105] have shown that of 17 monozygotic probands with an anxiety state, 47 per cent had twins with some psychiatric disorder, 41 per cent having an anxiety neurosis. The corresponding figures for the twins of 28 anxious dizygotic probands were 18 per cent for the presence of some psychiatric disorder and 4 per cent for an anxiety neurosis. Concordance rates for other neuroses were far smaller, the intrapair diagnostic specificity was lacking and there were no differences in concordance rates between monozygotic and dizygotic twins. The findings suggested that anxiety neuroses differed from other forms of neurotic illness in having some measure of genetic specificity.

The observations which suggest that anxiety states and depressions are relatively distinct forms of response have interesting biological implications. The bodily posture, expression and the physiological changes associated with the emotions of fear and anger led Cannon[7] to suggest that as the total response prepared the organism for violent exertion in combat or escape it had survival value. The capacity for anxiety reactions may therefore have been selected in the course of evolution and the fact that it is in some measure universal becomes understandable. From this point of view anxiety states may be regarded as the exaggerated and maladaptive prolongations of a response that has homeostatic and protective functions. Whether any corresponding biological role can be defined for depressive disorders has long been a subject of speculation and the question has recently attracted renewed interest[79]. The subject will be discussed further at a later stage.

Depression and Schizophrenia

The combination of depressive with schizophrenic or schizophrenia-like symptoms constitutes a third area of major nosological uncertainty. The conditions in this poorly charted borderland have received a variety of labels including schizo-affective psychosis, schizophreniform psychosis, cycloid psychosis and psychogenic psychosis. Although the aetiological concepts underlying these terms are different, the descriptions of the disorders given by the workers who have investigated this difficult territory have many common features.

One of the earliest writers in this field was Langfeldt[58, 59] who proposed that 'schizophreniform' psychoses should be classified separately from schizophrenia proper. This group of disorders was delineated by the presence of a precipitating factor, a relatively acute onset, initial clouding of consciousness and a florid symptomatology in which psychologically understandable themes could be found. Nuclear schizophrenic features were usually absent and a marked depressive colouring or an admixture of neurotic symptoms and hysterical features in particular were common. The psychoses were frequently reactive, following rapidly in the wake of a toxic state, physical illness or injury or psychological stress.

In the description of 'cycloid' psychoses given by Leonhard[60, 61] a number of these features recur. The illness is of sudden onset, precipitating factors are common and so are a strong depressive or manic colouring, disturbances of consciousness and florid delusions and hallucinations which are, however, devoid of specifically schizophrenic features. The prognosis is said to be favourable for, although the illnesses are recurrent, remissions between attacks are complete. The familial tendency is pronounced and Leonhard has advanced the suggestion that the condition should be regarded as a third form of psychosis, genetically independent of both schizophrenia and manic-depressive illness. In a recent study of a family[40] in which nine blood-related members had passed through 24 recorded psychotic periods, the consistency of the familial pattern of psychosis was striking. The disturbances of consciousness frequently reached almost delirious proportions. Despite depression and retardation, depressive thought content and hypochondriacal delusions were absent and so were autism and thought disorder. Hallucinations and delusions were florid and variable, agitation was pronounced and amnesia for the illness was a striking and consistent feature. Both psychological and physical stresses were prominent among the precipitants and five of the attacks were postpartum psychoses.

Kaij expresses the view that these physical and psychological factors act as mere triggers and the evidence suggests that in the Leonhard groups of cases it is the genetical predisposition that causes such mild or moderate stresses to exert such powerful effects. However, in the schizophrenia-like 'emotion' psychoses described by Labhardt[55], which have much in common with the concept of schizophreniform illness, the emotional stresses are of a drastic and overwhelming nature and the temporal connection with the psychiatric breakdown is impressive. Yet it is noteworthy that, in the whole of this borderland, physical illness and emotional stress are associated with the onset of psychotic illness and often appear to potentiate each other's effects. These stresses are non-specific in character and the psychological precipitants range over themes closely similar to those found in association with neuroses, depressions and indeed a proportion of schizophrenias.

The clinical features of the cases studied by Labhardt help to place the problems of classification in this area in a clearer perspective. The acute onset, florid clinical picture and clouding of consciousness, at times to the point of a delirious state, regularly occur. The psychological and physical stresses impinge on individuals who are often in a state of emotional exhaustion. There is severe anxiety in association with ideas of imminent death or disaster. However, perhaps the most significant and specific features of the illness are its strikingly short-lived nature and the evidence suggesting that it is an unusual response by neurotically predisposed subjects to stresses of an extreme nature. In more than 90 per cent of cases psychotic illnesses ended within a period of four weeks, and in nearly half, within a fortnight. Follow-up studies showed that relapse, which occurred in about half the cases observed, often took the form of a clearly neurotic or psychogenic disorder. The 'emotion' psychoses therefore have affinities not only with the 'schizophreniform' states but with those relatively rare and short-lived, acute psychoses of patients with anxious, obsessional or hysterical neuroses that usually develop in a step-like manner after stress and in which symptoms of anxiety or depression are usually prominent. It is, therefore, as well to be cautious about diagnosing schizophrenia when psychotic symptoms develop in a subject who has had a long-established neurotic illness.

Although there is some evidence[16, 39] that depressive, manic or mainly 'atypical' features in a schizophrenic illness portend a relatively good prognosis, there is little precise information about their predictive value. The degree of uncertainty that attaches to outcome in the individual case is well shown by Langfeldt's[59] study in which only 14 of 44 patients with schizophreniform psychosis were found on follow-up to have recovered: 16 were improved and 14 cases (almost a third) had undergone no change. In Faergeman's study[19] only 24 per cent of the paranoid syndromes initially judged to be psychogenic were still considered to be so at follow-up and well over half proved to be schizophrenic. On the whole the prognosis of 'reactive' psychoses with 'nuclear' schizophrenic features does not seem to differ from that of schizophrenia[36].

Notwithstanding the uncertainty about outcome, two broad

patterns of illness can be tentatively identified within this borderland between manic-depressive psychosis, schizophrenia and the neurotic disorders. The first is the psychosis of broadly endogenous type with a strong family history of identical illness described by Leonhard and others. This is a distinctive if uncommon phenomenon in clinical practice although strict evidence for its genetical independence from the two main forms of psychotic illness is lacking. Precipitating causes and a strong depressive colouring are usual. The second is more reactive in character, the stresses responsible being much more impressive in kind, but the term 'psychogenic psychosis' does not wholly convey their aetiological basis. In addition to the absence of any very clear hereditary tendency, these differ from the other group in the brief duration described in some studies and in being psychotic illnesses of neurotic or neurotically-predisposed individuals. Some preliminary evidence for the independence of these syndromes from generally recognized categories of psychiatric illness exists. However, much more evidence about the clustering of such features as severe stress at onset, clouding, anxiety and depressive symptoms, premorbid neurotic traits and 'nuclear' and other schizophrenic features and about their long-term outcome will be needed if they are to qualify for general acceptance as distinct entities.

Depressive States in Other Settings

Frommer[25] has indicated that depressive illness among children is not uncommon but that the true diagnosis may be masked by such presenting features as headache, enuresis, abdominal pain, a non-specific somatic malaise or anxiety symptoms. Agras[1] noted the frequency with which depression was present in school phobia and also in the mothers of children with this disorder. Frommer[24] has reported on the favourable response of children over the age of six with uncomplicated depression or a phobic anxiety state to treatment with monoamine oxidase inhibitors.

Depressive states occur relatively commonly in old age and account for between 30 and 50 per cent of admissions to mental hospitals after the age of 60. Most elderly depressives are below 70 and they form a very small proportion of persons admitted to psychiatric hospitals over the age of 80[78]. Although there is general agreement that patients with late onset depression tend to have been relatively stable, comparisons with middle-aged or elderly subjects with previous attacks have led to conflicting conclusions. Roth[88] found that the prognosis for late-onset depressives was better than for depressives with a previous history, while Post[77] found that the patients falling ill for the first time after 50 did less well than the early onset cases. Recent studies have, however, shown that depressions of late onset are not a homogeneous group so that such comparisons are not meaningful unless they refer to groups of cases selected by similar criteria.

Depressive episodes, usually of a florid type, are relatively common in patients suffering from progressive cerebrovascular disease. There is a distinctive variability of the symptoms and also a curiously fragmented quality to the clinical picture. Bizarre depressive ideas of guilt or nihilism are expressed in a flat or even euphoric mood, or ideas of hopelessness conveyed with little conviction. About a quarter of the cases show one or more episodes of this kind, usually in the early stages of the disease although some degree of intellectual impairment is almost invariable. Mild or moderate clouding of consciousness is not uncommon and may precipitate suicidal attempts which can be particularly serious. The instability of the affective state is reflected in the fact that some patients, within a few hours of such a bid, may be bland and euphoric and apparently unaware of what has happened. Many of these depressive episodes are short-lived, but sustained depressive states are seen in about ten per cent of cases. As the cerebral deterioration progresses, the depressive episodes gradually subside. A similar clinical picture may be found in association with other cerebral disorders such as cerebral tumour, cerebral syphilis and pernicious anaemia.

It has long been recognized that depressive states are liable to occur in the presence of physical disease. However, the contribution of the physical illness to the causation of the affective disorder in these cases has proved difficult to determine. Kay[43] has shown that aged patients with depressive symptoms in the setting of physical disease are closer to patients with neurotic depression than to those with manic-depressive illness both in their clinical picture and genetical basis. The recent finding[45] that the mortality in these cases is, among men, markedly in excess of expectation makes it clear that the association with physical illness cannot be fortuitous and is probably causal.

The relationship between carcinoma and depressive illnesses has been the subject of recent studies, Fras, Litin and Pearson[21] found that depression, anxiety, tension and anergia preceded the appearance of physical symptoms by about six months in half of a group of patients with carcinoma of the pancreas. Kerr, Schapira and Roth[48] have suggested that a mixed form of depressive illness with reactive and endogeneous features arising in late middle age, without previous psychiatric illness and without apparent cause, may be an early and direct manifestation of latent carcinoma.

Hillbom[34] studied many patients who sustained open head injuries in the last war and found that depression and neurotic reactions occurred in 38 per cent; there was also a high suicide rate of 1 per cent.

SUICIDE

In the recent Chichester studies a psychiatric diagnosis of depression was made in no less than 80 per cent of consummated suicides[4]. Helgason's survey[32] revealed that 17 per cent of manic-depressive patients committed suicide during the observation period of 60 years, while the study by Kessel and McCulloch[49] has indicated that psychopathic personalities with cyclothymic mood swings are also a high risk group.

Slater and Roth[69] have drawn up a predictive profile derived from published retrospective studies in which the presence of two of the following features indicates some suicidal risk and the presence of more than two indicates a serious risk; depression with guilt feelings; self-accusation; self-depreciation; nihilistic ideas and agitation; severe insomnia with disproportionate concern about it (regular early morning wakening with restlessness and the intrusion of distressing thoughts carries a high risk); severe hypochondriacal preoccupations associated with delusional and near delusional convictions of physical disease such as venereal disease, cancer, cardiac illness; a previous suicidal attempt; male sex and age over 55 years; a history of alcoholism or drug addiction; disabling, painful or serious physical illness particularly in a previously robust and energetic man; social isolation and an unsympathetic attitude of relatives which is either real or exaggerated by the patient; suicidal preoccupations and talk (unconfided preoccupations constitute a special risk); a history of suicide in the family; unemployment and financial difficulty, particularly if they represent a steep decline in fortune; towards the end of a period of depressive illness when the depressive mood persists but initiative and power of decision are recovering. Many of these items are either symptoms of depression or settings in which depressive states are particularly liable to develop.

Depression is a common side effect of certain hypotensive drugs, such as reserpine, methyldopa and guanethidine and Barraclough and Sainsbury (Personal communication, 1967) have shown that 23 per cent of suicides had been taking methyldopa or guanethidine.

SOME BIOLOGICAL ASPECTS OF DEPRESSION

Endogeneous depression and manic-depressive psychoses are relatively common disorders and the predisposition to them is even more wide-spread. Neurotic depression has an even higher prevalence. Indeed, if the evidence favouring transmission of manic-depressive forms of illness by a major dominant autosomal gene is accepted, this condition must be by far the commonest illness in the human race inherited in this manner. Since depressive illness may confer incapacity for long periods, carries an increased mortality from suicide, and possibly some decrease in fertility[42, 73] which may in earlier ages have been substantially greater, the question arises as to whether these ill-effects are counter-balanced, as in the case of other genetically determined conditions such as sickle cell anaemia, by compensatory advantages which are conferred on those who carry the predisposition to illness in attenuated form. It seems unlikely that a disorder determined in part by specific hereditary factors and causing such serious maladaption may merely be due to some inherent fault in the machine.

Attempts to define adaptive functions for depressive illness have been further stimulated by other observations. Some evidence exists that manic depression occurs with greater frequency in the upper than in the lower socio-economic segments of the population. In addition, it may be pertinent that suicide, as in the case of the Eskimo weakened by old age and disease, is sometimes an altruistic act that may in man's evolutionary past have helped social groups to survive; the underlying psychological characteristics would then have been perpetuated by natural selection between groups.

The oft-quoted association between manic-depressive illness or cyclical mood swings and outstanding creative gifts perhaps deserves mention. Goethe, Hugo Wolf and Samuel Johnson were cyclothymes; the poets Smart, Cowper and Clare as also Robert Meyer, who discovered the law of conservation of energy, had recurrent attacks of psychosis while Dickens and Balzac probably lived in a state of overactivity, elation and optimism broken by short periods of depression. However, the evidence for an increase in expectation of manic-depressive or depressive illness in men of genius is on the whole unconvincing. Havelock Ellis[17] estimated an incidence of only 4·2 per cent for all forms of insanity among 1030 British men of genius while Slater and Meyer[104] found the morbid risk for affective psychosis to be only slightly increased in Germans of outstanding creative gifts. Emotional instability of a less specific kind occurred with a frequency in excess of expectation.

Cannon's work[7] provided evidence for the view that anxiety states were exaggerated versions of the 'fight' or 'flight' reactions of animals. To make an equally good case for the survival value of depressive illnesses has proved much more difficult. Rodger[85] has suggested that depression may be regarded as a social biological reaction which, in animals, when linked with anxiety over separation from the herd, may perform the useful function of reducing motor activity, exploratory behaviour and food intake until the herd is rejoined. He speculates further that, in aged or unfit animals, acceptance of rejection by the herd may produce a state analogous to pathological depression.

Lange[57] put forward the idea that the counterpart of depression in man might be the state of hibernation found in certain animals and that features such as retardation, loss of appetite and diminished sexual interest could be related to the conservation of energy and the limitation of food intake. In other depressive states, motor restlessness and paranoid thinking could be conceived of as being advantageous to a nomadic people living in the less hospitable areas of the world[81]. Unfortunately for these theories there is no increase in incidence of depression or suicide in the winter and over-activity is probably more common in anxiety states than depressions which are quite as often inactive, retarded or stuperose.

The concept of dominance hierarchy, based on the social system of baboons and macaques, is derived from the work of comparative ethologists and relates to the complex behaviour which has evolved to maintain the stability of social groups. Price[80] has described how it is essentially an order of precedence based on individual recognition and appears to perform the function of allowing aggressive animals to live together in relative peacefulness. Each member is aware of his position in the hierarchy and, if an issue arises, the inferior submits before a fight occurs. Aggression and confidence are characteristic of behaviour towards subordinates, who respond with anxiety and withdrawal and might be said to pass their lives in a state of neurotic depression. Price[79] tentatively suggests that elated behaviour evolved in connection with a rise in the hierarchy and phasic endogenous depressive behaviour developed to facilitate peaceful adaptation to reduced states. He indicates that the clinical features of a depressive state are such as to permit a smooth descent without disruption of the social group by fighting. However, an excess of this behaviour manifest as depressive illness would be biologically disadvantageous and therefore limited by natural selection.

These features have to be taken together with the general advantages conferred by hierarchial systems which, by providing set positions in the social group for each individual, tend to promote concerted and effective action in the face of emergency.

There are other lines of speculation that suggest themselves. Perhaps the commonest morbid emotional reactions found in man, those of anxiety and depression, which are in some measure universal, may have been moulded to a pattern set by the exigencies of life among man's hominid ancestors: in the plains, escape or fight; in the jungle, concealment. The difficulty is to translate such speculations into hypotheses that can be submitted to critical tests. The need in the immediate future is for more precise evidence about the social status of the families of those who suffer from different forms of depressive illness. Several of these speculations outlined above demand that the first degree relations of subjects with manic-depressive and related forms of illness should manifest advantages in the form of increased fertility, intelligence, vigour or social effectiveness and this should be testable.

CONCLUSION

In this examination of the relationship between 'reactive' or 'neurotic' and endogenous depressions, anxiety states and other neuroses, certain forms of 'psychogenic' and 'emotion' psychoses and schizo-affective disorders, we have laid emphasis on the diversity rather than the unity of those disorders in which depressive symptoms can to some extent be attributed to exogenous causes. That unity as well as diversity exists is not in doubt. However, the time appears ripe for progress in the understanding of the aetiological basis of some forms of affective disorder. Progress has often been hastened in the past by the definition of demarcation lines within clinical phenomena formerly considered to merge by insensible gradations with one another. In the field of general medicine a good example is provided by the recognition of aldosteronism and phaeochromocytoma as causes of hypertension. Attention to the evidence for qualitative differences between the various forms of depression would open the way to exploring possible causes.

An underlying assumption in this chapter has been the view that the concept of disease, defined initially in descriptive terms, and at a later stage in terms of aetiology, is of value in psychiatry.

The subjects chosen for discussion reflect the many recent developments that have focused attention upon the biological foundations of depression. In the biochemical field interest has been reawakened by enquiries into catecholamines, among them the first substance to attract attention as possibly contributing to the symptomatology of psychiatric disorders. It will be recalled that in Cannon's concept of fear and anxiety some of the main features of this adaptive response were attributed to the effects of epinephrine. Moreover, in more recent enquiries all the brain monoamines concentrated almost entirely in the mid brain, hypothalamus and limbic system have come under scrutiny as being possibly concerned in the pathogenesis of some forms of depression. A good deal of evidence has accumulated to suggest that antidepressant drugs owe their effects to their influence upon the metabolism of one or more of these substances and the best biochemically-fashioned model of depressive disorder in the human subject is that produced by reserpine which brings about the depletion of the storage depots of monoamines in the brain.

The association of depressive states with some forms of cerebral disease and the contribution of physical illness to causation, particularly in men, has also helped to stimulate enquiry about the higher centres mediating depression and about their biological significance. However, in the association with physical illness as also in the peak incidence for depressive illness in middle or late life and their additional associations with isolation and suicide we are reminded that hypotheses about the causes of depression should take into account psychopathological as well as physical, biochemical and neurological observations. Stimulating and useful though they are, it does not appear as if current speculations about the biological significance of depression can be clearly expressed for the present in any readily testable form. This may prove possible after further progress in specific lines of scientific enquiry: perhaps as the result of systematic clinical, biochemical and therapeutic comparisons of neurotic depressions, neurotic anxiety and endogenous depression.

ACKNOWLEDGEMENT
We are grateful to Dr R. E. Kendell for permission to reproduce *Figure 1*.

ADDENDUM
(to section on Problems of Classification)

Pilowsky and collegues[76a] have recently applied the method of numerical taxonomy to an examination of the classification of depression. They studied the responses made by 200 consecutive psychiatric patients to a specially constructed depressive questionnaire, making the important point that this approach abolished observer bias. The authors found a significant association between the diagnostic and taxonomic classes and, more particularly, that there was strong support for the concept of endogenous depression. But perhaps their most striking finding was that 'of the 200 patients all but four have a probability of greater than 0·95 of belonging to the particular class in which they have been grouped. This is unequivocal evidence obtained from unbiased data, that patients suffering from depression form two distinct groups.

REFERENCES

1. Agras, S. (1959). 'The Relationship of School Phobia to Childhood Depression'. *Am. J. Psychiat.* **116,** 533

2. Ashcroft, G. W., Crawford, T. B. B., Eccleston, D., Sharman, D. F., MacDougall, E. J., Stanton, J. B. and Binns, J. K. (1966). '5-Hydroxyindole Compounds in the Cerebrospinal Fluid of Patients with Psychiatric or Neurological Diseases'. *Lancet* **2,** 1049

3. Astrup, C., Fossum, A. and Holmboe, R. (1959). 'A Follow-up Study of 270 Patients with Acute Affective Psychoses'. *Acta psychiat. neurol. scand.* **34,** Suppl. 135

4. Barraclough, B. M., Nelson, B. and Sainsbury, P. (1968). 'The Diagnostic Classification and Psychiatric Treatment of 25 Suicides'. *Proceedings of the Fourth International Conference for Suicide Prevention.* Los Angeles. October, 1967

5. Beck, A. T. Ward, C. H., Mendelson, M., Mock, J. and Erbaugh, J. (1961). 'An Inventory for Measuring Depression'. *Archs gen. Psychiat.* **4,** 561

6. Busfield, B. L. and Wechsler, H. (1961). 'Studies of Salivation in Depression'. *Archs gen. Psychiat.* **4,** 10

7. Cannon, W. B. (1928). *Feelings and Emotions.* The Wittenberg Symposium. Worcester, Massachusetts

8. Carney, M. W. P., Roth, M. and Garside, R. F. (1965). 'The Diagnosis of Depressive Syndromes and the Prediction of E.C.T. Response'. *Br. J. Psychiat.* **111,** 659

9. Carothers, J. C. (1947). 'A Study of Mental Derangement in Africans'. *J. ment. Sci.* **93,** 548

10. Coppen, A. and Shaw, D. M. (1963). 'Mineral Metabolism in Melancholia'. *Br. med. J.* **2,** 1439

11. —— and Farrell, J. P. (1963). 'Potentiation of the Anti-depressive Effect of a Monoamine Oxidase Inhibitor by Trypto-phan'. *Lancet* **1,** 79

12. —— Malleson, A., Eccleston, E. and Gundy, G. (1965). 'Trypt-amine Metabolism in Depression'. *Br. J. Psychiat.* **111,** 993

13. Crombie, D. L. (1957). 'The Prevalence of Psychogenic Illness in General Practice'. *Res. Newsl. Coll. gen. Practnrs* **4,** 218

14. Dencker, S. J., Malm, U., Roos, B.-E. and Werdinius, B. (1966). 'Acid Monoamine Metabolites of Cerebrospinal Fluid in Mental Depression and Mania'. *J. Neurochem.* **13,** 1545

15. Dewhurst, W. H. (1968). 'Cerebral Amine Functions in Health and Disease'. In *Studies in Psychiatry*, Chap. 14. Ed. by M. Shepherd and D. L. Davies. London: Oxford University Press

16. Eitinger, L., Laane, C. L. and Langfeldt, G. (1958). 'The Prognostic Value of the Clinical Picture and the Therapeutic Value of Physical Treatment in Schizophrenia and the Schizophreniform States'. *Acta psychiat. neurol. scand.* **33,** 33

17. Ellis, H. H. (1904). *A Study of British Genius*. London: Hurst and Blackett

18. Essen-Möller, E. and Hagnell, O. (1961). 'The Frequency and Risk of Depression within a Rural Population Group in Scania'. *Acta psychiat. scand.* **37,** Suppl. 162, 28

19. Faergeman, P. M. (1945). *Psychogenic Psychoses*. (Translated 1963). London: Butterworths

20. Field, M. J. (1958). 'Mental Disorder in Rural Ghana'. *J. ment. Sci.* **104,** 1043

21. Fras, I., Litin, E. M. and Pearson, J. S. (1967). 'Carcinoma of Pancreas Signalled by Appearance of Emotional Symptoms'. *Am. J. Psychiat.* **123,** 1553

22. Fraser, P. M. and Baron, D. N. (1968). 'Taxonomic Procedures Applied to Liver Disease'. *Proc. R. Soc. Med.* **61,** 1043

23. Fremming, K. H. (1947). *Morbid Risk of Mental Diseases and Other Abnormal Psychic States among the Average Danish Population*. Copenhagen: Munksgaard

24. Frommer, E. A. (1967). 'Treatment of Childhood Depression with Antidepressant Drugs'. *Br. med. J.* **1,** 729

25. — (1968). 'Depressive Illness in Childhood'. In *Recent Developments in Affective Disorders: A Symposium*, p. 117. Ed. by A. Coppen and A. Walk. British Journal of Psychiatry Special Publication No. 2. London: Royal Medico-Psychological Association

26. Garmany, G. (1956). 'Anxiety States'. *Br. med. J.* **1,** 943

27. — (1958). 'Depressive States: Their Aetiology and Treatment'. *Br. med. J.* **2,** 341

28. Gibbons, J. L. (1964). 'Cortisol Secretion Rates in Depressive Illness'. *Archs gen. Psychiat.* **10,** 572

29. Gillespie, R. D. (1929). 'The Clinical Differentiation of Types of Depression'. *Guy's Hosp. Rep.* **79,** 306

30. Grosz, H. J. (1968). 'The Relation between Neurosis and Psychosis: Observations on the Reliability of the Data Defining the Trouton and Maxwell Factors of Neuroticism and Psychotism'. *Br. J. Psychiat.* **114,** 189

31. Hamilton, M. (1960). 'A Rating Scale for Depression'. *J. Neurol. Neurosurg. Psychiat.* **23,** 56

32. Helgason, T. (1964). 'Epidemiology of Mental Disorders in Iceland: A Psychiatric and Demographic Investigation of 5395 Icelanders'. *Acta psychiat. scand.* **40,** Suppl. 173

33. Hemsi, L. K., Kendell, R. E. and McClure, J. L. (1968). Quoted by Kendell (1968)

34. Hillbom, E. (1960). 'After-effects of Brain Injuries'. *Acta psychiat. neurol. scand.* **35,** Suppl. 142

35. Hobson, R. F. (1953). 'Prognostic Factors in Electric Convulsive Therapy'. *J. Neurol. Neurosurg. Psychiat.* **16,** 275

36. Holmboe, R. and Astrup, C. (1957). 'A Follow-up Study of 255 Patients with Acute Schizophrenia and Schizophreniform Psychoses'. *Acta psychiat. neurol. scand.* **32,** Suppl. 115

37. Hopkinson, G. (1964). 'A Genetic Study of Affective Illnesses in Patients over 50'. *Br. J. Psychiat.* **110,** 244

38. Hordern, A., Burt, C. G., Holt, N. F. and Cade, J. F. J. (1965). *Depressive States: A Pharmacotherapeutic Study.* Springfield, Ill.: Charles C. Thomas

39. Jansson, B. and Alstrom, J. (1968). 'The Prognostic Significance of Certain Symptoms of Schizophreniform Psychoses in Young Adults'. *Proceedings of the Fourth World Congress on Psychiatry,* Vol. 4. Madrid, 1966. Ed. by J. J. López Ibor. London: Excerpta Medica Foundation

40. Kaij, L. (1967). 'Atypical Endogenous Psychosis: Report on a Family'. *Br. J. Psychiat.* **113,** 415

41. Kallmann, F. J. (1950). 'The Genetics of Psychoses: An Analysis of 1,232 Twin Index Families'. *Congrès International de Psychiatrie, Rapports VI Psychiatrie Sociale,* p. 1. Paris

42. — (1954). 'Genetic Principles in Manic-depressive Psychosis'. In *Depression.* Ed. by P. Hoch and J. Zubin. New York: Grune and Stratton

43. Kay, D. W. K. (1959). 'Observations on the Natural History and Genetics of Old Age Psychoses: A Stockholm Material, 1931– 1937'. (Abridged). *Proc. R. Soc. Med.* **52,** 791

44. — (1962). 'Outcome and Cause of Death in Mental Disorders of Old Age: a Long-term Follow-up of Functional and Organic Psychoses'. *Acta psychiat. scand.* **38,** 249

45. — and Bergmann, K. (1966). 'Physical Disability and Mental Health in Old Age'. *J. psychosom. Res.* **10,** 3

46. Kendell, R. E. (1968). 'The Problem of Classification'. In *Recent Developments in Affective Disorders: A Symposium,* p. 15. Ed. by A. Coppen and A. Walk. British Journal of Psychiatry, Special Publication No. 2. London: Royal Medico-Psychological Association

47. — (1968). *The Classification of Depressive Illnesses.* London: Oxford University Press

48. Kerr, T. A., Schapira, K. and Roth, M. (1969). 'The Relationship between Premature Death and Affective Disorders'. *Br. J. Psychiat.* **115,** 1277

49. Kessel, W. I. N. and McCulloch, W. (1966). 'Repeated Acts of Self-poisoning and Self-injury'. *Proc. R. Soc. Med.* **59,** 89

50. Kiloh, L. G. and Garside, R. F. (1963). 'The Independence of Neurotic Depression and Endogenous Depression'. *Br. J. Psychiat.* **109,** 451

51. — Ball, J. R. B. and Garside, R. F. (1962). 'Prognostic Factors in the Treatment of Depressive States with Imipramine'. *Br. med. J.* **1,** 1225

52. — Roy, J. R. and Carney, M. W. P. (1963). 'A Pilot Trial of G 33040 in the Treatment of Depressive Illness'. *J. Neuropsychiat.* **5**, 18

53. King, A. (1962). 'Phenelzine Treatment of Roth's Calamity Syndrome'. *Med. J. Austral.* **49**, 879

54. Kraepelin, E. (1904). 'Vergleichende Psychiatrie'. *Zentbl. Nervenheilk.* **15**, 433

55. Labhardt, F. (1963). *Die Schizophrenie ahnlichen Emotionspsychosen.* Berlin: Springer

56. Lambo, T. A. (1960). 'Further Neuropsychiatric Observations in Nigeria'. *Br. med. J.* **2**, 1696

57. Lange, J. (1928). 'The Endogenous and Reactive Affective Disorders and the Manic-depressive Constitution'. In *Handbook of Mental Diseases,* Vol. 6. Ed. by O. Bumke. Berlin: Springer

58. Langfeldt, G. (1937). 'The Prognosis in Schizophrenia and the Factors Influencing the Course of the Disease'. *Acta psychiat. neurol. scand.* **12**. Suppl. 13

59. — (1960). 'Diagnosis and Prognosis of Schizophrenia'. *Proc. R. Soc. Med.* **53**, 1047

60. Leonhard, K. (1937). *Involutive and Idiopathische Angstdepression in Klinik and Erblichkeit.* Stuttgart: Thieme Verlag

61. — (1961). 'Cycloid Psychoses–Endogenous Psychoses which are neither Schizophrenic nor Manic-depressive'. *J. ment. Sci.* **107**, 633

62. — Korff, I. and Schulz, H. (1962). 'Temperament in Families with Monopolar and Bipolar Phasic Psychoses'. *Psychiatria Neurol.* **143**, 416

63. Lewis, A. J. (1934). 'Melancholia: A Clinical Survey of Depressive 'States'. *J. ment. Sci.* **80**, 277

64. — (1950). 'Psychological Medicine'. In *A Textbook of the Practice of Medicine,* Section 20, 8th Ed. Ed. by F. W. Price. London: Oxford University Press

65. López Ibor, J. J. (1950). 'La Angustia Vital'. *Patologie General Psychosomatica.* Ed. by Paz Montalvo. Madrid

66. — (1962). 'The "Target" Symptoms in the Treatment of Depressions'. *Compreh. Psychiat.* **3**, 15

67. McConaghy, N., Joffe, A. D. and Murphy, B. (1967). 'The Independence of Neurotic and Endogenous Depression'. *Br. J. Psychiat.* **113**, 479

68. Mapother, E. (1926). 'Discussion on Manic-depressive Psychosis'. *Br. med. J.* **2**, 872

69. Mayer-Gross, W., Slater, E. and Roth, M. (1969). *Clinical Psychiatry,* 3rd Ed. London: Bailliere

70. Mendels, J. (1965). 'Electroconvulsive Therapy and Depression: I The Prognostic Significance of Clinical Factors'. *Br. J. Psychiat.* **111**, 675

71.   —   (1965). 'Electroconvulsive Therapy and Depression: II Significance of Endogenous and Reactive Syndromes'. *Br. J. Psychiat.* **111,** 682

72.   —   (1965). 'Electroconvulsive Therapy and Depression: III A Method for Prognosis'. *Br. J. Psychiat.* **111,** 687

73.   Ødegaard, Ø. (1959). Discussion. *Eugen. Q.* **6,** 137

74.   Palmai, G. and Blackwell, B. (1965). 'The Diurnal Pattern of Salivary Flow in Normal and Depressed Patients'. *Br. J. Psychiat.* **111,** 334

75.   — —   Maxwell, A. E. and Morgenstern, F. (1967). 'Patterns of Salivary Flow in Depressive Illness and During Treatment'. *Br. J. Psychiat.* **113,** 1297

76.   Perris, C. (1966). 'A Study of Bipolar (Manic-depressive) and Unipolar Recurrent Depressive Psychoses'. *Acta psychiat. scand.* **42,** Suppl. 194

76a   Pilowsky, I., Levin, S. Boulton, D. M. (1969).' The Classification of Depression by Numerical Taxonomy'. *Br. J. Psychiat.* **115,** 937

77.   Post, F. (1962). *The Significance of Affective Symptoms in Old Age.* Maudsley Monograph No. 10. London: Oxford University Press

78.   —   (1968). 'The Factor of Ageing in Affective Illness'. In *Recent Developments in Affective Disorders: A Symposium,* p. 105. Ed. by A. Coppen and A. Walk. British Journal of Psychiatry Special Publication No. 2. London: Royal Medico-Psychological Association

79.   Price, J. S. (1967). 'The Dominance Hierarchy and the Evolution of Mental Illness'. *Lancet* **2,** 243

80.   —   (1968). 'The Genetics of Depressive Behaviour'. In *Recent Developments in Affective Disorders: a Symposium,* p. 37. Ed. by A. Coppen and A. Walk. British Journal of Psychiatry Special Publication No. 2. London: Royal Medico-Psychological Association

81.   —   (1968). 'Genetics of the Affective Illnesses'. *Hosp. Med.* **2,** 1173

82.   Rainer, J. D. (1966). 'Genetic Aspects of Depression'. *Can. psychiat. Ass. J.* **11,** Suppl. 29

83.   Rawnsley, K. (1968). 'Epidemiology of Affective Disorders'. In *Recent Developments in Affective Disorders: A Symposium,* p. 27. Ed. by A. Coppen and A. Walk. British Journal of Psychiatry Special Publication No. 2. London: Royal Medico-Psychological Association

84.   Registrar-General (1964). *Statistical Review of England and Wales 1960. Supplement on Mental Health.* London: Her Majesty's Stationery Office

85.   Rodger, T. F. (1961). 'The Anglo-Saxon Approach to Depression'. *Acta psychiat. scand.* **36,** Suppl. 162, 201

86.   Rosenthal, S. H. and Gudeman, J. E. (1967). 'The Self-pitying Constellation in Depression'. *Br. J. Psychiat.* **113,** 485

87. —— (1967). 'The Endogenous Depressive Pattern: An Empirical Investigation'. *Archs gen. Psychiat.* **16,** 241

88. Roth, M. (1955). 'The Natural History of Mental Disorder in Old Age'. *J. ment. Sci.* **101,** 281

89. — (1969). 'The Classification of Affective Disorders'. In *Symposium on the Treatment of Depression,* p. 9. Ed by B. Cronholm and F. Sjöquist. Uppsala: Appelberg

90. — and Kay, D. W. K. (1956). 'Affective Disorder Arising in the Senium. II. Physical Disability as an Aetiological Factor'. *J. ment. Sci.* **102,** 141

91. — and Gurney, C. (1970). 'The Classification and Clinical Differentiation of Anxiety States from Depressive Disorders I'. In preparation

92. — Kerr, T. A. and Schapira, K. (1970). 'The Course of Affective Disorders'. In preparation

93. Sandifer, M. G., Pettus, C. and Quade, D. (1964). 'A Study of Psychiatric Diagnosis'. *J. nerv. ment. Dis.* **39,** 350

94. — Wilson, I. C. and Green, L. (1966). 'The Two-type Thesis of Depressive Disorders'. *Am. J. Psychiat.* **123,** 93

95. Sargant, W. (1961). 'Drugs in the Treatment of Depression'. *Br. med. J.* **1,** 225

96. Schildkraut, J. J. (1965). 'The Catecholamine Hypothesis of Affective Disorders: A Review of Supporting Evidence'. *Am. J. Psychiat.* **122,** 509

97. Schneider, K. (1955). *Klinische Psychopathologie,* 4th Ed. Stuttgart: Thieme Verlag

98. Shepherd, M., Cooper, B., Brown, A. C. and Kalton, G. W. (1966). *Psychiatric Illness in General Practice.* London: Oxford University Press

99. Shields, J. and Slater, E. T. O. (1966). 'La Similarité du Diagnostic chez les Jumeaux et la Problème de la Spécificité Biologique dans les Névroses et les Troubles de la Personnalité'. *L' Evolut. Psychiat.* No. 2, 441

100. Silverman, C. (1968). 'The Epidemiology of Depression—A Review'. *Am. J. Psychiat.* **124,** 883

101. Slater, E. (1936). 'The Inheritance of Manic-depressive Insanity'. *Proc. R. Soc. Med.* **29,** 39

102. — (1938). 'The Periodicity of Manic-depressive Insanity'. *Z. ges. Neurol. Psychiat.* **162,** 794

103. — and Slater, P. (1944). 'A Heuristic Theory of Neurosis'. *J. Neurol. Psychiat.* **7,** 49

104. — and Meyer, A. (1960).'Contributions to a Pathography of the Musicians: 2. Organic and Psychotic Disorders'. *Confinia psychiat.* **3,** 129

105.   — and Shields, J. (1967). 'Communication to Symposium on Anxiety'. *World Psychiatric Association Symposium*. London. November 1967. Documenta Geigy

106. Stainbrook, E. (1954). 'A Cross-cultural Evaluation of Depressive Reactions'. In *Depression*. Ed. by P. Hoch and J. Zubin. New York: Grune and Stratton

107. Stenbäck, A. (1963). 'On Involutional and Middle Age Depressions'. *Acta psychiat. scand.* **39,** Suppl. 169, 14

108. Stenstedt, A. (1952). 'A Study in Manic-depressive Psychosis'. *Acta psychiat. neurol. scand.* **27,** Suppl. 97

109.   — (1959). 'Involutional Melancholia: An Aetiological, Clinical and Social Study of Endogenous Depression in Later Life, with Special Reference to Genetic Factors'. *Acta psychiat. scand.* **34,** Suppl. 127

110. Strongin, E. I. and Hinsie, L. E. (1939). 'A Method for Differentiating Manic-depressive Depressions from Other Depressions by Means of Parotid Secretions'. *Psychiat. Q.* **13,** 697

111. Tait, A. C., Harper, J. and McClatchey, W. T. (1957). 'Initial Psychiatric Illness in Involutional Women'. *J. ment. Sci.* **103,** 132

112. Watts, C. A. H. (1966). *Depressive Disorders in the Community*. Bristol: John Wright

113. Wing, J. K., Birley, J. L. T., Cooper, J. E., Graham, P. and Isaacs, A. D. (1967). 'Reliability of a Procedure for Measuring and Classifying "Present Psychiatric State" '. *Br. J. Psychiat.* **113,** 499

114. Winokur, G. and Clayton, P. (1967). 'Family History Studies I. Two Types of Affective Disorders Separated According to Genetic and Clinical Factors'. *Recent Adv. biol. Psychiat.* **9,** 35

115. Yap, P. M. (1965). 'Phenomenology of Affective Disorder in Chinese and Other Cultures'. In *Ciba Foundation Symposium on Transcultural Psychiatry*, p. 84. Ed. by A. V. S. de Reuck and R. Porter. London: Churchill

CHAPTER 8

SCHIZOPHRENIA: TREATMENT AND OUTCOME

BERTRAM M. MANDELBROTE

INTRODUCTION

Schizophrenia is a syndrome of unknown aetiology in which a number of factors have been incriminated as causal. These include genetic and constitutional factors, factors associated with personality development and the close interpersonal relationship between parent and child, and factors which might be relevant in triggering off the disorder. It is well known that a similar syndrome of symptoms may be triggered off in relation to drug intoxication such as in amphetamine psychosis and in relation to cerebral injury or disease as occurs in temporal lobe epilepsy. It is conceivable that as knowledge progresses this syndrome may be divided into a group of conditions with specific aetiology, but for the present aetiology remains relatively undefined. Equally, there are differences in the course of the disorder unrelated to treatment and consequent upon treatment. Some patients appear to recover completely whilst others show a relapsing course with or without impairment of personality, affect and volition. Some of these patients will be able to spend most of their life outside of hospital whilst others will spend most of their life in hospital. This will depend on the attitude of the hospital authorities, the assets of the individual, his capacity for employment and the tolerance and capacity for support which is present in his family and from the community at large. Up to the present time we are unable to state clearly the contribution of aetiological factors to the syndrome and equally we are unable to predict with certainty which patients suffering from this syndrome will recover completely and which patients will show a deterioration. With these deficiencies in the understanding of the natural history of the disorder, it is not surprising that treatment is essentially empirical and the effects of treatment on the individual are difficult to assess. This does not mean, however, that a very wide range of research investigation is not being carried out in order to evaluate treatment procedures and elucidate social and clinical factors relevant to prognosis and outcome.

200

REVIEW OF THE MANAGEMENT OF SCHIZOPHRENIA

Moral Era

The moral era of treatment (*c.* 1825 to 1875) is relevant to the treatment of schizophrenia in that many aspects of its philosophy relating to the social setting in which treatment takes place is reflected in recent changes in the social setting of mental hospitals. Greenblatt, York and Brown[35] summarized it 'as therapy that emphasized close and friendly association with the patient, intimate discussions of his difficulties and the daily pursuit of purposeful activity'.

Bockoven[13] analysed follow-up reports from the Worcester State Hospital (U.S.A.) covering the 20 year period from 1833 to 1852. Out of 2,267 first admissions to the hospital, ill for less than one year prior to hospitalization, 70 per cent were discharged as recovered or improved. For chronic patients, with illnesses of longer than one year, out of 1852, 45 per cent were discharged as recovered or improved. It is not possible to make any real assessment of schizophrenia from these results because of the problem of diagnostic categories. Nevertheless, as schizophrenia represented a fair proportion of hospital admissions, this reflects an extraordinarily high rate of favourable discharge from hospital.

Custodial Era

The custodial era refers to a later period between the end of the nineteenth century and early part of the twentieth century. It reflected the rapid increase in the patient population of mental hospitals and the administrative emphasis on certification with prevention of escape of patients for the protection of the public. Although it is not possible to distinguish clearly the extent of moral or custodial treatment in the various hospitals, it is not unreasonable to generalize that in many hospitals a custodial setting predominated. The emphasis was placed on institutional care and supervision and regimentation rather than friendly participation in intimate discussion and purposeful activity. In the Worcester State Hospital during this period the number of discharges of recovered patients dropped to 4 per cent[13] and there was a steady rise in the population of chronic patients.

A review of surveys of schizophrenic patients in the United States exposed to non-specific custodial care[84] showed that roughly 30–40 per cent acute schizophrenics recovered or improved during the custodial era over a five year period. This was presumed to be the spontaneous remission rate whilst the remaining 60–70 per cent

PM—*H**

became chronic patients. Drasgow[22] plotted the discharge rates of 100 randomly selected patients in order to assess the effects of custodial care on chronically ill schizophrenic patients and found that the discharge rates of patients who had been in hospital three years was balanced by relapse rates so that the net discharge rate approached zero.

Insulin Coma and Electroconvulsive Therapy

Between the two wars a number of energetic treatment measures such as insulin coma, electroconvulsive therapy and more intensive occupational therapy were introduced in the treatment of schizophrenia. Administrative procedures with the passing of the 1930 Mental Treatment Act made entry to the mental hospital easier by enabling voluntary and temporary admissions in addition to certification. There was a time when a full course of insulin coma was considered essential for every schizophrenic patient of recent onset. It was also considered by Kalinowsky and Hoch[50] essential for schizophrenics to have 20 treatments of electroconvulsive therapy before they could be considered adequately treated. Insulin coma and electroconvulsive therapy have now been superseded by the phenothiazine drugs and are rarely used except in the case of electroconvulsive therapy for catatonic patients in states of withdrawal or stupor[48].

Prefrontal Leucotomy

The operation of prefrontal leucotomy was introduced originally by Moniz[73] in Portugal, followed by Freeman and Watts[28] in the United States, and McKissock[59] in the United Kingdom. Freeman's series certainly showed a more favourable outcome than previously. Of those patients who had been in hospital from one to two years, 52 per cent were out of the hospital one year after operation[27]. The review of the American studies and British studies did not tally in their assessment of successful outcome. Paul and Greenblatt[80] said that psychosurgical techniques were the first treatment methods capable of preventing chronic hospitalization in acute patients and of leading to significant and sustained improvement and discharge rates even in patients who were already chronically ill. Pippard's[82] findings were less dramatic. In the American studies the bimedial operation showed the most significant improvement. Because of the degree of personality change which occurred with the early patients and the not very satisfactory results in the British series, drug treatment has also very much replaced the use of prefrontal leucotomy in schizophrenia and this is a procedure which is rarely used in the United Kingdom.

Inevitably, the period during World War II resulted in a reversion to custodial management for those schizophrenics remaining in hospital with minimum skilled staff available and emphasis on treatment of psychiatric problems in the Forces. Many experiments in the rehabilitation of psychiatric casualties were developed which initially had no relevance to problems of schizophrenia but which at a later date influenced the setting in which schizophrenic patients were treated. These had to do with group and community methods based on psychoanalytic theories which highlighted the extent to which the dependency needs of the individual interfered with therapy—a fore-runner to therapy changes in relation to problems of institutionalism.

Psychotherapy—Individual and Group

Psychotherapy in schizophrenia has ranged from psychotherapy on a strictly psychoanalytical basis to modifications dependent on the personality of the therapist and his dynamic beliefs. In the main, psychoanalytically oriented psychotherapy was a feature of private clinics in the United States, well described by Freda Fromm-Reichmann[29] at Chestnut Lodge, Maryland. Work with schizophrenics there came under serious criticism[85] because of the lack of awareness of aspects of behaviour and interpersonal relationships outside the analytical hour.

Appel and colleagues[4], in an attempt to assess the hospital out-come of schizophrenics treated with psychotherapy, analysed 'seven of the more carefully evaluated studies' and came to the conclusion that approximately 39 per cent of these patients had made a good recovery and that this reduced to 27 per cent if followed up over a five year period. Although little better than the spontaneous remis-sion rate, comment would depend on the prognosis of the cases treated. Betz and Whitehorn[10] came to the conclusion that classical psychotherapy techniques were less appropriate than active inter-pretation and involvement with the patient. They came to this con-clusion after studying the relationship between therapeutic success and the personality and methods of approach of the therapist. Stephens and Astrup[86] tested this hypothesis on doctors at the Phipps Clinic and disagreed with the findings. In Britain psycho-therapy for schizophrenia has been mainly in the context of sup-portive psychotherapy designed to develop a relationship with the patient leading to an increased feeling of trust and confidence. This in turn is helpful in maintaining contact with the patient over a long period of time and encouraging the acceptance of appropriate drug regimes. In a few instances more psychoanalytic procedures have been used cautiously, more especially in patients after initial recovery, but no evaluation of results has been adequately carried out. Gilligan[30] concludes from a review of the literature that group psychotherapy, whilst facilitating social rehabilitation, does not produce any basic psychodynamic change.

Social Treatment and Administrative Changes

The change over to the National Health Service provided scope for more money and skills to be directed toward the problem of the treatment of people in mental hospitals. Schizophrenia had remained the disorder least amenable to treatment if this is judged by the extent to which schizophrenic patients tended to remain indefinitely in hospital. More than 60 per cent of the mental hospital population consisted of people suffering from schizophrenia whose prospects at that time of discharge from hospital were remote. Developments took the form of establishing a more liberalizing regime in psychiatric hospitals thereby re-discovering many of the philosophies of treatment practised during the moral era. These changes have been well described[20, 64]. This development was greeted with a mixture of strong enthusiasm and pessimistic criticism which nevertheless led to dramatic changes in the social setting of some hospitals. There was more concern about the welfare of the large number of schizophrenic patients in hospital. Efforts were made to run the hospitals along 'open-door' lines and to do away with seclusion and restraint by means of better classification of patients. The more disturbed patients were grouped together in small groups with a higher complement of skilled nursing staff. Emphasis on habit training and work therapy produced hospitals in which there was less incontinence and less aggressive and disturbed behaviour[61, 68]. The sexes began to mix more freely and programmes of education for the public resulted in a freer acceptance of the mental hospital with an influx of voluntary patients. Diagnoses were made earlier and the acute schizophrenic was treated enthusiastically with social and physical measures. Subsequently, greater emphasis was placed on the screening of all patients prior to admission. A small number of schizophrenic patients could be treated as out-patients. Continuity of care programmes with planned follow-up procedures including out-patient attendance and follow-up visits from psychiatric nurses, social workers and mental welfare officers were designed.

In Britain[8] and Norway[76] there is evidence to suggest that reduction in the hospital population and disturbed behaviour within the hospital had already begun to occur before the advent of the new drugs. Comments by sociologists[7, 18, 85] about the adverse social setting for treatment in mental hospitals profoundly influenced certain psychiatrists with consequent efforts to change the setting of treatment in an attempt to avoid some of the damaging effects of custodial care on the long-stay schizophrenic patient. This led to experiments with group psychotherapy and community therapy and active work programmes designed toward the social rehabilitation and resettlement of the long-stay patient. The advent of the phenothiazine drugs has helped considerably in effecting the changed setting for the treatment of the long-stay schizophrenic patient. This has probably occurred for a multiplicity of reasons. The drugs have reduced the degree of disturbed behaviour and have also assisted the nursing staff in altering their attitudes toward an enthusiastic approach[9]. In an appraisal of papers dealing with phenothiazine drugs in the treatment of long-stay patients, Hughes and Little[45] imply that social changes in themselves have been mainly responsible for improvement in chronic schizophrenia and that prolonged drug therapy may have adverse effects. An apparently irreversible syndrome of choreiform movements in brain damaged elderly patients following prolonged medication with phenothiazines has been described[46]. There are papers[40, 58] which demonstrate that drug therapy has had no effect on the chronic schizophrenic and other papers which show evidence of considerable improvement in chronic schizophrenics treated with drugs. The comparative study of Greenblatt and colleagues[36] in the U.S.A. leaves little doubt about the improvements in chronic schizophrenia that can occur with the use of phenothiazine drugs in patients previously treated in large custodial mental hospital settings and the extent to which this can be complemented by treating the patient in a more satisfactory milieu.

The Mental Health Act of 1959 gave legal sanction for the admission of patients on an informal basis and encouraged the development of community care programmes. These include facilities for sheltered work and sheltered living, but the developments which have occurred so far either through the enthusiasm of the hospital staff or by dint of the Local Authority have been patchy and work effectively in only a few areas. The social treatment programme can be divided into:

(1) programmes of work therapy and rehabilitation
(2) programmes of social and domestic rehabilitation
(3) milieu therapy.

Work Therapy and Rehabilitation Programmes

The work therapy and rehabilitation programmes have been of

predominant importance to the long-stay schizophrenic who, by dint of a combination of illness and hospital stay, could not readily be placed in outside employment. Patients were grouped together for work projects instead of the more traditional occupational therapy. These varied from projects within the hospital of a gardening and building nature to a wide range of industrial remunerative projects. In some instances these occurred in hospital workshops devised to do imple assembly work with sub-contracting arrangements covering a wide range of procedures involving plastics, dismantling of apparatus and toy making. These have been extended from the hospital into the community through Local Authority sheltered workshops and voluntary bodies such as industrial training organizations[23] with factory schemes based on standard factory working conditions both inside and outside of hospital.

In several experiments it was shown that different encouragements such as goal setting, acknowledgement of results, failed to make much impact on schizophrenic patients. Wing and Freudenberg[93] investigated the effect of controlled social pressure brought to bear by familiar staff-nurse supervisors in the workshops and found that under these conditions performance was maintained. Wing and Giddens[92] also assessed the effect of the admission of chronic schizophrenic men from Long Grove Hospital to a course at an industrial rehabilitation unit. These were compared with a controlled sample who remained working as previously within the hospital. The outcome, after six months experiment, indicated that considerable improvement in attitude to work was possible in the moderately ill group attending the unit but was less possible in the more severely ill. Seven of the 20 patients attending were employed and self-supporting one year later. Since then a wide range of experience has been gained in the placement of chronic schizophrenics in work situations. Leopoldt[56] at Littlemore Hospital, Oxford, has described sub-contracting schemes with the Local Authorities for road sweeping and with the Post Office which have been successful in rehabilitating chronic schizophrenic patients to enable regular participation in full-time or part-time employment situations. There is a good deal of evidence to suggest that patients discharged into the community who are unemployed carry a poor prognosis and efforts toward training for practical employment makes the possibilities of establishing the patient outside of the hospital setting much more realistic. Chronic schizophrenics trained in work situations at Littlemore have tended to reach their maximum level of function within the space of a few weeks and it is only rarely that more progress is made at a subsequent date. The greatest difficulty they present is associated with their slowness and diminished capacity for attention in selective tasks. Encapsulated symptoms do not seem to affect work capacity much where adequate social improvement has occurred. Experiments with chronic schizophrenics in the main reflect a fairly rapid initial progress to a level of maximum function with very little subsequent improvement[56]. This is contrary to the findings of Wing[90] and may apply to only some schizophrenics. Whilst these comments apply predominantly to chronic schizophrenic patients, many schizophrenic patients with relapsing illness, out of work for some time, fall into the same category. Brown and his colleagues[16], in their investigation of schizophrenics in the community, assessed the amount of time that the patient is occupied and found a direct relationship between time occupied and family burden, relapse and return to hospital.

Domestic and Social Function

In terms of social programmes this area is less well defined. Many of the groups are designed to deal with the problems of personal relationships and in some hospitals the patients have elected their own foreman and have been responsible for their own assessments in order to encourage participation in decision making and a capacity to tolerate critical judgments[26].

Housewives with disabilities in domestic and home management have participated in programmes which involve re-education in household duties. Social assignments have been devised both within the hospital and in relation to community centres outside of the hospital. There have been many experiments with long-stay schizophrenic patients who have gone to camps for holidays where they and the staff have participated in an experiment in living together[77]. At Littlemore Hospital the most damaged group of schizophrenic patients attend a summer camp each year for a period of one month. Certain hospitals have arranged exchanges of patients to enable them to gain fresh experiences and see different surroundings[11, 12].

Milieu Therapy

This has been well described by many authors[47, 62, 89]. Patients participate in a planned programme consisting of large community meetings, small group therapy meetings and planned work settings. The emphasis is toward total community participation in decision making. There is scope for community understanding of acting out behaviour and personal distress. Emergencies are dealt with by community discussion with a view to learning ways of talking about feelings rather than acting out these feelings. A good description of one such unit is given by a sociologist[87] who spent several months on the Phoenix Unit at Littlemore Hospital. Schwartz and Schwartz[83] describe the changes which took place at the Yale Psychiatric Institute. Attempts were made to alter the milieu from a traditional setting in which a programme of individual psychotherapy took place to that of a community setting with greater participation in the total function of the community. They discuss in detail some of the problems which change presented to the various different disciplines working in the setting and the extent to which there was a shift in the balance of power for decision making. Laing and his colleagues base their programme of milieu and family orientated therapy on the theory that people diagnosed as schizophrenic show a network of disturbed and disturbing communication with those in their immediate environment. They have attempted to produce a milieu within the hospital which is informal and unstructured, avoiding situations producing psychotic behaviour as judged by their studies of schizophrenics and their families[53]. Each patient is assured of a relationship with at least one person significant to him. Treatment is focused on the group of people with whom the patient has to communicate either within the family or within the hospital[24].

PROGRAMMES FOR COMMUNITY CARE

Assessments made in relation to the social outcome of discharged schizophrenic patients indicate that in a varying number of families difficulties arise which reflect problems in tolerance of patient behaviour. In some instances relatives have complained of feeling less well themselves or that the incidences of emotional complaints from the children in the household are more marked[15, 34, 66]. In the latter study a relatively small number of family burdens were found in relation to a follow-up of 171 schizophrenic patients living in the community. Grad and Sainsbury[33] indicate that the problems which are most difficult for the family relate to the demands of the patient where the man is unemployed or the patient stays in bed and is constantly making demands on the relatives. Mandelbrote and Folkard[65] found that parental families tolerate sons better than daughters and that there were more disturbed conjugal than parental families of male patients, but more disturbed parental than conjugal families of female patients. There were also more unemployed male patients in the disturbed parental families. Brown and colleagues[16] found that the degree of emotional stress within the family setting was related to relapse and return to hospital.

As it has become apparent that for many long-stay patients return to the family is unsatisfactory for both patients and relatives, various forms of sheltered accommodation have been developed. In some instances these have taken the form of a hostel with a warden; in others there have been experiments with small group homes consisting of patients known to one another in hospital. These experiments suggest that idiosyncracies and eccentricities are well tolerated. Relapse is infrequent and problems for the community have been minimal. Such group homes have been set up in conjunction with Littlemore Hospital and Severall Hospital psychiatric community services[81]. At Littlemore Hospital[56] group homes have been supported effectively, initially with psychiatric nurse support and subsequently with the help of volunteers, until the patients are eventually self-sufficient.

ASPECTS OF INSTITUTIONALISM

Goffman[31] and others have indicated the effect of a barren life setting on people as a whole and especially on the schizophrenic patient. This may apply to life in prisons and concentration camps but also in relation to large hospitals and welfare settings. It may even have relevance to the family and home if the individual is lacking in initiative and sufficiently withdrawn not to have much contact with other members living in the same setting[6]. The problems of personality change involved and the degree of dependence on the setting militate against satisfactory functioning. The changes effected by social treatments have done much to undo the problems of institutionalism, but these treatments are necessary both within the hospital and the community in vulnerable individuals.

SOCIAL BREAKDOWN SYNDROME

Gruenberg[38], who for a long time has been interested in public health and the reduction of psychiatric disability, has coined the phrase 'social breakdown syndrome' to describe the disordered personal and social relationships which occur in people suffering from psychiatric illnesses. He maintains that the degree of social breakdown is the predominant syndrome which leads to concern on the part of the family and/or community for hospital treatment and pressures on the psychiatrist to admit to hospital. This syndrome usually is present in all the major psychiatric disorders and many people feel that the extent to which this is altered is the true index of change with treatment. Thus in schizophrenia treatment needs will vary in accordance with the degree of social breakdown. Where this is minimal, drugs of the phenothiazine and butyrophenones group may well contain the problem adequately. These are patients who can be treated as out-patients. When the degree of social breakdown is more marked, pressures from the family and community usually lead to hospital admission. Psychiatrists concerned with the concept of social breakdown and its amelioration have attempted to develop a treatment setting which they hope will reduce the degree of social breakdown. In some instances, especially in the initial schizophrenic breakdown, this can be achieved with the use of drugs alone. In the majority of schizophrenics with relapsing illnesses or with poor assets, personality problems and psychosocial difficulties which militate against return to family or community, the treatment setting and social treatments will affect the extent to which the patient will be able to function.

DRUG TREATMENT

By far the commonest phenothiazine drug used is chlorpromazine. This has been followed by an increased use of trifluoperazine (Stelazine), thioridazine (Melleril), perphenazine (Fentazine), prochlorperazine (Stemetil) and, more recently, fluphenazine hydrochloride (Moditen). So far no study has shown unequivocal evidence demonstrating superiority over chlorpromazines. The use of the drugs have very much depended on the therapist's choice and the side effects produced in the patient which may determine whether he will continue with drugs or not. Side effects have been predominantly in the autonomic nervous system and extrapyramidal system, but sensitivity responses, hepatic damage and blood dyscrasias have also occurred. Chlorpromazine has had the disadvantage of photosensitivity which has led to its substitution by thioradazine which does not produce these effects. For the extrapyramidal symptoms antiparkinsonian drugs have been used, predominantly orphenadrine hydrochlor (Disipal) 50 mgm t.d.s. and benzhexol (Artane) 5 mgm t.d.s. Especially in the treatment of acute schizophrenia large doses of phenothiazines have been given, an average dose being chlorpromazine 600 mgm/day, whilst in the maintenance treatment of schizophrenia the dosage has been reduced to the minimum which is not associated with relapse. Chlorpromazine, perphenazine and fluphenazine can be given in liquid form and more recently fluphenazine enanthate by intramuscular injection meets the needs of a long-acting phenothiazine and is a more certain way of ensuring that the patient definitely receives his medication. Unfortunately, it is the most potent of the phenothiazines and careful initial regulation is essential with prompt treatment for the unpleasant extrapyramidal side effects which might occur in some patients. Its dosage varies from 0·25 cm³ to 1 cm³ and more, given initially in weekly dosage and subsequently at intervals of two to four weeks depending on the patient's needs. Reserpine first introduced with the phenothiazines is now rarely used, but the butyrophenones, especially haloperidol, has its exponents and appears to be equally useful as a tranquillizer in schizophrenia.

Osmond and Hoffer[78] claimed that Niacin (nicotinamide adenine dinucleotide N.A.D.) was successful in the treatment of acute and chronic schizophrenic patients, but this has been refuted in a carefully controlled trial by Kline and colleagues[52] who found no consistent differences with a matched group treated with placebo.

CLINICAL AND SOCIAL OUTCOME OF SCHIZOPHRENIA

Because this disorder is not an homogeneous syndrome and the course may be so variable in terms of recovery, relapse, or deterioration, it is appropriate to assess outcome both in clinical and social terms. Follow-up studies can be divided into studies dealing with schizophrenia in its early or late stages. Some of these studies refer to the outcome of first admission schizophrenia as opposed to patients with recurring admissions. Other studies attempt to define early onset patients who have been admitted to hospital within a year of the development of the syndrome as opposed to patients who have been in the hospital for more than two years continuously. Very few papers published before 1945 report any clinical examination of long-stay patients—it was assumed that these patients were unimproved.

ASSESSMENT OF RESULTS OF TREATMENT

The problem of assessing the results of empirical treatment in a syndrome which is non-homogeneous and ill defined is considerable. Nevertheless, much research investigation has been carried out in relation to the outcome of schizophrenia in order to assess the effects of the various treatments outlined. Bannister[5] has criticized many of these investigations on the grounds that they may not be comparing likes and has suggested that in every case of schizophrenia it would be more correct to assess outcome in relation to standard symptoms, or groups of symptoms, rather than make a global diagnostic appraisal.

Clinicians have varied in their diagnostic criteria for schizophrenia depending on the emphasis of Bleulerian or Kraepelinian concepts.

Langfeldt[54, 55] attempts to differentiate schizophrenia syndromes by dividing them into nuclear and process schizophrenia linking these with a good and bad prognosis—concepts not acceptable to many psychiatrists because of the varied prognosis findings[1]. Some psychiatrists, e.g. Fish[25] utilizing Langfeldt's concepts, have implied that statistics dealing with hospital in-patients refer predominantly to a process form of schizophrenia, whilst schizophreniform syndromes are less likely to be referred to the mental hospital. In an attempt to assess the differences between prevalence rates of discharge and referred incidence, Mandelbrote and Monro[69] studied two small communities in Oxfordshire of 8,000 population. In this small but intensive study evidence does not substantiate Fish's belief in that no patient suffering from schizophrenia was discovered who had not had a referral to the hospital service. These reservations need to be borne in mind in relation to the comments made about the results of treatment.

In the early follow-up studies attention was mainly directed toward assessing the hospital outcome of schizophrenia. These studies showed that about 60 per cent of schizophrenics who were admitted to hospital remained there and the assumption was that they were seriously handicapped by reason of illness; 20 per cent recovered relatively quickly and another 20 per cent made a fair social adjustment although they had long-term disabilities of moderate severity and frequent exacerbations of illness[43, 60]. One of the most extensive studies carried out in relation to schizophrenia pre-World War I was that of Mayer-Gross[72]. He followed up the outcome of schizophrenic patients admitted to the Heidelburg Clinic in 1912 and 1913 sixteen years later and found that 38 per cent were outside of hospital (30 per cent well; 8 per cent handicapped by symptoms) whilst 62 per cent had either died or were still in the institution. The proportion of these deaths were attributed to conditions in German mental hospitals during World War I.

During the next 30 years the hospital course of the illness showed some improvement, but the studies carried out were not comparable with Mayer-Gross's study in that the length of follow-up was much shorter. Long-term hospital care became associated with a much lower death rate, shorter stay in hospital and greater likelihood of discharge from hospital[44, 67]. Guttman, Mayer-Gross and Slater[39] followed up schizophrenic patients of less than one year duration, under the age of 46, who were discharged from the Maudsley in 1934–35, found three years later that 43 per cent were functioning moderately well in the community and 6 per cent had died. Harris and colleagues[42] studied schizophrenic patients admitted to the Maudsley for insulin therapy between 1945 and 1946 and found five years later that 50 per cent were socially independent and managing well. Ackner and Oldham[2], following up patients between the age of 18 and 40 at the Maudsley who were treated either with insulin or barbiturate induced coma, found that 58 per cent were socially independent three years after follow-up and 44 per cent of these showed good clinical recovery. Kelly and Sargent[51] compared the results of two groups of schizophrenic patients of recent onset, treated with insulin coma and with phenothiazine drugs. A two year follow-up study showed that of the patients treated with phenothiazine drugs 67 per cent were socially independent whilst only 31 per cent were symptom free. Although Kelly and Sargent expressed the opinion that the present treatment with phenothiazines is far superior to that shown in the insulin coma treatment group, the improvements they showed were mostly in the sphere of social independence rather than in the clinical field. Clinically there was a shift of emphasis from psychotic to residual symptoms but no statistical difference in the number of patients who were symptom free.

The value of insulin coma in the treatment of schizophrenia was seriously questioned in the study of Ackner and Oldham[2] when it was found that there was virtually no difference in the outcome of two groups of people between the ages of 18 and 40 with early schizophrenia treated at the Maudsley Hospital with either insulin or induced barbiturate coma and assessed three years after termination of treatment. Ackner and Oldham's conclusions were that insulin coma appeared to have no specific effect in the treatment of schizophrenia. Markowe, Steinert and Heyworth-Davis[71] in a ten year follow-up of matched patients treated with insulin coma and phenothiazines, did not find any marked difference in the social or clinical outcome of the patients; women patients improved significantly more than men; 45 per cent were free of symptoms; 53 per cent were rated as having a normal social life and 71 per cent were in employment over the last 12 months of the ten year follow-up. Changes in attitude toward compulsory detention and enthusiastic use of drug therapy and social therapy have led to a marked alteration in the pattern of hospital stay of the schizophrenic patient. Whereas Vera Norris[75] indicated that 50–60 per cent of patients admitted to hospital remained for more than one year, and subsequently almost indefinitely, more recently the figure is of the order of 10–15 per cent and, in at least one hospital, 0–5 per cent[62].

In an attempt to assess the therapeutic efficacy of phenothiazine drugs Goldberg, Klerman and Cole[32] compared patients with recent onset schizophrenia treated with chlorpromazine and placebos. They found that whilst 30–40 per cent showed some improvement on placebos after six weeks of treatment, 95 per cent showed some improvement with chlorpromazine. Both sets of patients were treated in the same setting. Perhaps the best evidence of the value of drugs is seen in studies of continuous treatment[37, 79]. Gross and colleagues withdrew phenothiazine drugs in one group of patients and replaced them with a placebo of identical appearance. Of these patients 54 per cent relapsed compared with only 14 per cent of the subjects who continued with phenothiazines. Pasamanick and colleagues, in a double blind study, demonstrated that over 18 months 83 per cent of schizophrenic patients treated with phenothiazines remained continuously in the community compared with 55 per cent of those given a placebo. Both communities were under the careful supervision of public health nurses. In both studies half the schizophrenic patients remained well without drugs and one-sixth relapsed in spite of continuous administration of phenothiazines—highlighting two aspects of the problem of schizophrenia. The natural history of spontaneous remission and the question of determining whether patients took their drugs adequately to enable a reliably valid experiment to be carried out. Schizophrenics share the reluctance of many other psychiatrically and physically ill patients to take drugs over short or long periods irrespective of their efficacy.

Hare and Wilcox[41] have shown that even with in-patient management a substantial proportion of patients do not take their drugs as prescribed and that this problem is more marked in relation to day-patient and out-patients[88]. The use of intramuscular long-acting fluphenazine enanthate may overcome this difficulty and preliminary work suggests that relapsing patients treated in this way show a much better response than would be anticipated on statistical grounds[17, 21].

The studies described deal with the supposedly best prognostic group of schizophrenic patients, i.e. recent onset with acute symptoms and good previous personality, or patients who had not been treated previously for schizophrenia. The general impression in relation to the follow-up study of this group of patients indicate that less patients became permanently hospitalized, more made a good social recovery, but that the number free of symptoms on clinical assessment is still less than 50 per cent.

For the long-stay schizophrenics and the schizophrenics who have spent long continuous spells in hospital as part of the legacy of past management the position has also changed by dint of the social treatments and drug therapies. Whereas previously very few patients who had stayed in hospital for more than two years were discharged from hospital, at Littlemore, in a unit dealing with the rehabilitation of long-stay moderately ill schizophrenics, whose average duration of illness is ten years, out of an original group of 90 patients only 27 are still in hospital. Out of these 27 ten have remained continuously in hospital and the remainder have spent varying periods in sheltered accommodation and sheltered work but at the time of assessment were back in hospital. A seven year follow-up shows that seven patients have died (two suicides) 56 are in the community—28 of these are functioning independently; 16 of them are in group homes and 12 are living in hostel accommodation but functioning satisfactorily. Clinical evidence of schizophrenic illness is, however, apparent in the majority of the patients. Of a further 185 patients suffering from schizophrenia who have passed through the unit, at present only one has remained continuously in hospital for more than 12 months. However, many have had relapsing ill-nesses and have been treated in the out-patient clinics or readmitted at intervals to hospital.

Criticisms about the extent to which the changed management has led to increase of readmissions, premature discharge from hospital with inadequate treatment and heavier burdens for family and community cannot be dismissed lightly. In the main, despite re-admissions, schizophrenic patients are spending much less total time in hospital and show a much greater degree of social recovery and competence. Family and community burdens are present, but this does not necessarily mean that the position would best be resolved by hospitalization. The conclusion of Wing[91] in a five year follow-up study of patients treated in three psychiatric hospitals were that the course of schizophrenia since patients were treated with pheno-thiazines and an improved treatment setting resulted in an increase in the recovered group from 35 to 55 per cent. It remains for us to discover ways of alleviating family and community burdens by better follow-up services, better control of the taking of pheno-thiazine drugs, and the provision of supervised accommodation in group homes or hostels in cases where the relationships with the family are incompatible.

FUTURE INVESTIGATIONS

With the possibility of a more satisfactory control of drug taking with long acting intramuscular preparations it should be easier to assess the clinical outcome of the syndrome in relation to factors which are reputed to be indicators of good prognosis:

(1) The illness of acute onset as opposed to insidious onset.

(2) The predominantly paranoid illness as opposed to the predominantly hebephrenic.

(3) Unsatisfactory premorbid personality as opposed to good previous personality.

(4) Good work record pre-illness as opposed to poor work record pre-illness.

(5) Family accepting with facilities for accommodation of patient as opposed to unfavourable psychosocial setting with no real placement in the community apart from hostel or group homes.

The clinical parameter and the social parameter affecting the outcome of the illness do not necessarily go side by side. There are some patients who, despite delusions and hallucinations and evidence of moderate clinical illness, make independent social adjustment and have good work records. In a recent study Mandelbrote and Trick[70] compared patients with schizophrenia, who had remained in the community for more than two years after discharge from hospital, with patients who had remained continuously in hospital and found that whilst they do not show striking differences in their clinical rating they do show striking differences in social outcome. In the one instance the patient is able to be socially independent in the community and in the other the patient is socially dependent on the hospital setting.

The concept of social breakdown and its implication, despite the work of Gruenberg[38], has not yet been adequately assessed in relation to different treatment settings with standardized drug procedure. Evidence is suggestive that the long-term morbidity of schizophrenia has been considerably reduced when treated with drugs in an improved social milieu. With the use of well supervised group homes and long acting phenothiazine drugs given by injection it will be interesting to see whether the adverse social and psychological factors that produce difficulty in returning the patient to the family or community will continue to apply.

The enigma of schizophrenia however remains. Is this a group of syndromes like epilepsy which will eventually become a smaller and smaller segment of unclear aetiology? Can we still delineate schizophrenia into:

(a) A condition which remits completely spontaneously?

(b) A relapsing condition amenable to drug treatment and social and psychological influence?

(c) A condition inevitably becoming chronic in nature with serious impairment of personality and functional capacity.

How can we predict which of these courses the initial illness will take? These are questions which future research should eventually answer.

REFERENCES

1. Achte, K. A. (1961). 'The Course of Schizophrenic and Schizophreniform Psychoses'. *Acta psychiat. neurol. scand.* Suppl. 155
2. Ackner, B. and Oldham, A. J. (1962). 'Insulin Treatment of Schizophrenia: A Three Year Follow-up of a Controlled Study'. *Lancet* **1,** 504
3. Appel, K. E., Myers, J. M. and Scheflen, A. E. (1953). 'Prognosis in Psychiatry: Results of Psychatric Treatment'. *A.M.A. Archs Neurol. Psychiat.* **70,** 459
4. — Lhamon, W. T., Myers, J. M. and Harvey, W. A. (1953). Long-term Psychotherapy in Psychiatric Treatment'. *Res. Publs Ass. Res. nerv. ment. Dis.* **31,** 21
5. Bannister, D. (1968). 'The Logical Requirements of Research in Schizophrenia'. *Br. J. Psychiat.* **114,** 181
6. Barton, R. (1959). *Institutional Neurosis.* Bristol: John Wright
7. Belknap, I. (1956). *Human Problems of a State Mental Hospital.* New York: McGraw-Hill
8. Bell, G. M. (1955). 'A Mental Hospital with Open Doors'. *Int. Soc. Psychiat.* **1,** 42
9. Bennett, D. H. (1967). *New Aspects of the Mental Health Services.* Ed. by H. Freeman. Oxford: Pergamon Press
10. Betz, B. J. and Whitehorn, J. C. (1956). 'The relationship of the Therapist to the Outcome of Therapy in Schizophrenia'. *Psychiat. Res. Rep.* No. 5
11. Bickford, J. R. (1961). 'The Rehabilitation of Schizophrenics'. *Lancet* **2,** 1082
12. — and Millar, H. J. B. (1959). 'Exchange of Patients by Mental Hospitals'. *Lancet* **2,** 96
13. Bockoven, J. S. (1956). 'Moral Treatment in American Psychiatry', *J. nerv. ment. Dis.* **124,** 167
14. — (1956). 'Moral Treatment in American Psychiatry'. *J. nerv. ment. Dis.,* **124,** 292
15. Brown, G. W., Monck, E. M., Carstairs, G. M. and Wing, J. K. (1962). 'Influence of Family Life on the Course of Schizophrenic Illness'. *Br. J. prev. soc. Med.* **16,** 55
16. — Bone, M., Dalison, B. and Wing, J. K. (1966). *Schizophrenia and Social Care: A Comparative Follow-up Study of 339 Schizophrenic Patients.* Maudsley Monograph No. 17. London: Oxford University Press

17. Capstick, N. and Oliver, J. E. (1966). 'Fluphenazine Enanthate in the Maintenance Treatment of Schizophrenia'. *Br. med. J.* **2,** 1962
18. Caudill, W. (1958). *The Psychiatric Hospital as a Small Society.* Cambridge, Mass.: Harvard University Press
19. Cerletti, U. and Bini, L. (1938). 'Electroshock'. *Boll. Atti Accad. Med.* **64,** 36
20. Clark, D. H. (1965). 'The Therapeutic Community—Concept, Practice and Future'. *Br. J. Psychiat.* **111,** 947
21. Dillon, J. B. and Bates, N. T. J. (1966). 'Fluphenazine Enanthate in the Maintenance Treatment of Schizophrenia'. *Br. Med. J.* **2,** 1328
22. Drasgow, J. (1957). 'A Criterion for Chronicity in Schizophrenia'. *Psychiat. Q.* **31,** 454
23. Early, D. F. (1965). 'Economic Rehabilitation'. In *Psychiatric Hospital Care*, p. 176. Ed. by H. Freeman. London: Baillière, Tindall and Cassell
24. Esterson, A., Cooper, D. G. and Laing, R. D. (1965). 'Results of Family-orientated Therapy with Hospitalized Schizophrenics'. *Br. med. J.* **2,** 1462
25. Fish, F. J. (1962). *Schizophrenia.* Bristol: John Wright
26. Freeman, J., Mandelbrote, B. and Waldron, J. (1965). 'Attitudes to Discharge Among Long-stay Mental Hospital Patients and Their Relation to Social and Clinical Factors'. *Br. J. soc. clin. Psychol.* **4,** 270
27. Freeman, W. (1965). *Frontal Lobotomy (1936–1956): A Follow-up Study of 3,000 Patients from One to Twenty Years.* Presented at the Annual Meetings of the American Psychiatric Association. Chicago
28. — and Watts, J. W. (1942). *Psychosurgery, Intelligence Emotion and Social Behaviour Following Prefrontal Lobotomy for Mental Disorder.* Springfield, Ill.: Charles C. Thomas
29. Fromm-Reichmann, Freda (1948). 'Notes on the Development of Treatment of Schizophrenics by Psychoanalytic Psychotherapy'. *Psychiatry* **11,** 263
30. Gilligan, J. (1965). In *Drug and Social Therapy in Chronic Schizophrenia.* Ed. by M. Greenblatt, H. H. Solomon, A. S. Evans and G. W. Brooks. Springfield, Ill.: Charles C. Thomas
31. Goffman, E. (1961). *Asylums.* New York: Doubleday
32. Goldberg, S. C., Klerman, G. L. and Cole, J. O. (1965). 'Changes in Schizophrenic Psychopathology and Ward Behaviour as a Function of Phenothiazine Treatment'. *Br. J. Psychiat.* **111,** 120
33. Grad, J. C. and Sainsbury, P. (1963). 'Mental Illness and the Family'. *Lancet* **1,** 44
34. — — (1966). 'Problems of Caring for the Mentally Ill at Home'. *Proc. R. Soc.* **59,** 20
35. Greenblatt, M., York, R. H. and Brown, E. L. (1955). *From Custodial to Therapeutic Care in Mental Hospital.* New York: Russell Sage Foundation

36. — Solomon, M. H., Evans, A. S. and Brooks, G. W. (Eds) (1965). *Drugs and Social Therapy in Chronic Schizophrenia*. Springfield, Ill.: Charles C. Thomas

37. Gross, M. (1961). Discussion of Kris, Else B. (1961). Children Born to Mothers Maintained on Pharmocotherapy During Pregnancy and Postpartum: *Recent Adv. biol. Psychiat.* **4**, 180, 186

38. Gruenberg, E. M. (1967). 'The Social Breakdown Syndrome—Some Origins'. *Am. J. Psychiat.* **123**, 1481

39. Guttmann, E., Mayer-Gross, W. and Slater, E. T. O. (1939). 'Short-distance Prognosis of Schizophrenia'. *J. Neurol. Psychiat., Lond.* **2**, 1

40. Hamilton, M. (1965). 'Ten years of Chlorpromazine'. *Compreh. Psychiat.* **6**, 291

41. Hare, E. H. and Wilcox, D. R. C. (1967). 'Do Psychiatric In-patients take their Pills?' *Br. J. Psychiat.* **113**, 1435

42. Harris, A., Linker, I., Norris, V. and Shepherd, M. (1956). 'Schizophrenia: A Prognostic and Social Study'. *Br. J. prev. soc. Med.* **10**, 107

43. Hastings, D. W. (1958). 'Follow-up Results in Psychiatric Illness'. *Am. J. Psychiat.* **114**, 12

44. Hoenig, J. and Hamilton, M. W. (1965). 'Social Agency Care of Schizophrenic Patients'. *Med. Offr.* **114**, 303

45. Hughes, J. S. and Little, J. Crawford (1967). 'Tranquillising Drugs for Long Stay Patients: An Appraisal'. *Br. J. Psychiat.* **113**, 867

46. Hunter, R., Earl, C. J. and Thornicroft, S. (1964). 'An Apparently Irreversible Syndrome of Abnormal Movements Following Pheno-thiazine Medication'. *Proc. R. Soc. Med.* **57**, 758

47. Jones, M. (1962). *Social Psychiatry in the Community, in Hospitals and in Prisons*. Springfield, Ill.: Charles C. Thomas,

48. Kalinowsky, L. B. (1958). 'Appraisal of the "Tranquillizers" and Their Influence on Other Somatic Treatments in Psychiatry'. *Am. J. Psychiat.* **115**, 294

49. — (1958). 'Physical Treatments in Psychiatry'. *J. ment. Sci.* **104**, 553

50. — and Hoch, P. H. (1952). *Somatic Shock Treatments, Psycho-surgery and other Treatments in Psychiatry*, 2nd edn. New York: Grune and Stratton; London: Heinemann

51. Kelly, D. H. W. and Sargant, W. (1965). 'Present Treatment of Schizophrenia'. *Br. med. J.* **1**, 147

52. Kline, N. S. Barclay, G. L., Cole, J. O., Esser, A. H., Lehmann, H. and Wittenborn J. R. (1967). 'Controlled Evaluation of Nicotin-amide Adenine Dinucleotide in the Treatment of Chronic Schizo-phrenic Patients'. *Br. J. Psychiat.* **113**, 731

53. Laing, R. D. and Esterson, A. (1964). 'Sanity, Madness and the Family'. *Families of Schizophrenics*, Vol. 1. London: Tavistock Publications

54. Langeldt, G. (1952). 'Some Points Regarding the Symptomatology and Diagnosis of Schizophrenia'. *Acta psychiat. scand.* Suppl. 80

55. — (1956). 'The Prognosis of Schizophrenia'. *Acta psychiat. scand.* Suppl. 110

56. Leopoldt, H. K. (1967). 'Schizophrenia'. *Rehabilitation* **60,** 48

57. — (1967). 'New Approach to Psychiatric Care'. *Nurs. Mirror* **125,** 10

58. Letemendia, F. J. J. and Harris, A. D. (1967). 'Chlorpromazine and the Untreated Schizophrenic—A Long-term Trial'. *Br. J. Psychiat.* **113,** 950

59. McKissock, W. (1943). 'Technique of Pre-frontal Leucotomy'. *J. ment. Sci.* **89,** 194

60. Malamud, W. and Render, I. N. (1939). 'Course and Prognosis in Schizophrenia'. *Am. J. Psychiat.* **95,** 1039

61. Mandelbrote, B. M. (1958). 'An Experiment in the Rapid Conversion of a Closed Mental Hospital into an Open-door Hospital'. *Ment. Hyg.* **42,** 3

62. — (1964). *Mental Illness in Hospital and Community: Developments and Outcome,* p. 267. (For the Nuffield Provincial Hospitals Trust—Essays on current research.) London: Oxford University Press

63. — (1965). 'The Use of Psychodynamic and Sociodynamic Principles in the Treatment of Psychotics: A Change from Ward Unit Concepts to Grouped Communities'. *Compreh. Psychiat.* **6,** No. 6

64. — (1965). *Therapeutic Aspects of Organization. Factors Associated with the Rapid Conversions of a Custodial Institution into a Therapeutic Community.* Ed. by H. Freeman. London: Baillière, Tindall and Cassell

65. — and Folkard, S. P. (1961). 'Some Factors Related to Outcome and Social Adjustment in Schizophrenia'. *Acta psychiat. scand.* **37,** 223

66. — — (1961). 'Some Problems and Needs of Schizophrenics in Relation to a Developing Psychiatric Community Service'. *Compreh. Psychiat.* **2,** 6

67. — — (1963). 'The Outcome of Schizophrenia in Relation to a Developing Community Psychiatric Service'. *Ment. Hyg.* **47,** 43

68. — and Freeman, H. L. (1963). 'The Closed Group Concept in Open Psychiatric Hospitals'. *Am. J. Psychiat.* **119,** 763

69. — and Monro May (1964). 'The Prevalence of Psychiatric Morbidity, and its Relevance to Future Planning'. Presented at Spring Meeting, R. M. P. A., Oxford. Unpublished

70. — and Trick, K. L. (1969). 'Social and Clinical Factors in the Outcome of Schizophrenia'. *Acta psychiat. scand.* In press

71. Markowe, M., Steinert, J. and Heyworth-Davis, F. (1967). 'Insulin and Chlorpromazine in Schizophrenia'. *Br. J. Psychiat.* **113,** 1101

72. Mayer-Gross, W. (1932). In *Handbuch der Geisterkrankheiten,* Vol. 9, p. 534. Ed. by O. Bumke. Berlin: Springer

73. Moniz, E. (1936). *Tentatives Operatoires dans le Traitement de Certaines Psychoses'.* Paris: Masson et Cie

74. Monro, May (1965). *A Contribution to Psychiatric Epidemiology—A Comparative Study of Neurotic Illness. Unpublished M. D. Thesis.* University of Aberdeen

75. Norris, Vera (1959). *Mental Illness in London.* Maudsley Monograph No. 6. London: Oxford University Press

76. Odegaard, O. (1964). 'Pattern of Discharge from Norwegian Psychiatric Hospitals Before and After the Introduction of the Psychotropic Drugs'. *Am. J. Psychiat.* **120,** 772

77. Ortega, M. J., Williams, M,. Bewick, J. H. and Cherry, D. N. (1964). 'Psychiatric Patients at Camp'. *Nurs. Mirror* **125,** 75

78. Osmond, H. and Hoffer, A. (1962). 'Massive Niacin Treatment in Schizophrenia. Review of a Nine Year Study'. *Lancet* **1,** 316

79. Pasamanick, B. (1964). 'Home Versus Hospital Care for Schizophrenia'. *J. Am. med. Ass.* **187,** 177

80. Paul, N. L. and Greenblatt, M. (1958). 'Psychosurgery and Schizophrenia'. In *Schizophrenia: A Review of the Syndrome*, p. 501. Ed. by L. Bellak. New York: Logos Press

81. Phoenix Group Homes (1967). *People Without Homes. First Annual Report.* Colchester, Essex: Manor Press

82. Pippard, J. (1955). 'Rostrol Leucotomy. A Report on 240 Cases. Personal Follow-up After 1½–5 Years. Volume for 1955'. *J. ment. Sci.* **101,** 756

83. Schwartz, M. S. and Schwartz, C. G. (1964). *Social Approaches to Mental Patient Care.* New York, London: Columbia University Press

84. Standt, V. M. and Zubin, J. (1957). 'A Biometric Evaluation of the Somatotherapies in Schizophrenia—A Critical Review. *Psychol. Bull.* **54,** 171

85. Stanton, A. H. and Schwartz, M. S. (1954). *The Mental Hospital: A Study of Institutional Participation in Psychiatric Illness and Treatment.* New York: Basic Books

86. Stephens, J. H. and Astrup, Ch. (1965). 'Treatment Outcome in Process and Non-process Schizophrenics Treated By "A" and "B" Types of Therapists'. *J. nerv. ment. Dis.* **140,** 449

87. Sugarman, B. (1968). The Phoenix Unit: Alliance Against Illness. In *The New Society.* London: New Science

88. Willcox, D. R. C., Gillan, R. and Hare, E. H. (1965). 'Do Psychiatric Out-patients Take Their Drugs?' *Br. med. J.* **2,** 790

89. Wilmer, H. A. (1958). 'Toward a Definition of a Therapeutic Community'. *Am. J. Psychiat.* **114,** 824

90. Wing, J. K. (1961). 'Attitudes to the Employability of Chronic Schizophrenic Patients'. *Occup. Psychol.* **35,** 58

91. — (1965). 'Community Services for Schizophrenic Patients'. *Proceedings of the Leeds Symposium on Behavioural Disorders*, Chap. 19. Dagenham: May and Baker

92.　　— and Giddens, R. G. T. (1959). 'Industrial Rehabilitation of Male Chronic Schizophrenics'. *Lancet* **2,** 507
93.　　— and Freudenberg, R. K. (1961). 'The Response of Severely Ill Chronic Schizophrenic Patients to Social Stimulation'. *Am. J. Psychiat.* **118,** 311

CHAPTER 9

THE THERAPEUTIC COMMUNITY

JOHN HARDING PRICE

INTRODUCTION

There are for the general psychiatrist two initially distinct therapeutic communities, the hospital community and the general community. Until recent years the psychiatrist was solely concerned with the hospital—to-day his role has been enlarged and he is becoming equally concerned with the structure of society in the general community. There are three main reasons for this change. The first reason is the extension of psychoanalytic techniques. A patient undergoing modern psychotherapeutic treatment lives in the community. His visits to the psychiatrist do not separate him from the community. They are as routine as his visits to the general practitioner. A second cause may be found in the advance of physical treatments. Patients who would formerly have stayed many years in hospital now benefit from modern treatments and soon return to the community. In the United Kingdom there is a third reason for the change in the psychiatrist's role—the 1959 Mental Health Act[121, 154] which requires that the community (i.e. the local authorities) shall make provision for patients who are mentally ill and can be contained in the community but do not need treatment in hospital. It is required, for instance, that the local authorities shall appoint mental welfare officers and provide training centres and residential hostels.

In this review the psychiatrist's roles and responsibilities will be considered in hospital, the ward and the community.

Most general communities in peacetime are themselves therapeutic[135, 183] because they provide a suitable environment in which the personalities can develop. The community is established either naturally by genetic, family and geographical considerations or by a process of self selection where a common psychological bond exists, as occurs in music circles or trade union movements. All hospital communities are drawn together artificially; their common factor is illness, but in the case of the psychiatric hospital this factor divides the community. Therefore, if the patient is to benefit by his stay in hospital the psychiatric unit must provide a counter-balance to these divisions. It is important to realize that the role of the psychiatrist in the hospital and ward cannot be divorced from his role in the community.

THE HOSPITAL THERAPEUTIC COMMUNITY

Changes in Hospital Policy

Great changes have taken place in most hospital communities following the work of Rees during the 1950s[141, 142]. The old uncompromising totalitarian approach[5, 43, 47, 75, 80, 115, 158] has been swept away and patients are encouraged to take part in the life of the community[79, 80, 81, 82]. This participation reduces both personal anxieties and such general community anxieties as, for example, the fear of entering hospital. When these anxieties are reduced, the patient's chance of adjusting satisfactorily to his environment on his discharge is greatly increased.

Under the former authoritarian system, also, it was very difficult for the patient to establish therapeutic contact between himself and other patients or between himself and any member of the staff, except the one in whose care he had specifically been placed. The Medical Superintendent was personally responsible for everything that happened to every patient and the patient therefore became subject to immutable rules as soon as he entered hospital. Now the patient has regained a large measure of the personal freedom that he enjoyed outside the hospital. Recent developments have made possible a wider intermingling of patients and staff and therefore the patient can avoid antagonistic situations and make contact with the persons who have most to offer him in resolving his crises and aiding his recovery[74, 116, 117, 145]. These therapeutic advances are common to most mental hospitals[56, 111] although each hospital community will develop its own characteristic patterns. Nevertheless, there are certain basic features which should be present in every hospital community which includes psychiatric patients in its care. These features, together with any specific treatment required, are essential for the development of the patient's personal occupational and social life.

Organization of the Psychiatric Firm and Ward Policy

The organization[103] of the wards often presents a major problem. Patients should be admitted to the ward which corresponds most closely to their state of health and to their personal and social condition. The psychiatrist therefore requires the following minimum facilities in order to provide his patients with both the service which they need and the continuing care of a personal doctor which is an integral part of any psychiatric relationship.

(1) Infirmary wards

(2) Psychogeriatric wards—these wards themselves must also have infirmary facilities.

(3) Neurosis wards—these units also require facilities for a mother and baby unit—such a unit is preferably directly attached. The function of these wards is to provide specific treatment for disease processes but also, more fundamentally, to enable the patient to learn from his illness. He has to come to recognize those factors which he could previously not understand and which, in consequence, directly affected his decompensation.

(4) Acute psychotic wards—the purpose of these units is to treat those patients whose illness renders them out of touch with reality.

(5) and (6) At least two Residential wards—these units are divided into those housing patients mainly at work in the hospital community and those housing patients normally at work in the general community. This latter group have acquired economic independence and they require only the minimum nursing supervision. They often attain a degree of freedom which is not practical in most homes.

(7) Deteriorated wards—for the presenile dementias, post-encephalitics, and severe brain damaged patients.

(8) Character disorder (Social rehabilitation ward)—this unit is for the stabilized psychopath who is acquiring the grace necessary to establish himself safely with other people in a home.

Access to the above facilities enables every psychiatrist to look after all the cases referred to him and to make appropriate admission arrangements. *Figures 1, 2* and *3*, illustrations of modern hospital treatment, contrast with the old textbook pictures illustrating schizophrenia and institutionalization which showed patients sitting about listlessly on benches.

The ideal size of each ward is 25–30 beds. The sexes normally mix and these wards should, therefore, be integrated. Each psychiatric clinical firm requires 400–600 beds. The minimum medical staff necessary to operate the firm with its outside commitments are two consultants, four senior doctors with considerable psychiatric experience and four other full-time medical staff. In addition one psychologist is required. The number of psychiatric social workers and their location will depend on whether the firm serves primarily an urban or a rural district. Much of the routine work, especially in the social rehabilitation ward and the outworkers wards, is done by patients. Nevertheless, the calibre of nurses available as charge nurses and ward sisters is most important, for in the therapeutic community they have direct responsibilities to their patients. The sisters are aided and supported in this work by the nursing staff whose constant presence is more than an important and stabilizing factor in the treatment of the patient. The daily contact provides the basis for the social intercourse which is a necessary basis for the development of the therapeutic community. Decisions about leave and exeats, for instance, can invariably be left to the ward sister. She can also deal with the question of locking the ward[11, 114, 156, 157, 164]

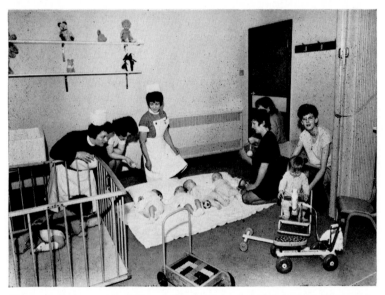

Figure 1. Patients and children in the nursery of the Mother and Baby Unit, St. John's Hospital, Lincoln

although there is rarely any need for this measure nowadays. Visiting is also left to the ward sister's discretion. It is normally unrestricted except that it is subject to the patient's personal condition and the medical state of the patients in the ward.

Upon admission, patients can be provided with a brochure outlining the hospital's function and duties and drawing their attention to their importance[81] not only in the domestic running of the ward but also as active participants in the social milieu. They are required to bring their own clothes and personal requisites into hospital and to be responsible for them and their laundry arrangements.

Each set of wards should be a unit and develop as far as possible its own potential as a therapeutic community[49]. Thus the hospital provides a diverse experience for different people, but without forcing patients to live intimately with those with whom they have no common bond. This policy is enhanced by having smaller units or subdivisions within each ward and this is particularly desirable when the wards have other functions for day patients or serve as night hostels.

The physical conditions of each ward and its decor require constant review. Particular attention should be paid to adequate day space, quiet and noisy rooms and privacy in both sleeping and toilet accommodation. Each patient needs a private lockable wardrobe and dressing table. Nevertheless, morale is always more important than decor.

The changes in psychiatric treatment have reduced the number of beds required. Most estimates show that 1·8 beds per 1000 of the population are required for the mentally ill and certainly hospitals based on this figure can provide properly for their catchment area[167].

In the future, provision will have to be made for some inadequate families[69] to be housed upon the hospital campus. The principle here is no different from that of any other subsidized housing and indeed many of these problem families are potentially economically viable. However, such a scheme affords the necessary opportunities for family therapy amongst problem families.

Two or three clinical psychiatric firms can then share the ancillary services which are necessary for the patient's rehabilitation.

Rehabilitation Services

The majority of people spend a large part of their time at work. Therefore, if patients are to be successfully rehabilitated into the general community, it is essential that they should continue to work whenever this is possible[187, 190]. Some patients are able to follow their own occupation during their hospital treatment; for others, the hospital itself must make provision.

The rehabilitation services consist of those available at ward level, traditional occupational therapy and individual therapy units[172, 173]. The domestic work of the ward should, wherever possible, be done by the patients as though they were in their own homes. Hospitals are not hotels: enforced periods of useless idleness serve no therapeutic purpose and do not equip people to take part in life. The domestic work of the infirmaries and deteriorated wards can be undertaken by patients from other units and excellent opportunities for integration of the sexes are thus presented. Psychopaths particularly benefit from domestic work in the senile unit where they show great tenderness and care. Male neurotics learn of the drudgery attached to much home life and often see more clearly the effects of their own behaviour mirrored upon other women. All patients learn of the distress of others and then put their illness into perspective.

The traditional occupational therapy department can provide basket work, embroidery, rug making, knitting, sewing and weaving, as well as minor carpentry, art classes and pottery. These classes, apart from preventing lethargy, are invaluable as a stimulus towards the industrial unit and they have particular value if they stimulate an interest which the patient can continue after discharge. The articles produced can be used in the hospital community or sold to the general public. In these units the work is not done with a commercial end in view, but the patients do receive pocket money.

Patients can be seconded to the hospital departments either to work or to receive a training from the artisan staff who should themselves receive a reward for these re-educative duties. The hospital catering, tailoring and shoe repairing, gardening, farm, clerical and engineering departments should all be prepared to receive patients. Patients who are nurses can be employed in the infirmary wards of the hospital or in the neighbouring general hospitals.

The patients are rewarded initially on a flat rate according to their abilities. In assessing the reward, account must be taken of the cost of maintaining the patient. Too large a reward will leave the patient more pocket money than he would have if he worked competitively and the domestic and occupational rewards must themselves provide graded financial incentive. Additional incentive is provided by the companionship available in the residential wards.

It is advisable to have at least one hospital department providing services for other hospitals and establishments. The hospital laundry, tailoring, printing department or catering services are admirably suited to this. Patients can now graduate on to the hospital paid staff and so further their training. They can then choose where they will live—in the hospital staff residences or in the general community.

Many patients today move through a different sequence of progress on the way to economic independence. In order to achieve this progression, hospitals have developed industrial therapy departments[3, 67, 172] and two distinct patterns of development are occurring in hospitals.

The Industrial Therapy Organization (I.T.O.) at Bristol aims to provide a unit in the general community which is itself economically viable, but which provides patients with a sheltered occupation[65, 66, 67]. This programme has been successfully copied and expanded by the St. Bernard's Hospital programme (I.T.O. Thames).

The Lincolnshire scheme consists of establishing a multi-purpose factory within the hospital and, in addition, providing access to a large amount of employment in the general community. The multi-purpose factory contracts for work in the open market and pays patients according to the work done and normal standards. Hospital industrial units are now paying attention to the working conditions of their employees including the lighting, the installation of machines, industrial seating, and continuous belt processes. General factors such as canteen facilities, vending machines, music while you work, and time sheets and clocks, are also being studied. Of the patients working in the industrial unit 35 per cent were discharged from the

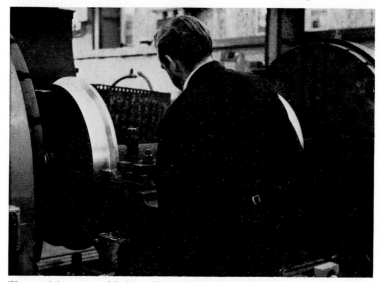

(Photograph by courtesy of Redbourn Works, British Steel Corporation)

Figure 2. Long-stay patient (chronic schizophrenic) trained as a skilled centre lathe turner

hospital in each of the years 1965 and 1966. When the patient is considered ready to work outside the hospital the rehabilitation staff, which includes charge nurses and factory personnel officers, are responsible for securing suitable employment for the patient and then continuing his medical stabilization. This last task is completely supervised by the works medical officer and his staff. The industrial medical officer must also have direct access and communication with the hospital and the authority to return patients to the hospital in an emergency. At the same time industry have the assurance that if they are worried by any employee they can call in the psychiatrist.

Formerly it was felt that the remote location of many hospitals precluded industrial rehabilitation. It has now been shown that with modern transport this is no longer an important factor[138]. When the local employers accept the value of patient labour, diverse facilities are immediately available to suit their abilities. Prejudice is further reduced when patients admitted from industry are able to continue

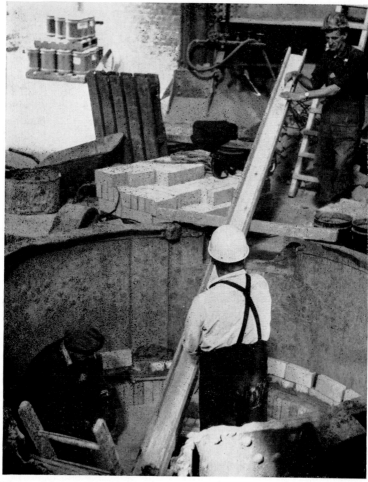

(Photograph by courtesy of Redbourn Works, British Steel Corporation)

Figure 3. Three schizophrenic patients laying bricks in a ladle

at their work and these patients are, moreover, often instrumental in obtaining employment for their less fortunate colleagues. Great care is necessary on the part of the medical staff in selecting patients, particularly in selecting the first patients who work in open industry. The interaction between the patients and their workmates creates a healthy and productive tension, which is enhanced by the tolerance and understanding of both management and labour in the works.

The new-found economic freedom encourages the patient to develop his independence. He is able to provide his own personal requisites and clothing and he is able to pay towards his maintenance costs. The hospital continues to provide working clothes if the patient requests them. These hospital clothes, although hardly fashionable, are very strong and hard-wearing and these qualities have even been known to cause envious comment amongst their fellow workmen! As many as 20 per cent of the hospital community's patients can be at work outside the hospital[63], a further 10–20 per cent may be employed in the hospital industrial unit, whilst 20–30 per cent of the remainder are employed on the hospital artisan units, the wards and the occupational therapy departments. Work therapy constitutes a part of the life and rehabilitation for about a half of the hospital population. Furthermore, patients are referred into the hospital for retraining by the general hospitals and the community on a daily basis.

Another variant of this scheme has been set up in the Birmingham region, where St. Wulstan's Hospital has been specially designed for the rehabilitating of patients[127, 128]. All the patients from the region which it serves are sent to St. Wulstan's when they have reached the rehabilitation stage of their treatment. The chief innovation in this scheme has been the successful establishment of a system whereby patients are paid for piecework.

The Government has also developed a series of training centres intended to equip patients with a trade. Entry to these centres is secured through government industrial rehabilitation units. This system is particularly advantageous for patients who, having established themselves in the community, now seek further advancement.

Many psychiatrists feel that industrial work has a therapeutic effect on patients. It has been shown that the duration of unemployment is a greater bar to the patient's rehabilitation than is the length of his stay in hospital[138]. There is no reason why large hospitals should not develop original ideas and produce their own goods[180] but they would be unwise to copy local industry and attempt to compete with it.

Recreational Activities

Greater attention is now directed towards the pleasurable use of leisure time. The doctor in charge of the ward is responsible for ensuring that each ward is responsible for its own social functions, musical evenings and whist drives[160]. These activities should preferably be developed by the patients[148]. Hospital activities are best organized so that they can be enjoyed both by patients and members of the public. The local community will be glad to share the hospital cinema, social club and swimming pool. There is an enormous fund of goodwill for the sick and many bands, musicians and entertainers will give their services freely.

Sports activities are particularly valuable for younger patients. Tennis, rugby, squash, cricket and football matches can be played against the staff, other hospitals and local teams. Croquet and bowls should be available for older patients. The proper organization of the sports department requires a competent charge nurse or patient to ensure that the facilities are available when required.

The valuable interaction between the community and the hospital is enhanced when the patients utilize the outside facilities efficiently and properly. In this way the hospital is further integrated into the city's life. Patients are welcomed for their patronage in the shops and at the hotels, theatres, cinemas, restaurants, dances and social functions. They are especially welcome in the Cathedral, the churches and chapels and in the libraries. The initial introduction of patients into the community is made by the social worker or the voluntary workers from the hospital League of Friends. It is not long before patients are invited into people's homes. The social worker will also arrange for the holidays of individual patients. Exchange visits of whole wards with other hospitals[4, 18] provide useful stimulation for deteriorated patients.

These contacts, and indeed all social relationships[151] are especially helpful to patients who are faced with a lengthy illness (for instance severe post-traumatic head injuries) and who thereby find it difficult to re-establish their confidence. They receive further stimulus from their contact with patients suffering from short-term illnesses who usually succeed in re-establishing themselves firmly in the general community within a short time of leaving hospital.

Domestic Rehabilitation

Patients living in the hospital should take a full part in the community's responsibilities. Nevertheless patients should, wherever they are fit, be discharged into the community. This domestic re-settlement often involves a step-by-step programme. Some patients will go to lodgings, others into hotels. The Church Army and the Salvation Army provide hostels for both young and old men and women which offer comradeship as well as shelter. Many of the single patients will marry and establish their own homes and local authorities will readily provide council housing accommodation.

Some hospitals have established their own hostels in the community[48, 105, 179]. This pattern is useful where the main hospital complex is remote from much of its catchment area[51, 85, 86], as in parts of Canada and North America, but great care must be taken to ensure that these hostels are an effective part of their community and not remote chronic wards without proper psychiatric supervision[28].

A different development has been the provision of residential accommodation by factories (for example the Richard Thomas and Baldwin Steel Company Ltd. of Scunthorpe) for their workers. These hostels with all their attendant facilities are also available to patients who are ready for discharge. Such hostels are invaluable because they provide patients with residence where it is needed.

Patients who have spent many years working in the hospital community may, when they reach a suitable age, be transferred to the accommodation provided for the elderly by the local authority[108, 118] (Part 3 accommodation). Patients whose major disability is organic and causes chronic illness, for example, disseminated sclerosis or parkinsonism, are transferred to the appropriate ward in a general hospital when their mental condition permits it. This resettling of patients into the accommodation most suited to their needs ensures that the mental hospital or the psychiatry department in the general hospital always has room for the patients who are in need of its specialized services. The ideal is always, where it is reasonable, to discharge the patient to his family, but it is necessary to make certain that the relevant home nursing or welfare after-care is available in order to prevent relapse and to make the patient's life worth while.

Children's Unit

This is best organized as a separate unit. The most suitable staff consists of a child psychiatrist and his own team. There are, however, great social and economic advantages to be gained by siting this unit within the hospital precinct.

Adolescent Unit

Adolescents are helped to see their problems in perspective when admitted to the ward appropriate to their social state[181]. There is no justification for placing adolescent patients in wards containing

233

senile or deteriorated patients. The special problems of adolescence and psychopathy are discussed later. The importance of adolescents as a stimulus to the whole community cannot be overstated.

Addiction

Addicts fall into two groups. There are those who have established themselves in life and therefore have something to lose, but who have nevertheless succumbed to addiction because of life's stresses. These patients, frequently alcoholic and with a good premorbid personality, have a relatively good prognosis and can if they desire be treated voluntarily or in private units. The second group are the inadequate personalities who, in addition to needing specific treatment for their primary or secondary mental illnesses, require the full resources of the therapeutic community. (There is no evidence that addicts living together as in the Haight Ashbury district of San Francisco will spontaneously generate into a therapeutic community. This Haight Ashbury district development did show how indifferent or aggressive the community can become to mental illness.)

All the hospital's facilities are available to patients on a day or night hospital basis[19] according to their needs. If a special day unit is not established[83], each day-patient's progress should be the responsibility of the mental welfare officer appointed by the community and this is particularly true for psychogeriatric patients.

THE WARD COMMUNITY

Discussion groups, known as ward meetings, form an important part of the life of any ward. They fall into two groups—social meetings involving all patients and staff and clinical meetings involving relevant staff and individual patients.

Ward Meetings (Social)

The essence of these informal meetings involves the free expression of all members of the community, both staff and patients[49, 117]. The aims are to permit abreaction of emotions and evaluation of community problems but above all to generate activities. In the hospital community the activities generated will often be of a temporary nature because of the rapidly changing patient population and for the same reason too great a degree of autonomy is not possible. The meetings should not, therefore, replace the energy and drive required from the medical staff.

These meetings give an opportunity to discuss and remedy grievances[2], for example the meals, their content, presentation and cooking. The patient's behaviour in the ward community is studied and he can see how his personality and behaviour act and react on other patients. Any incidents can be analysed. In the neurosis unit these meetings tend to be community meetings discussing personality and community problems. Disturbance by malicious damage need not be tolerated any more than it would be allowed within a family unit. Control can be effective without an authoritarian approach or the existence of rules. The reasons for a ward policy should be self-evident—it will certainly be discussed at the meeting—if it is wrong it can then be corrected. It is amazing how much deviant behaviour and personality variation patients will tolerate and frequently transfer of patients or staff to other wards can be avoided.

These community meetings can be held by as many as 70 people, although smaller units are preferable. Group discussions with carefully selected nurses and psychiatric social workers are also valuable. The main aim of all community therapy is to replace the custodial atmosphere with an active social culture, but meetings should not be held for their own sake or as a distraction from the proper running of the community.

Ward Meetings (Clinical)

At the formal case conference (ward round) the patient's clinical record is presented by his doctor. The related clinical ward sister, psychiatric social worker or mental welfare officer, industrial rehabilitation officer and, if possible, the general practitioner should be present. The relatives are invited and will be seen either with the patient or on their own. They can discuss their difficulties and any problems expected when the patient is discharged. This helps them to know and have a relationship with the team responsible and to assist in the planning of the patient's future.

The aim is to secure a better clinical balance and to prepare the patient for his discharge from the hospital. It is advisable to inform those responsible for the patient's daily care of any impulsive tendencies, for example suicide, whilst it is necessary for the psychiatrist to receive a first-hand objective account of the patient's attainment. The patient's future treatment is then discussed with him and thus everyone involved is appraised of the medical policy to be followed for the case. This ensures a consistent and reliable attitude towards the patient's occupational, social and domestic life in the hospital community and also prepares him to undertake responsibility for the conduct of his own affairs upon discharge. For instance he is able to handle his drugs responsibly without supervision.

Frequently the patient or his relatives will ask for a case conference in order to learn of the patient's current position. All long-stay patients should be reviewed by the consultant every six months whilst acute cases need to be seen weekly at least. After discharge the patient, his relatives, the local mental welfare officer or general practitioner may come back to the case conference for further help.

Ward rounds are held during normal working hours. They should not replace individual discussion by the patients with the ward doctor or the consultant of his personal difficulties and problems. Neither of these doctors should alter the agreed clinical policy unless all the other members of the firm are aware of the intended change.

Henderson Hospital Unit at Belmont Hospital

The term therapeutic community was formerly limited to the social rehabilitation unit[92] [101] designed by Maxwell Jones in 1947. The wider application of the term to the whole hospital community and to the general community is a later development. The Maxwell Jones pattern remains important not only because of its value in the treatment of mental disorders especially character disorders (psychopathic disorders) but also because the analysis and understanding derived from the study of interpersonal difficulties is applicable to other communities.

In order to establish these personal living and learning studies, it is necessary to have a social (therapeutic) culture. This is achieved by the patients living together communally in the ward and having free opportunity to both react and interact according to their own desires and needs. The culture is enhanced by regular (daily) ward meetings at which the personality interactions are reviewed and evaluated. The aim of this type of community is to establish its own norms, which are under constant examination and review. The group therefore evolves its own society rather than plans it, but rules emerge in the light of experience and the community is then required to abide by these rules.

During the evolution of the therapeutic culture's norms there is a living learning situation. The patient, often for the first time, becomes aware of the existence of others and then of their thinking and finally of their feeling. He can question everyone else in the group, including the leader. The importance of the leader's ability to accept public examination cannot be over-emphasized, equally important is his ability to accept extreme variations in behaviour from the social norms. This is, of course, not so different from the varieties of change which the general community itself has more recently tolerated.

An important feature is the opportunity for the patient to abreact and so feel his emotions that he can learn to understand and control them, thereby reducing his own intrapersonal tensions. The realization that the staff's problems and disturbances may exceed their own helps to provide a common social basis. It does not appear to undermine their confidence in the ability of the staff to help with their problems.

The development of the Maxwell Jones unit as an example of social understanding and toleration, coupled with his results in re-establishing patients whom no one else would accept, stands as a landmark in modern psychiatry.

Homestead Unit at St. John's Hospital

This programme is intended for the resocialization of psychopaths. Most psychopaths are either so disturbed or come from such abnormal backgrounds that treatment within the family is not practical.

Examination of the behaviour of many psychopaths shows one of three main patterns. Firstly, an adverse reaction to frustrating situations with a correspondingly low tolerance to frustration; or secondly a severe impulse reaction to instinctual demands; or thirdly an inadequacy to choose in environmental situations with a resulting mental decompensation. In the case of the psychopath the reaction is usually antisocial either with acts of aggression or the development of the parasitic attitude. The reaction which develops is not volitional and most patients are therefore treated on Orders under the Mental Health Act.

The Order permits control of the patient's reactions and then provides an opportunity for examining the behaviour pattern in a social setting. Thus, if a patient absconds or commits an offence, he is returned to the hospital for further evaluation of the situation. Much antisocial psychopathic behaviour is so obviously disordered that even momentary reflection by the patient shows its effect upon the individual and society. Hitherto the tendency has been to pass along or to confine psychopaths depending upon the patient's reaction and the individual studying it. The hospitals tend to pass patients on, whilst judges confine patients. Those patients who are confined in prison tend to become institutionalized and are certainly not fitted to return to society. In many cases the patients actively learn other evil practices.

In Lincoln a psychopathic patient, like all other patients, is admitted (irrespective of his legal status) to the most suitable ward in the hospital. He is then clinically assessed. He is required to be of reasonable behaviour, to take a part in the community and, in due course, to occupy himself usefully. During this period he learns to understand his actions and discusses them with other patients and the staff but he also sees and assesses the available possibilities for his social and economic advancement within the hospital community. At this stage the advancement made, whether social or in work or in his ward, is the responsibility of the ward charge nurse. In practice the energy, drive and direction is selected by the patient and provided this is either reasonable or not dangerous, it is normally permitted. Shortage of nursing staff and their lack of clinical experience has always tended to allow too precipitous an advancement by the patient—exposing him to stresses which he could not yet manage—with a consequent failure to establish himself at the next level of development. As the experience of the staff increases, however, this failure is slowly becoming less common.

A second cause of failures occurs after the patient's discharge. This nearly always involves his social and personal relationships. When the patient's confidence in the hospital community increases, he tends to return volitionally to the hospital in times of stress—either because of a simple feeling of inadequacy or because of anxiety or depression. There is, therefore, need to equip patients with the ability to organize and evaluate their domestic lives. It was for this reason that the Homestead Social Rehabilitation Unit was established.

This self-governing unit of 25 mixed beds is run by the community; it is in the nominal charge of only a warden and his wife—no additional staff have been engaged. The warden and his wife live in a self-contained flat within the Homestead and since they live with the patients they both feel and take part in the interpersonal tensions. The unit is run as a home. Regular meetings are held to deal with problems generated within the community, between the Homestead and the parent hospital or the Homestead and society.

These meetings give an additional opportunity to evaluate society's standards and responsibilities and to discuss those changes which are taking place. The meetings give opportunity for abreaction and for the patient to alter the social pattern[144, 145] of the unit. Living together with people of diverse backgrounds and occupations supplies an extremely wide range of conversation and a fund of knowledge not available in the usual household.

The meetings last for many hours in the evenings and full, frank and free discussion takes place. The consultant normally upholds the community's views.

New patients may present themselves for admission at the community meeting, but more frequently either the hospital staff or the patient's relatives apply for the patient to join the Homestead. The intended patient then presents himself at the patients' evening meeting, the recommendations and bed situation are considered and the appropriate admission arrangements made. All patients are attending full-time employment or education in the city before being admitted.

At this stage the patient has virtually complete freedom. Whilst he takes his own decisions he may always refer to the medical or nursing staff. As in normal households no formal rules are produced. Patients sooner or later accept a reasonable code of behaviour. It is rare for patients to abuse the freedom accorded them although frequently, as a part of the learning process, they extend the society's established norms.

The community, which is self-contained, looks after itself except that the meals are provided from the main hospital. All the patients (except children and adolescents who are attending full-time education) make a contribution for their board and lodging. Patients at their meetings organize their own social activities and outings either in their own or the hospital's grounds or outside, and they mix fully with the city community not only at work but socially in the youth clubs, theatres, Cathedral and hotels. Members frequently go to friends' homes and people from outside come in to join the activities of the community.

Patients are first taught to establish their interpersonal relations and to master social and work problems. They are then subjected to this more definite social milieu and relate themselves to it. They now learn verbal techniques. This social and verbal mastery enables the patient to have some control over his environment and so to reduce the effects of chance upon his life. By these techniques the psychopath becomes a member of a psychotherapeutic group and he enjoys the relationship and protection such a group affords. By this stage psychopaths have acquired considerable social and occupational grace, they have provided for their instinctive needs and have developed considerable control and tolerance of frustrating situations. Together they no longer form an explosive mixture.

During his stay in the unit the patient will usually ask to be regraded to informal status. Subsequent discharge occurs when the patient is himself satisfied with his ability to organize his own life. The normal period of hospitalization for character disorders is two to three years.

THE GENERAL COMMUNITY

The psychiatrist is responsible for the organization and running of the psychiatric services in the community. He therefore meets the community at out-patient clinics, on domiciliary consultations and at their work. He is also responsible for the psychiatric care of the psychogeriatric patients[6, 108] and for the education of the public on matters of mental health.

Out-patient Clinics

The out-patient department should provide a comprehensive area service for both referrals and after-care[102]. Clinics should be held at the nearest hospital in order to prevent patients requiring follow-up appointments from losing work and so putting their employment in jeopardy. The area served by the district hospital should correspond with the psychiatric firm in order to effect continuity of consultant care. Too many patients pass on to other doctors so that neither patient nor doctor see and learn from their own mistakes. Nevertheless, modern treatment does reduce the number of admissions, so every clinic should also provide facilities for individual and group psychotherapy.

Out-patient social clubs are particularly valuable for patients discharged[182] from hospital and other institutions[126]. These can be run by the local authority mental welfare officer or the hospital psychiatric social worker, who then have direct access to a consultant if they are worried. Psychiatrists will normally accept referrals from general practitioners. They must be prepared to see patients referred by clergymen, lawyers, courts, mental welfare officers or the patient himself or his relatives. In every case the detailed report should go to the general practitioner who is responsible for the patient's community care.

An interesting experiment has recently been successfully established in Plymouth with the opening of the Nuffield Centre[182]. In this centre psychiatric out-patients and day patients, psychologist, child psychiatric and local authority integrate their services. The value of these centres is more obvious where the district psychiatric hospital is remote from its population catchment area.

Domiciliary Consultations

Domiciliary consultations are the most efficient way of dealing with emergencies, understanding domestic situations and providing the best opportunity for family therapy[1, 8, 76, 77].

Domiciliary consultations enable the psychiatrist to separate psychiatric, medical and social emergencies. In this way he can direct the admission of the patient to the appropriate psychiatric ward or to a general hospital. In the case of social emergencies he can discuss the problems with the general practitioner and establish rapport with the family. In all cases he can advise on the community's facilities and arrange for them to be called upon when necessary. If the patient is not achieving a useful level of function or if the family is becoming decompensated because of the patient, then the patient can be returned to lead a useful life in the hospital community.

In a number of police cases a psychiatric opinion will prevent unnecessary investigation.

Local Authorities

Forward-looking community authorities have now established useful services for the patients. The most important development is the appointment of capable mental nurses or psychiatric social workers as mental welfare officers. These officers run the local services, care for patients and organize them with all the additional aids which they may need, such as domestic help, meals on wheels, the aid of voluntary groups and home nursing. In this way the reduplication of social services is avoided. The better officers are devoted and realize that clinical care is not confined to office hours. These mental welfare officers are normally responsible to the consultant psychiatrist and work with the general practitioner although they are paid by the community.

Some local authorities are now developing hostels for the mentally ill. These must be clinically supervised and their function decided[125] before they are built. It is essential that there should be consultation between the local authority and the hospital consultant staff on the location and siting of the hostels before they are built, for some authorities are already closing hostels because of their prohibitive cost and the lack of demand for places[127, 178].

Education

It is advisable to have the public's confidence before developing a therapeutic community. The most effective way of destroying the old asylum image is by the interaction between the hospital and the general community[59, 131]. The constant movement of people (the fact that patients get well and lead a normal life) roots out the attitude that asylums are in reality prisons. The psychiatrist should himself live in the general community. In this way he feels the stresses and strains which occur and he can make the appropriate corrections. The tendency to attach greater importance to community psychiatry has been fully recognized in the United States and the University of Pennsylvania has established a special division of community psychiatry. This department is not solely concerned with academic teaching but rather with a centre and the organization necessary to develop the community services and to integrate these into the University Department. The consortium which runs the centre also includes the local social workers and all who are interested in any aspect of community care for the mentally ill. This interesting development, showing yet another way in which the community plan can be organized, brings the University out of medieval isolation and into the life of the general community.

The general practitioner is trained to recognize the symptoms relating to illness; he is not trained to appreciate his role in the after-care of the patients and the patient's family in the community, yet the community thrusts this responsibility upon him. Recent studies have shown that the rate of relapse of patients under the care of the psychiatric services is less than that of those under the care of general practitioners. Furthermore, it has been shown that standard medical care does not really affect the morbidity caused by chronic psychiatric illnesses in the community[52].

Whilst the need for community therapy is clear the additional responsibilities, particularly mortality, must be recognized[190]. No clear change in the suicide statistics has been shown since the introduction of community care although the tendencies are at present encouraging[149, 150, 177] especially with regard to people over 60.

The effect of this policy is reflected in the suicide figures as given by the Registrar General and this shows a fall of three per cent in this area compared with a rise of three per cent for the whole of England and Wales. Although not statistically significant this is encouraging.

TABLE 1

Death by Suicide at All Ages

	England and Wales			Lindsey, Grimsby and Lincoln		
	Males	Females	Total	Males	Females	Total
1954–9	18,897	12,248	31,145	202	95	297
1961–6	18,536	13,687	32,223	181	107	288
Difference	−361	+1439	+1078	−21	+12	−9
Percentage change	−2	+12	+3	−10	+12	−3

Therefore, the postgraduate education of both the doctors and the social workers is the responsibility of the local psychiatric firm or hospital. In addition to welcoming the general medical practitioner into the hospital and to the ward rounds, regular postgraduate lectures, seminars and discussions should take place.

School teachers frequently still discourage students from entering mental nursing. Student nurses feel very relieved when they discover the actual conditions that exist in mental hospitals. They had feared far worse. Prejudice can be overcome when mature students (community service volunteers) enter the wards.

An attempt was made in 1957 to influence public attitudes[162] to psychiatry by an intensive education programme[55] which lasted for six months and included articles in the local newspaper and television programmes. It failed to influence the public attitudes and in fact evoked anxiety and open hostility.

Nevertheless, there is a great demand for psychiatrists to speak at local meetings and these are often organized by bodies such as Alcoholics Anonymous. People attending these lectures are probably also more receptive to television broadcasts than are the general public who cannot be bulldozed into accepting changes overnight.

The most effective way to influence the public is by calling on their own personal experience of any given problem. At all times the psychiatrist's approach must be rational and he must explain to the patient and his relatives what he is trying to do and why. Above all he must be honest, particularly with regard to the possible early signs of a relapse. The psychiatrist has, also, a personal responsibility to re-educate the patient so that he can mature, develop pride in his work and, wherever possible, control his environment.

Communication

Much emphasis has been laid on the opening up of communication inside the hospital[62, 132]. Equal opportunity must now be given for the opening up of communications to the psychiatrist from the patient, his relatives, the factory and all the other outside agencies and bodies such as the Church and the Law. Each psychiatrist must organize a suitable system so that someone is available for urgent advice and particularly so that emergencies can be dealt with expeditely, irrespective of the source of referral. The over-all responsibility, however, is vested in the general practitioner and the psychiatrist jointly and they must determine together the necessary care for their patient. Since it is not possible to separate the hospital services from the community services, it would probably be better if they had a unified administration to serve them.

The psychiatrist must realize that social disorganization can lead to breakdown as effectively as mental disease may produce social disaster. It is no help to a pregnant girl to refuse to terminate the

TABLE 2

Facilities Necessary for the Comprehensive and Co-ordinated Treatment of General Psychiatric Patients

	Medical Facilities	Social Facilities	Domestic Facilities
Services predominantly and best orientated around the hospital complex	Medical and biochemical assessment of patients Emergency admission procedures Psychosurgery	Ward social activities Hospital social activities Special ward arrangements for the personal rehabilitation of character disorders	Comprehensive provision of different ward communities to meet different patients' needs including provision for subnormality patients Units for character disorders Mother and baby units
Facilities which must be available both to the hospital and the general community	Psychiatric assessment of patients Medical assessment of patients Modern psychiatric therapies Educational facilities Psychological assessment of the patient Out-patients Occupational and industrial rehabilitation units Group or individual psychotherapy programme X-ray and laboratory services and physiotherapy Conferences and communication between general practitioners and hospital staff Legal control	Religious activities Hospital social activities Special ward arrangements for the personal rehabilitation of character disorders	Night hostels Day facilities with particular provision for geriatric cases
Services which should be available in the community	Domiciliary, mental and social assessment of both patient and family External (local authority) services including nursing and mental welfare officers Hospital, domiciliary, educational, nursing and social services	Social clubs (including such groups as Alcoholics Anonymous and Gamblers Anonymous Financial arrangements for those genuinely no longer able to provide for themselves	Homes Lodgings Hostels Hotels Separate provision for the elderly including the senescent (e.g. flats and Part 3), senile and elderly infirm

pregnancy on moral grounds unless one can provide the care and services which she needs. The psychiatrist must not only be aware of all the community's resources—he must also feel its needs, for he has a responsibility to assist in organization of requisite services.

Voluntary Work

The value of voluntary work to the psychiatric services has not yet been fully explored. No definite all-embracing system has been developed. But, the assistance given to hospital authorities by such bodies as the League of Friends, the St. John's Ambulance Brigade, the Red Cross Society and the Women's Voluntary Services is of great help in enabling the patient to take his place in the community[58]. A voluntary services organizer is desirable to correlate all the available help effectively, particularly in the community.

Planning the Future

The general community has slowly come to realize that it is important to be sympathetic towards mental disease and to neither ignore nor ridicule it as has occurred in the past[60]. It is essential that this community concern should be extended beyond mere sympathy into more practical measures. For instance, the community should consider whether large blocks of flats are a suitable method of housing people; whether more leisure facilities should be provided (playing fields, tennis courts, swimming pools and recreation centres, for example); whether cities should be made more restful by the provision of parks and pedestrian precincts; whether modern and noisy transport facilities should be sited so close to centres of population; whether a comprehensive co-ordinated system should be formulated, under which every member of the community can receive help if he should wish it. These are but a few examples of the many ways in which society should generate its own well-being from within itself and so forestall illness arising from unnecessary stresses which are produced by living in a modern community.

SUMMARY

The value of the hospital community lies in its ability to produce a pattern which is stable and yet not rigid. The ability of the hospital community to generate and vary its personal, social, productive, and moral standards enables the patient to evaluate his position and contribution to the community.

The interactions and experiences inside the hospital community and between the hospital and the outside community create helpful tensions which avoid stagnation, lethargy and indifference. This activity avoids chronicity and is as necessary for the medical and nursing staff as it is vital for the patients recovery.

The psychiatrist must assess the patient's present potential capabilities, just as he must assess what opportunities the community can offer. If these advantages are fully pursued and developed, the patient is much less likely to relapse.

Modern medication (particularly the long acting tranquilizer drugs) has enabled even the most seriously disturbed patient with character disorder to make full use of the open hospital and the world beyond.

REFERENCES

1. Ackerman, N. W. (1958). *The Psychodynamics of Family Life.* New York: Basic Books
2. Annesley, P. T. (1961). 'A Rehabilitation Unit on Group Therapy Lines for Long-stay Patients'. *Psychiat. Q.* **35,** 231
3. Baker, A. A. (1956). 'Factory in a Hospital'. *Lancet* **1,** 267
4. — and Freudenberg, R. K. (1957). 'Therapeutic Effect of Change in the Pattern of Care for the Long-stay Patient'. *Int. J. Soc. Psychiat.* **3,** 22
5. Barton, R. (1959). *Institutional Neurosis.* Bristol: John Wright
6. — (1965). 'Developing a Service for Elderly Demented Patients'. In *Psychiatric Hospital Care.* Ed. by H. Freeman. London: Bailliere, Tindall and Cassell
7. Barton, W. E. (1962). *Administration in Psychiatry.* Springfield, Ill.: Charles C. Thomas
8. — and Davidson, E. M. (1961). 'Psychotherapy and Family Care'. *Current Psychiatric Therapies,* Vol. 1. Ed. by J. Masserman. New York: Grune and Stratton
9. Bastoe, O. (1960). 'Environmental Therapy of Chronic Schizophrenic Patients and a Social Psychiatric Study of Problems of Nursing Staff'. *Int. J. soc. Psychiat.* **5,** 281
10. Bateman, J. F. and Dunham, H. W. (1948). 'The State Mental Hospital as a Specialised Community Experience'. *Am. J. Psychiat.* **105,** 445
11. Belknap, I. (1956). *Human Problems of a State Mental Hospital.* New York: McGraw-Hill
12. Bell, G. M. (1955). 'A Mental Hospital with Open Doors'. *Int. J. soc. Psychiat.* **1,** 42
13. Bennett, D. H. (1961). *The Rehabilitation of the Chronic Patient.* Unpublished observations
14. — and Robertson, J. P. S. (1955). 'Effects of Habit Training on Chronic Schizophrenic Patients'. *J. ment. Sci.* **101,** 664

15. — Folkard, S. and Nicholson, A. (1961). 'Resettlement Unit in a Mental Hospital'. *Lancet* **2,** 539

16. Bickford, J. A. F. (1954). 'Treatment of the Chronic Mental Patient'. *Lancet* **1,** 924

17. — (1960). 'Rehabilitation of Schizophrenics'. *Lancet* **2,** 1802

18. — and Miller, H. J. B. (1959). 'Exchange of Patients by Mental Hospitals'. *Lancet* **2,** 96

19. Bierer, J. (1951). *The Day Hospital.* London: Lewis

20. Bion, W. R. (1961). *Experiences in Groups.* London: Tavistock Publications

21. — and Rickman, J. (1943). 'Intra-group Tensions in Therapy'. *Lancet* **2,** 678

22. Blair, D. (1966). 'Industrial Units for the Rehabilitation of Psychiatric Patients'. *Current Psychiatric Therapies VI.* Ed. by J. Masserman. New York: Grune and Stratton

23. Board of Control (1933). *Memorandum on Occupational Therapy for Mental Patients.* London: Her Majesty's Stationery Office. 37051

24. Bockoven, J. S. (1956). 'Moral Treatment in American Psychiatry'. *J. nerv. ment. Dis.* **124,** 167, 292

25. — (1963). *Moral Treatment in American Psychiatry.* New York: Springer

26. Bovet, L. (1951). 'Psychiatric Aspects of Juvenile Delinquency'. *Monograph Ser.* W.H.O. **1**

27. Bowen, A. and Crane, C. B. (1953–1957). *York Mental Health Service Reports.* Unpublished observations

28. Brooks, G. W. (1959). 'Opening a Rehabilitation House'. In *Rehabilitation of the Mentally Ill,* p. 127. Washington, D.C.: American Association for the Advancement of Science

29. Browne, W. A. F. (1937). *What Asylums Were, Are and Ought to Be.* Edinburgh: Black

30. Burdett, H. C. (1891). *Hospitals and Asylums of the World.* London: Churchill

31. Cameron, J. L., Laing, R. D. and McGhie, A. (1955). 'Patient and Nurse; Effect of Environmental Changes in the Care of Chronic Schizophrenia'. *Lancet* **2,** 1384

32. Caplan, G. (1959). *Concepts of Mental Health and Consultation.* Washington, D.C.: U.S. Government Printing Office

33. — (1964). *Principles of Preventive Psychiatry.* London: Tavistock Publications

34. Carmichael, D. M. (1961). 'Community After Care Services'. *Current Psychiatric Therapies I.* Ed. by J. Masserman. New York: Grune and Stratton

35. Carse, J., Panton, N. and Watt, A. (1958). 'A District Mental Health Service'. *Lancet* **1,** 39

36. Carstairs, G. M. (1961). 'Research in Social Psychiatry'. *Scott. med. J.* **6,** 391

247

37.   —   Clark, D. H. and O'Connor, N. (1955). 'Occupational Treatment of Chronic Psychotics—Observations in Holland, Belgium and France'. *Lancet* **2**, 1025

38.   —   O'Connor, N. and Rawnsley, K. (1956). 'Organization of a Hospital Workshop for Chronic Psychotic Patients'. *Br. J. prev. soc. med.* **10**, 136

39.   Caudill, W. (1958). *The Psychiatric Hospital as a Small Society.* Cambridge, Mass.: Harvard University Press

40.   —   Redlich, F. C., Gilmore, H. R. and Brody, E. B. (1952). 'Social Structure and Interaction Processes on a Psychiatric Ward'. *Am. J. Orthopsychiat.* **22**, 314

41.   Clark, D. H. (1958). 'Administrative Therapy: Its Clinical Importance in the Mental Hospital'. *Lancet* **2**, 805

42.   —   (1960). 'Principles of Administrative Therapy'. *Am. J. Psychiat.* **117**, 506

43.   —   (1963).'Administrative Psychiatry'. *Br. J. Psychiat.* **109**, 178

44.   —   (1964). *Administrative Therapy.* London: Tavistock Publns

45.   —   (1965). 'The Therapeutic Community Concept, Practice and Future'. *Br. J. Psychiat.* **111**, 947

46.   —   (1965). 'The Ward Therapeutic Community and its Effects on the Hospital'. In *Psychiatric Hospital Care.* Ed. by H. Freeman. London: Bailliere, Tindall and Cassell

47.   —   and Hoy, R. M. (1957). 'Reform in the Mental Hospital; A Critical Study of a Programme'. *Int. J. soc. Psychiat.* **3**, 211

48.   —   and Cooper, L. W. (1960). 'Psychiatric Halfway Hospital— A Cambridge Experiment'. *Lancet* **1**, 588

49.   —   Hooper, D. F. and Oram, E. G. (1962). 'Creating a Therapeutic Community in a Psychiatric Ward'. *Hum. Relat.* **15**, 123

50.   Colwell, C. and Post, F. (1963). 'Community Needs of Elderly Psychiatric Patients'. In *Trends in the Mental Health Service.* Ed. by H. Freeman and J. Farndale. Oxford: Pergamon Press

51.   Community Psychiatry (1967). *Supplement to American Journal of Psychiatry* **124**, 4

52.   Cooper, B. (1965). 'A Study of One Hundred Chronic Psychiatric Patients Identified in General Practice'. *Br. J. Psychiat.* **111**, 595

53.   Crocket, R. W. (1960). 'Doctors, Administrators and Therapeutic Communities'. *Lancet* **2**, 359

54.   Crutcher, H. B. (1959). 'Family Care'. In *American Handbook of Psychiatry*, Vol. 2. Ed. by S. Arieti. New York: Basic Books

55.   Cumming, E. and Cumming, J. (1957). *Closed Ranks.* Cambridge, Mass.: Harvard University Press

55.   —   Clancy, R. W. and Cumming, J. (1956). 'Improving Patient Care Through Organizational Changes in the Mental Hospital'. *Psychiatry* **19**, 249

57.   Cumming, J. and Cumming, E. (1962). *Ego and Milieu.* New York: Atherton Press

58. Cummings, R., Grant, I. and Karl, V. (1957). 'Foster Home and other Trial Visits for Psychotic Patients'. *Development in the V.A. in 1954 and 1955*, Part I, Bull. 10–90. Washington, D.C.: Psychiatry and Neurology Service, Veterans Administration
59. Dax, E. C. (1961). *Asylum to Community*. Melbourne, Vict.: Cheshire
60. Dean, W. N. (1963). 'Democracy and Rehabilitation of the Mentally Ill'. *Archs gen. Psychiat.* **9**, 1
61. Denber, H. C. B. (1960). *Research Conference on Therapeutic Community*. Springfield, Ill.: Charles C. Thomas; Oxford: Blackwell
62. Dolgoff, T. and Sheffel, I. (1958). 'Communication—The Pulse of the Mental Hospital'. *Ment. Hosps* **9**, 25
63. Douglas, A. D. M., Conway, S. and Beeby, G. J. (1966). 'Survey of Industrial Therapy in the Sheffield Region'. *Br. J. Psychiat.* **112**, 1013
64. Dunham, W. and Weinberg, S. K. (1960). *The Culture of the State Mental Hospital*. Detroit: Wayne State University Press
65. Early, D. F. (1960). 'The Industrial Therapy Organization (Bristol)'. *Lancet* **1**, 754
66. — (1963). 'The Industrial Therapy Organization (Bristol)—The First Two Years'. *Lancet* **1**, 435
67. — and Magnus, R. V. (1968). 'The Industrial Therapy Organization (Bristol) 1960–65'. *Br. J. Psychiat.* **114**, 508, 335
68. Edwards, A. H. (1961). *The Mental Health Services*. London: Shaw
69. Elles, Gil. (1961). 'The Closed Circuit—The Study of a Delinquent Family'. *Br. J. Criminol.* **2**, 23
70. Freeman, H. L. (1959). 'Psychiatric Day Hospitals'. *Oxf. med. Sch. Gaz.* **12**, 119
71. — (1968). 'Community Psychiatry'. *Br. J. Psychiat.* **114**, 481
72. Freudenberg, R. K., Bennett, D. H. and May, A. R. (1957). 'Relative Importance of Physical and Community Methods in the Treatment of Schizophrenia'. *Report of the Second International Congress for Psychiatry*, Vol. 1. Zurich. 1957
73. Garcia, Leonardo B. (1960). 'The Clarinda Plan. An Ecological Approach to Hospital Organization'. *Ment. Hosps.* **30**, 1
74. Glatt, M. M. and Weeks, K. F. (1957). 'Experiences of the Community Treatment of Neurosis in a Mental Hospital Unit'. *Int. J. soc. Psychiat.* **3**, 203
75. Goffman, E. (1958). 'The Characteristics of Total Institutions'. *Symposium on Preventive and Social Psychiatry*. Walter Reed Army Institute of Research. Washington, D.C.: U.S. Government Printing Office
76. Grad, J. C. and Sainsbury, P. (1963). 'Mental Illness and the Family'. *Lancet* **1**, 566
77. — — (1966). 'Problems of Caring for the Mentally Ill at Home'. *Proc. R. Soc. Med.* **59**, 20

78. Gralnick, A. and D'Elia, F. (1961). 'Role of the Patient in the Therapeutic Community: Patient-participation'. *Am. J. Psychother.* **15,** 63

79. Greenblatt, M. and Simon, B. (1959). *Rehabilitation of the Mentally Ill.* Washington, D.C.: Am. Ass. Advmit Sci.

80. — York, R. H. and Brown, E. L. (1955). *From Custodial to Therapeutic Patient Care in Mental Hospitals.* New York: Russell Sage Foundation

81. — Levinson, D. J. and Williams, R.H. (1957). *The Patient and the Mental Hospital.* Glencoe, Ill.: The Free Press

82. — — and Klerman, G. L. (1961). *Mental Patients in Transition.* Springfield, Ill.: Charles C. Thomas

83. Haider, I. (1967). 'A New Day Hospital Service'. *Br. J. Psychiat.* **113,** 173

84. Hansard (1959). House of Commons. Mental Health Bill (17 March 1959, Col. 480–500). (1962). House of Lords (4 July 1962, Col. 1235–1339)

85. Huseth, B. (1958). 'Halfway Houses; A New Rehabilitation Measure'. *Ment. Hosp.* **9,** 5

86. — (1960). *Halfway Houses in England.* Unpublished observations

87. John, A. L. (1961). *A Study of the Psychiatric Nurse.* Edinburgh: Livingstone

88. Joint Commission on Mental Illness (1961). *Action for Mental Health.* New York: Basic Books

89. Jones, Kathleen (1955). *Lunacy, Law and Conscience, 1744–1845.* London: Routledge

90. — (1960). *Mental Health and Social Policy, 1845–1969.* London: Routledge

91. — (1963). 'The Role and Function of the Mental Hospital'. *Trends in the Mental Health Services.* Ed. by H. Freeman and J. Farndale. Oxford: Pergamon Press

92. Jones, Maxwell (1942). 'Group Psychotherapy'. *Br. med. J.* **2,** 276

93. — (1952). *Social Psychiatry (A Study of Therapeutic Communities).* London: Tavistock Publications

94. — (1952). *Rehabilitation in Psychiatry.* WHO/Ment/30, Geneva

95. — (1953). *The Therapeutic Community.* New York: Basic Books

96. — (1954). 'The Treatment of Character Disorder in a Therapeutic Community'. *Wld ment. Hlth* **6,** 1

97. — (1954). 'The Treatment of Psychopathic Personalities'. *Proc. R. Soc. Med.* **47,** 636

98. — (1962). *Social Psychiatry.* Springfield, Ill.: Charles C. Thomas

99. — (1963). *Social Psychiatry in the Community, in Hospitals and in Prisons.* Springfield, Ill.: Charles C. Thomas

100. — (1966). 'Group Work in Mental Hospitals'. *Br. J. Psychiat.* **112,** 1007

101.　— Baker, A., Merry, J. and Pomryn, B. (1953). 'A Community Method of Psychotherapy'. *Br. J. med. Psychol.* **26,** 222

102.　Kessel, N. Hassell, C., Blair, R., Gilroy, S,M., Pilkington, F. and Weeks, K.F. (1965). 'Psychiatric Out-patients in Plymouth. An Area Service Analysed'. *Br. J. Psychiat.* **111,** 10

103.　Kidd, H. R. (1965). 'The Team System and Integration of Staff'. In *Psychiatric Hospital Care.* Ed. by H. Freeman. London: Bailliere, Tindall and Cassell

104.　Lancet (1956). (a) Hunter, R. H. 'Rise and Fall of Mental Nursing'. *Lancet,* **1,** 98; (b) Jones, M., Pomryn, B. H. and Skellen, E. 'Work Therapy'. *Lancet* **1,** 343

105.　Landy, D. (1960). 'Exploration in Residential After-care of Psychiatric Patients; A Men's Halfway House'. *Int. J. soc. Psychiat.* **6,** 132

106.　Linn, L. (1955). *A Handbook of Hospital Psychiatry.* New York: International Universities Press

107.　Macmillan, D. (1956). 'An Integrated Mental Health Service'. *Lancet* **2,** 1094

108.　— (1967). 'Problems of a Geriatric Mental Health Service'. *Br. J. Psychiat.* **113,** 175

109.　Main, T. F. (1946). 'The Hospital as a Therapeutic Institution'. *Bull. Menninger clin.* **10,** 66

110.　— (1953–58). Cassel Hospital Reports.

111.　Mandelbrote, B. (1958). 'An Experiment in the Rapid Conversion of a Closed Mental Hospital into an Open Door Hospital'. *Ment. Hyg.* **42,** 3

112.　— (1959). 'Development of a Comprehensive Psychiatric Community Service Around the Mental Hospital'. *Ment. Hyg.* **43,** 368

113.　— (1965). 'Therapeutic Aspects of Organization. Factors Associated with the Rapid Conversion of a Custodial Institution into a Therapeutic Community'. In *Psychiatric Hospital Care.* Ed. by H. Freeman. London: Bailliere, Tindall and Cassell

114.　— and Freeman, H. (1963). 'The Closed Group Concept in Open Psychiatric Hospitals'. *Am. J. Psychiat.* **119,** 763

115.　Martin, D. V. (1955). 'Institutionalization'. *Lancet* **2,** 1188

116.　— (1962). *Adventures in Psychiatry.* Oxford: Bruno Cassirer

117.　— (1965). 'Importance of Free Communication'. In *Psychiatric Hospital Care.* Ed. by H. Freeman. London: Bailliere, Tindall and Cassell

118.　Mason, A. S., Cunningham, M. K. and Tarpy, E. K. (1963). 'The Quarter-way-house—A Transitional Programme for Chronically Ill Geriatric Mental Patients'. *J. Am. geriat. Soc.* **11,** 574

119.　Masserman, C. M. G. (1964). 'Teaching is Learning'. *Am. J. Psychiat.* **121,** 221

120.　May, A. R. (1956). 'Changes in Social Environment; Their Effect on Mentally Deteriorated Patients'. *Lancet* **1,** 500

121. Mental Health Act (1959). London: Her Majesty's Stationery Office

122. Mercier, C. A. (1894). *Lunatic Asylums, Their Organization and Management*. London

123. Mercier, O. von and King, S. H. (1957). *Remotivating the Mental Patient*. New York: Russell Sage Foundation

124. Miller, D. (1954). 'Rehabilitation of Chronic Openward Psychiatric Patients'. *Psychiatry* **17**, 347

125. Mikels, E. and Gumrukcum, P. (1963). 'A Therapeutic Community Hostel'. *J. Rehabil.* **29**, 20

126. Morgan, G. D. and Tylden, E. (1957). 'The Stepping Stones Club'. *Lancet* **1**, 877

127. Morgan, P. (1964). 'A Local Authority Psychiatric Rehabilitation Hopital'. *Mon. Bull. Minist. Hlth* **23**, 224

128. Morgan, R., Cushing, D. and Manton, N S. 1965). 'A Regional Psychiatric Rehabilitation Hospital'. *Br. J. Psychiat.* **111**, 955

129. Morrissey, J. and Sainsbury, P. (1959). 'Observations on the Chichester and District Mental Health Service'. *Proc. R. Soc. Med.* **52**, 1061

130. Nicholas, M. (1967). 'The Rehabilitation of Long Stay Schizophrenic Patients'. *Br. J. Psychiat.* **113**, 155

131. Nunnally, J. C. and Bobren, H. M. (1959). 'Variables Governing the Willingness to Receive Communications on Mental Health'. *J. Personality* **27**, 38

132. Osmond, H. and Clancy, I. L. W. (1958). 'Communications and Expression of Administration'. *Ment. Hosps.* **9**, 15

133. Ozarin, L. D. (1954). 'Moral Treatment and the Mental Hospital'. *Am. J. Psychiat.* **111**, 371

134. Peabody, G. A. (1961). 'Campus Psychiatry'. In *Current Psychiatric Therapies*, Vol. 1. Ed. by J. Masserman. New York, London: Grune and Stratton

135. Pilkington, F. (1969). 'Twenty Years A-growing'. *Br. J. Psychiat.* **115**, 1

136. Pinel, P. (1801–1809). Translated from *Traite Medico-Philisophique Sur L'Alienation Mentale*. (Paris) by D. D. Davies. As *A Treatise on Insanity*. (1962) History of Medicine. Series No. 14. New York Academy of Medicine. New York: Hafner

137. Pinsker, H. (1966). 'Fallacies in Hospital Community Therapy'. *Current Psychiatric Therapies*, Vol. 6. Ed. by J. Masserman. New York, London: Grune and Stratton

138. Price, J. H., Bleaden, F. A., Thomas, J. D. and Kerridge, D (1969). 'The Lincoln Rehabilitation Scheme'. *Br. J. Psychiat.* **115**, 1043

139. Rapoport, A. (1960). *Community as Doctor*. Springfield, Ill.: Charles C. Thomas

140. Ratcliff, R. A. W. (1962). 'The Open Door; Ten Years' Experience in Dingleton'. *Lancet* **2**, 188

141. Rees, T. P. (1957). 'Back to Moral Treatment and Community Care'. *J. ment. Sci.* **103**, 303

142. — and Glatt, M. M. (1955). 'The Organisation of a Mental Hospital on the Basis of Group Participation'. *Int. J. Grp Psychother.* **5**, 157

143. Roberts, E. L. and Lindsay, J. S. B. (1962). 'The Mental Hospital: Structure, Function and Communication'. *Br. J. med. Psychol.* **35**, 155

144. Rowland, H. (1938). 'Interaction Processes in the State Mental Hospital'. *Psychiatry* **1**, 323

145. — (1939). 'Friendship Patterns in the State Mental Hospital'. *Psychiatry* **2**, 363

146. Sainsbury, P., Costain, W. R. and Grad, J (1966). 'The Effects of a Community Service on the Referral and Admission Rates of Elderly Psychiatric Patients',. In *Psychiatric Disorders in the Aged,* p. 23, Manchester: Geigy Publications

147. — Walk, D. and Grad, J. (1966). 'Evaluating the Graylingwell Hospital Community Psychiatric Service in Chichester Suicide and Community Care'. *Millbank Mem. Fund Q.* Suppl. **44** No. I, Part 2, 243

148. Sanders, R., Weinman Smith, R. S. B., Smith, A. and Kenny, J, (1962). 'Social Treatment of the Male Chronic Mental Patient'. *J. nerv. ment. Dis.* **134**, 244

149. Schmidt, E. H., O'Neal, P. (1954). 'Evaluation of Suicide Attempts as a Guide to Therapy'. *J. Am. med. Ass.* **155**, 549

150. Schwartz, C. G. (1953). 'Rehabilitation of Mental Hospital Patients'. *U.S. Public Health Monograph No. 17.* Washington, D.C.

151. Schwartz, M. S. and Stanton, A. H. (1950). 'A Social Psychological Study of Incontinence'. *Psychiatry* **13**, 399

152. Sheldon, A. (1964). 'An Evaluation of Psychiatric After-care'. *Br. J. Psychiat.* **110**, 662

153. Shoenberg, E. and Morgan, R. (1958). 'Starting a Schizophrenic Unit'. *Lancet* **2**, 412

154. Short-Doyle Act for Community Mental Health Services (1957). Sacramento, State of California Department of Mental Hygiene

155. Simon, H. (1927, 1929). 'More Active Treatment of Mental Patients in Hospital'. *Allg. Z. Psychiat.* **87, 81** and **90, 69**

156. Snow, H. B. (1959). 'Open Door Policy at St. Lawrence State Hospital'. *Am. J. Psychiat.* **115**, 779

157. Sofer, C. (1955). 'Reactions to Administrative Change: A Study of Staff Relations in Three British Hospitals'. *Hum. Relat.* **8**, 291

158. Sommer, R. and Osmond, H. (1961). 'Symptoms of Institutional Care'. *Social Prob.* **8**, 254

159. Southwest Metropolitan Regional Hospital Board (1959). *Worthing Experiment, London.* Southwest Metropolitan Regional Hospital Board

160. Stanton, A. and Schwartz, M. (1949). 'Medical Opinion and the Social Context in the Mental Hospital'. *Psychiatry* **12**, 243

161. —— (1954). *The Mental Hospital*. London: Tavistock Publications

162. Star, Shirley A. (1955). *The Public's Ideas About Mental Illness*. Paper presented at the annual meeting of the National Association of Mental Health, Indianapolis, Indiana. November 5

163. Stearns, L. (1957). 'A Therapeutic Community; As A Nurse Sees It'. *Milit. Med.* **121**, 121

164. Stern, E. S. (1959). 'Open Wards in Large Mental Hospital'. *Int· J. soc. Psychiat.* **4**, 299

165. Sullivan, H. S. (1931). 'Socio-psychiatric Research'. *Am. J. Psychiat.* **10**, 977

166. Taylor, F. K. (1958). 'A History of Group and Administrative Therapy in Great Britain'. *Br. J. med. Psychol.* **31**, 153

167. Tooth, G. C. and Brooke, E. (1961). 'Trends in the Mental Hospital Population and their Effect on Future Planning'. *Lancet* **1**, 710

168. Tuke, D. H. (1882). In *History of the Insane of the British Isles*. London: Kegan Paul

169. Tuke, S. (1813). *A Description of the Retreat*. York: Alexander

170. Tylden, E., Morgan, T. D. and Bates, M. E. (1956). *The Stepping Stones*. WHO/Ment/118, Geneva

171. —— and Salisbury, H (1961). *First Report on Work of Stepping Stones Club*. Bromley Hospital Management Committee

172. Wadsworth, W. V. and Wells, B. W. P. (1962). 'The Organization of a Sheltered Workshop'. *J. ment. Sci.* **108**, 780

173. —— Scott, R. F. and Tonge, W. L. (1958). 'A Hospital Workshop'. *Lancet* **2**, 896

174. —— (1958). *Further Thoughts on the Hospital Workshop*. Address to the Royal Medico-Psychological Association. July 1958 meeting

175. Walk, A. (1954). 'Some Aspects of the 'Moral Treatment' of the Insane up to 1854'. *J. ment. Sci.* **100**, 807

176. —— (1961). 'The History of Mental Nursing'. *J. ment. Sci.* **107**, 2

177. —— (1967). 'Suicide and Community Care'. *Br. J. Psychiat.* **113**, 1381

178. Walker, D. L. (1958). 'The Pattern of Post War Psychiatric Practice'. *Unpublished M.D. Thesis*, University of London

179. —— (1967). 'A Hostel for Mentally Ill Patients Run by a Psychiatric Hospital'. *Br. J. Psychiat.* **113**, 167

180. Wansbrough, N. and Miles, A. (1968). *Industrial Therapy in Psychiatric Hospitals*. King Edward Hospital Fund for London

181. Weeks, H. A. (1958). *Youthful Offenders at Highfields*. Ann Arbor, Mich.: University of Michigan Press

182. Weeks, K. (1965). 'A Community Mental Health Centre'. In *Psychiatric Hospital Care*. Ed. by H. Freeman. London: Bailliere, Tindall and Cassell

183. Wilkinson, J. C. M. (1965). 'Mental Illness in London: A Horton Profile, 1963'. *Br. J. Psychiat.* **111,** 429

184. Wilmer, H. A. (1958). *Social Psychiatry in Action*. Springfield, Ill.: Charles C. Thomas

185. —— (1968). 'Towards a Definition of the Therapeutic Community'. *Am. J. Psychiat.* **144,** 824

186. Wilson, A. T. M., Doyle, M. and Kelnar, J. (1947). 'Group Techniques in a Transitional Community'. *Lancet* **1,** 735

187. Wing, J. K. (1963). 'Rehabilitation of Psychiatric Patients'. *Br. J. Psychiat.* **109,** 635

188. —— (1965). 'Long-stay Schizophrenic Patients and Results of Rehabilitation'. In *Psychiatric Hospital Care*. Ed. by H. Freeman. London: Bailliere, Tindall and Cassell

189. —— and Giddens, R. G. T. (1959). 'Industrial Rehabilitation of Male Chronic Schizophrenic Patients'. *Lancet* **2,** 505

190. —— Monck, E., Brown, G. W. and Carstairs, G. M. (1964). 'Morbidity in the Community of Schizophrenic Patients'. *Br. J. Psychiat.* **110,** 10

191. Wolf, S. (1964). 'Group Discussion with Nurses in a Hospital for Alcoholics'. *Int. J. nurs. Stud.* **1,** 131

192. Wootton, Barbara (1956). *Sickness or Sin*. The Twentieth Century.

193. —— (1959). *Social Science and Social Pathology*. London: Allen and Unwin

194. World Health Organization (1953). *Third Report of the Expert Committee on Mental Health*, Geneva

195. —— (1956). *First Report of the Expert Committee on Psychiatric Nursing*, Geneva

CHAPTER 10

BEHAVIOUR THERAPY

JOHN PAUL BRADY

INTRODUCTION

Psychotherapy refers broadly to the treatment of psychiatric and general medical disorders by psychological means. The present chapter deals with a particular psychotherapeutic approach, variously called behaviour therapy, conditioning therapy or learning therapy. Over the last few years interest in this approach has rapidly increased as its application has extended to a wide range of clinical problems and its efficacy amply demonstrated.

It will be helpful to delineate behaviour therapy from other psychotherapeutic approaches such as dynamic (psychoanalytically-oriented) psychotherapy and supportive psychotherapy. The reason for this is not to discredit other forms of psychotherapy but to aid the reader to understand what is essentially different about behaviour therapy. An often cited distinction concerns the focus of the treatment. Typically, the focus in behaviour therapy concerns the principal symptoms which the patient presents and the modification of his symptomatic behaviour pattern. In contrast, the focus in dynamically-oriented therapy is usually the patient's character structure or the unconscious conflicts which are presumed to give rise to the patient's neurotic behaviour. This is not an absolute distinction, however[14]. For example, homosexuality and other sexual disorders may sometimes be effectively treated by a behaviour therapy technique called 'assertive training' (described below) on the assumption that the deviant sexual behaviour is a by-product of failure of appropriately aggressive behaviour in a variety of social situations. Conversely, there is a growing tendency for dynamically-oriented therapists to focus more on the patient's presenting symptoms.

A second distinction concerns the theoretical basis of the various approaches. Behaviour therapists conceptualize clinical problems in terms of learning theory. Many behaviour therapy techniques involve the direct application of principles derived from experiments in learning. Some procedures have a strong empirical basis. In contrast, other psychotherapeutic approaches tend to emphasize one or another theory of personality. In the case of 'dynamic' psychotherapy, psychoanalytic psychology is the main conceptual framework. However, close examination of the behaviour of therapists of various schools reveals much overlap in actual practice[14]).

The third and most important distinction concerns the manner of analysis of the problem the patient presents. Behaviour therapy begins with a behavioural analysis of the patient's adjustment difficulties. The therapist asks questions such as 'what are the antecedent events which occasioned the patient's symptoms?' 'When the patient displays symptomatic behaviour, what changes occur in his social and physical environment which might provide clues as to why the seemingly maladaptive behaviour persists?' It is a functional analysis in the sense that questions like the above are directed at ascertaining the variables of which the symptoms or adjustment difficulties are a function. The behavioural analysis is the first and essential step in designing a behavioural treatment. Of course, questions of this kind are often asked by practitioners who favour other treatment approaches. However, dynamically-oriented therapists are often more concerned with the patient's unconscious conflicts. These are not directly observable but to a large extent are inferred from the patient's present behaviour and past experience with the aid of psychoanalytic theory.

In this chapter it is not possible to describe all the psychotherapeutic procedures which are subsumed under the rubric of behaviour therapy. Nor can any be described in sufficient detail to serve as an adequate guide to treatment for the inexperienced. Rather the scope of behaviour therapy will be indicated by describing some clinical applications of the more common procedures. The reader will be referred to other sources for more detailed information.

SYSTEMATIC DESENSITIZATION

The treatment of neurotic disorders by systematic desensitization is the single most widely used behaviour therapy technique. It will be described from the standpoint of its experimental basis, clinical application, results and variations of the basic procedure.

Experimental Basis

This treatment grew out of studies of Professor Joseph Wolpe and others on experimental neuroses in animals. Consider, for example, an experimental animal that has been given a number of painful electric shocks in a particular cage in a particular room. Following this procedure the animal will show increasingly intense fearful behaviour as he is brought closer and closer to the cage. This may be understood in terms of classical (Pavlovian) conditioning. Previously neutral stimuli, such as the sight and smell of the cage, have become conditioned stimuli and elicit a conditioned emotional response (fear). The animal will try also to avoid the cage and other cages and rooms with similar physical characteristics (stimulus generalization). This may be regarded as an experimental analogue of a clinical phobia in which the patient may avoid a particular object or situation in order to reduce the fear or anxiety which approaching it generates. Working with cats, Wolpe[50] demonstrated an effective procedure for eliminating experimentally induced phobias of this kind. He brought the cat toward the anxiety-provoking cage from a distance in a series of small, discreet steps. The first step on this 'anxiety hierarchy' was sufficiently removed from the original situation that only a small amount of anxiety was apparent. By feeding the animal at this location the fear associated with this situation disappeared. The cat was then moved to the second step of the fear hierarchy and again fed to neutralize the anxiety previously associated with this degree of closeness to the feared object. This procedure was continued until the cat was able to remain in the original cage with apparent equanimity. Wolpe reasoned that the anxiety associated with each step in this procedure was inhibited or counterconditioned by the psychophysiological responses which accompany eating. Borrowing a term which Sherrington applied to spinal reflexes, he termed this process *reciprocal inhibition* and suggested a general psychotherapeutic principle as follows: 'If a response inhibitory to anxiety can be made to occur in the presence of anxiety-evoking stimuli, it will weaken the connection between these stimuli and the anxiety responses'[51]. This principle is also refered to as 'counterconditioning'.

Clinical Application

In the treatment of human neuroses by systematic desensitization, the experimental procedure described above is modified in several ways. Usually, deep muscular relaxation is used instead of eating as a means of inhibiting anxiety. Also, rather than actually approach the anxiety-provoking object or situation, the patient imagines a series of situations in which the feared object or situation is gradually approached. This will be first illustrated with a monosymptomatic acrophobia.

The patient is taught to acquire a state of deep muscular relaxation. This is a modification of a technique originally described by Jacobson[33] which usually takes about 20 minutes of each of five or six sessions. During this period the therapist and patient construct a list or hierarchy of fear-producing situations involving heights. This list usually contains 10 to 20 items or 'scenes' which are arranged from one which elicits only minimal anxiety—perhaps that he is standing near a closed window on the second floor of a building—to one that elicits intense anxiety—perhaps that he is leaning out a window on the 20th floor of the same building. In the deconditioning sessions the patient first becomes deeply relaxed in the manner he has learned. Then he is instructed to vividly imagine the first or least anxiety-evoking scene on the hierarchy. This first scene is presented two or three times for 5 to 20 seconds' duration each or until no further anxiety is elicited by the scene. Then the second scene is presented in the same manner and so forth until the last or previously most anxiety-provoking scene can be vividly imagined without discomfort. The number of sessions required to accomplish this varies greatly but most therapists report a mean of 10 to 15 sessions. The therapist's expectation is that situations which are desensitized in imagination will be desensitized in reality. This carry-over to real world situations is usually prompt and complete. The reader is referred to other sources for further procedural details of this treatment[38, 53].

Often a patient's inappropriate anxiety is not confined to a single category such as heights but occurs in a variety of situations. In this case the patient's various fears are grouped into two or more thematic categories. For example, the patient may report inappropriate anxiety in situations involving heights, being physically confined or restricted, and being exposed to ordinary criticism. Then a hierarchy would be constructed for each of these three themes. Systematic desensitization would then be applied to each, either treating them in order or working on all three at the same time.

Although the mechanism of systematic desensitization therapy is most easily described in the context of classical phobias, the procedure is by no means limited to these disorders. In general, any neurotic disorder in which the stimulus antecedents of the anxiety which mediates the neurotic response can be identified is suitable for desensitization therapy. For example, the technique has been successfully applied to stuttering by deconditioning the anxiety associated with specific speaking situations in which the patient habitually stutters[15]. Similarly it has been applied to the treatment of sexual frigidity to decondition the anxiety elicited by sexual approaches by the patient's husband[37].

Clinical Results

Wolpe and Lazarus[53] report a 90 per cent improvement rate in unselected patients with phobias and related anxiety response habits treated with systematic desensitization. This is a much higher improvement rate than is usually reported for other forms of treatment with the same criteria of improvement. However, a limitation of these data is the absence of appropriate control groups treated by other methods. Such comparative prospective studies have been carried out on patients with phobias[29, 30]. Although the percentage improvement was not so high in these studies, systematic desensitization proved to be generally superior to the control treatment of brief re-educative psychotherapy.

A number of more experimental comparative studies have been carried out in which subjects with particular irrational fears were asked to participate in treatment. Although the subjects of these studies were not patients in the usual clinical sense, the experimental control possible in these researches makes them of interest. Thus Paul[43] divided volunteer subjects with severe fears of public speaking into three treatment groups and two control groups. The treatment procedures were systematic desensitization, insight-oriented psychotherapy, and an 'attention-placebo' procedure to examine the effects of non-specific factors such as emotional support and suggestion. The control groups consisted of a 'wait-list' group that anticipated later treatment and a 'no-contact' group. Of the treatment procedures desensitization therapy was clearly superior. Least improvement was seen in the two no-treatment control conditions. Similar results were obtained in reducing chronic anxiety in college students[44] and eliminating snake phobias[36].

It should be mentioned that on the basis of psychoanalytic theory some would predict that the elimination of neurotic symptoms by desensitization therapy would result in the emergence of new symptoms—so-called 'symptom substitution'. From the now very considerable experience with desensitization therapy it is clear that this is not in fact a problem; new symptoms occur no more frequently than in untreated controls or patients successfully treated by other means[53].

Clinical Variations and Innovations

Many therapists use hypnosis as an adjunct in desensitization therapy. In susceptible patients, hypnosis appears to facilitate the relaxation process and may enhance the vividness of imagined scenes. Orally administered phenothiazines such as chlorpromazine and barbiturates such as phenobarbital are also used adjunctively in systematic desensitization. They are especially useful with patients who have difficulty achieving adequate relaxation during the early sessions. Usually these drugs can be discontinued as the patient feels more comfortable in the treatment situation. In instances where pervasive and intense anxiety prevents desensitization therapy, Wolpe and Lazarus[53] advocate the use of a mixture of 65 per cent carbon dioxide and 35 per cent oxygen. The patient makes a single full-capacity inhalation of the mixture. This may be repeated up to three times with a few minutes rest in between. This procedure often produces a marked diminution in anxiety and makes it possible to begin desensitization therapy.

Recently the use of subanaesthetic doses of intravenous methohexitone sodium (Brietal) has been introduced into desensitization therapy. The technique consists of injecting 20–30 mg of the drug at the beginning of the session and then, by leaving the needle in the vein, injecting an additional 20 to 50 mg as needed over the course of the 20-minute session. This quantity of the drug produces drowsiness without sleep and enhances relaxation and calm. Because of its very rapid action, the patient is able to leave the treatment room and return home or to work within 10 to 15 minutes after the treatment session. By the use of this drug in desensitization therapy, preliminary training in relaxation can be largely done without delay and the deconditioning of anxiety responses appears to proceed more rapidly. The technique has been successfully applied to the treatment of phobias[27, 28], sexual frigidity[11], chronic stuttering[15] and other disorders. Originally the drug was thought to aid desensitization therapy by enhancing physical relaxation. However, it has been argued that it functions as an inhibitor of anxiety *sui generis* and may facilitate the counterconditioning of anxiety responses by the state of emotional calm it induces[12].

Anxiety responses can also be eliminated by having the patient approach the actual feared situation or object in a graded, systematic manner under conditions of an emotional state which is inhibitory of anxiety. For example, the acrophobic patient, who feels calm and secure in the presence of a therapist with whom there is good mutual rapport, may actually go through the steps on the anxiety hierarchy in the presence of the therapist. This is often termed *in vivo* desensitization or practical retraining. Related to this is the procedure of having the phobic patient observe another person approach the feared object or situation with equanimity. This procedure, often called modelling, has been used extensively by Bandura for the treatment of common fears in children[7].

ASSERTIVE TRAINING

A common impediment to satisfying interpersonal relationships and a good personal adjustment seen in neurotic persons is an inability to be adequately assertive in appropriate situations. This is seen particularly in the patient with a 'passive-aggressive' personality in whom the expression of resentment, irritation and anger may take only indirect forms which are generally ineffectual and self-defeating. Such difficulties usually have their origin in parental influences during the formative childhood years. Typically the direct expression of negative affects and normal aggressivity was repeatedly and excessively punished in some manner. As a result the direct expression of these affects is perceived by the person as dangerous and provokes guilt and anxiety. However, the habitual inhibition of appropriate assertiveness itself leads to anxiety, in part because of the fear of loss of self-control in provoking situations.

Assertive training often proves of value in these problems. The basic technique is to have the patient practice assertiveness in appropriate situations. As in desensitization therapy, this is best done systematically, beginning with situations that require only a minimum of assertiveness. For a particular patient this might be a minor complaint to the waiter about the service in a restaurant. When the patient feels comfortable being assertive in this and other situations which provoked a small amount of anxiety, he is encouraged to go on in a graded series of progressively more difficult situations until a level of assertiveness is obtained which facilitates better relationships in general. Lack of self-esteem and other derivatives of excessive submissiveness usually improve as a result.

It should be mentioned that an increase of assertiveness in a usually very submissive member of a marital couple may disrupt the equilibrium which had existed between them—as mutually neurotic or unsatisfactory as this may have been. This is not necessarily a contraindication to assertive training but rather points up the necessity of a complete behavioural analysis before the total treatment is planned—an analysis which may have to include the marital relationship itself.

The mechanism of this treatment may be viewed as follows. The encouragement and 'emotional support' offered by the therapist may allow the patient to be assertive in situations of minimal difficulty. Once the assertive behaviour is emitted the accompanying positive affect may operate to inhibit the weak anxiety associated with this behaviour (counterconditioning). At the same time the assertive behaviour has several rewarding consequences; its usefulness in dealing effectively with others, the satisfaction which results from reasonable assertiveness and the later approval of the therapist. All these positive consequences make the assertive behaviour more likely in the future (the 'operant-reinforcement' principle to be described later).

A variation in this procedure is to have the patient rehearse or role-play assertive behaviour with the therapist. In this the therapist takes the part of the person toward whom the patient is to be assertive. This role-playing may also be done in a systematic, graded manner in anticipation of similar real life situations outside the therapist's office[53].

Although the technique has been applied especially to the problem of inadequately assertive behaviour, it can be used to help patients learn to express other habitually inhibited emotions as well. Thus Salter[46] has applied the technique to patients who inhibit expressions of affection and concern.

AVERSIVE CONDITIONING

Treatment of Alcoholism

The prototype of these procedures is the conditioned aversion treatment of alcoholism with emetine, apomorphine or other nausea-producing drugs. Efforts to develop an aversion to alcohol date back to at least Pliny the Elder[26], but the development of systematic programmes of treatment, spirited by Pavlov's conditioning studies, first appeared about a quarter of a century ago. The basic procedure consists of pairing cues associated with the drinking of alcoholic beverages (conditioned stimuli) with the unpleasant experience of nausea and vomiting (unconditioned response) induced by an emetic drug (unconditioned stimulus). After several such pairings the alcohol itself comes to elicit nausea and vomiting (conditioned response) and thus prevents or at least deters drinking behaviour. Timing is very important in this procedure. To obtain strong conditioning in a few trials it is essential that the drinking-related cues (the sight, odour and taste of alcohol) immediately precede and overlap the onset of the nausea and vomiting.

In the author's experience treatment results with this procedure alone are often disappointing. A likely reason for this limited success is that the chronic alcoholic is usually a behaviourally restricted person. Indeed, the long reliance on alcohol as the principal means of reducing the anxiety and frustrations associated with life's stresses and conflicts leads to a constriction of the patient's repertoire of means of dealing with problems. Thus the temporary suppression of drinking may not be sufficient treatment. In a short time the behaviourally constricted alcoholic may again turn to alcohol and persist in attempts to drink until the conditioned response of nausea and vomiting weakens and finally disappears (extinction). Accordingly, it is good practice to make use of the period of suppressed drinking to aid the alcoholic to learn or relearn alternative ways of dealing with his anxieties and adjustment problems. General emotional support and counselling may be of great help as well as specific psychotherapeutic procedures such as assertive training. However, the details of the complementing psychotherapy will depend on the patient's individual needs as ascertained from a behaviour analysis. If additional time is required to carry out these other procedures, the conditioned aversion may be periodically strengthened by having the patient undergo reinforcing trials in which drug-induced nausea and vomiting is again paired with drinking-related cues.

An important innovation in the conditioned aversion treatment of alcoholism is the substitution of painful electric shock for drug-induced nausea and vomiting[26]. Electric shock has many technical advantages in aversion therapy[45]. It is safer than nausea-inducing drugs and easier to use. Further, the therapist has greater control over the onset, duration and intensity of the aversive stimuli which permits conditioning with high resistance to extinction to be efficiently induced. A number of authors have described electric shock units suitable for clinical use[23, 41].

Treatment of Other Disorders

The conditioned aversion procedure with either nausea-inducing drugs or electric shock can be applied to a wide variety of clinical disorders. The common denominator of most of these is an obsessional attraction to a situation, object or idea. Thus these procedures have been successfully applied to sexual disorders such as transvestism, fetishism and homosexuality[21]. Here the procedure is to pair the nausea and vomiting or electric shock with the cues associated with performance of the deviant sexual behaviour. Similarly, compulsive eating or excessive smoking may be treated by pairing electric shock with eating particular foods or the behaviour of beginning to smoke. Such disparate clinical conditions as narcotics addiction[52] and compulsive gambling[31] have been treated by this method. It should be stressed, however, that conditioned aversion therapy may not be the treatment of choice in all these conditions. First, the therapist should ascertain whether the behaviour is being maintained by anxiety reduction. For example, a male patient with disturbing homosexual ruminations and behaviour may experience intense anxiety when he finds himself in an imminently sexual situation with a woman. The homosexual behaviour may be a means of reducing this anxiety. In such a case dealing with the anxiety, for example by desensitization therapy, would be the better choice of procedure. If the homosexual problem persisted after the heterosexual anxiety was largely removed, a course of aversion therapy might be instituted at that time. In instances where the obsessional behaviour is not associated with anxiety *ab initio*, aversion therapy is properly the initial treatment[53].

Covert Sensitization

A promising innovation in aversion therapy consists in presenting both the conditioned stimuli and the unconditioned stimuli in imagination only. This procedure, developed largely by Cautela[17] has been applied to alcoholism, homosexuality, excessive smoking and other disorders. First the patient is trained in deep muscular relaxation as in systematic desensitization therapy. In treating an alcoholic, the patient is then instructed to vividly imagine reaching for his usual kind of alcoholic drink, smelling it and tasting it. As soon as he signals obtaining a clear image of this situation, he is instructed to abruptly discontinue this image and instead vividly imagine a situation which is designed to provoke intense anxiety, revulsion or disgust. For example, the patient might suddenly imagine he is eating something he finds especially revolting and repugnant. Actual nausea and vomiting may be induced in the cooperative patient with good imaginal ability. As in drug-induced nausea and vomiting, after a time attempts to actually drink will elicit a strongly disagreeable visceral reaction. An advantage of this innovation is that the motivated patient can practice the whole procedure by himself between treatment sessions with the therapist. Thus periodic reinforcement of the conditioning can be easily carried out.

NON-AVERSIVE ELECTRIC SHOCK

Recently, techniques have been developed which employ a level of electric shock which is clearly not painful. Two distinct procedures will be briefly described.

Desensitization with Galvanic Shocks

This procedure is useful for patients with phobic-like disorders who are unable to obtain sufficient physical and emotional relaxation for the systematic desensitization procedure described earlier. The procedure employs a battery-operated device which can deliver one-second galvanic pulses through electrodes attached to the patient's wrist and below the elbow. By means of a variable resister in the circuit, the current is adjusted on a trial-and-error basis so as to be clearly felt without being aversive. Then the therapist presents the first scene on the anxiety hierarchy to the patient's imagination. As soon as the patient has a clear image of the scene, as signalled to the therapist by lifting a finger, two or three galvanic pulses are delivered. This is repeated until the first scene no longer elicits anxiety. The therapist then proceeds to the next scene and so forth as in the desensitization therapy. Some patients fail to report decrements in anxiety to imagined scenes with this procedure. Wolpe and Lazarus[53] suggest in these cases that the intensity of the shock be increased to the point of producing vigorous contractions of the forearm muscles. This level of shock, still not painful to most patients, appears to be more efficacious in some instances.

Various theoretical explanations have been offered to account for the deconditioning of anxiety in this procedure. However, the mechanism is still obscure.

Habit Elimination with Galvanic Shocks

This procedure is used chiefly with obsessional disorders and does not involve the use of an anxiety hierarchy. For example, a patient with the recurrent thought of an automobile accident in which he was involved would be instructed to signal the occurrence of the disturbing scene by raising his finger. At each such signal a non-aversive shock is delivered. The patient may be instructed to intentionally think of the disturbing thought during treatment sessions so that many thought-shock pairings can be administered. In addition, the patient may be supplied with a small self-shocking device which fits into the hand. With this device he may deliver shocks to himself outside the treatment session when the obsessional thought occurs. This procedure would constitute a form of conditioned aversion therapy if the shock level were in fact painful. It is stressed, however, that the procedure does not operate on this basis since very mild and clearly non-aversive levels of shock are used. The psychophysiological mechanism by which this procedure disrupts or interferes with obsessional thought patterns is not known.

OPERANT-REINFORCEMENT PROCEDURES

A number of powerful procedures are best conceptualized within the framework of operant or instrumental conditioning. The basic paradigm in this kind of conditioning may be illustrated by the common laboratory preparation of an experimental animal, such as a rat, pressing a lever for a food reward in a 'Skinner box'. The characteristics of the 'operant' behaviour generated in this kind of experimental situation have been extensively studied in animals as well as in man. The essential difference between operant and classical (Pavlovian) conditioning is the temporal relationship between reinforcement and the response being conditioned. In classical conditioning the reinforcement precedes the conditioned response; in operant conditioning the reinforcement follows the conditioned behaviour. For example, in classically conditioning salivation in a dog, the bell is sounded (conditioned stimulus), food is presented (unconditional stimulus or reinforcement) and the dog salivates (conditioned response). In contrast, in the operant conditioning of barpressing behaviour, the animal presses the bar (conditioned response) and then food is presented (reinforcement). A second distinction is that classical conditioning is concerned chiefly with involuntary (autonomically mediated) behaviour whereas operant conditioning is concerned almost entirely with voluntary (skeletal muscle) behaviour. However, the two kinds of conditioning are closely related and interact. Both can be seen to be operating in many experimental situations and in many clinical applications.

Schizophrenia

The first extensive clinical application of operant conditioning techniques was to chronic psychosis. Working in a mental hospital setting, Ayllon and colleagues[3, 4, 5] demonstrated the striking degree to which the socially disruptive, disorganized and 'regressive' behaviour of many chronic schizophrenic patients can be favourably modified by the systematic application of reinforcement principles. Their first efforts were with patients with eating problems, a frequent source of medical concern with hospitalized chronic psychiatric patients. Following a period of observation, they suggested that the eating disturbances exhibited by many of these patients were being inadvertently reinforced by the medical and nursing staff as well as by some of the other patients. A common occurrence, for example, was the patient whose principal social contact with the nurses occurred at mealtime when coaxing, assistance with the utensils, and other forms of reinforcing social stimulation occurred as a consequence of the patient's apparent inability to eat unaided. To corroborate this hypothesis and solve the eating problems of such patients, Ayllon simply reversed the reinforcement contingencies. More independent and socially adaptive behaviour was reinforced with praise, attention or tangible rewards such as cigarettes and candy while apparent inability to eat unaided was simply ignored. In a short time virtually all patients responded to this regimen with adequate food intake without assistance. In a similar fashion Ayllon was able to modify many other maladaptive behaviours previously ascribed to the patients's psychoses but which proved to be largely a product of the unwitting reinforcement of abnormal behaviour in a hospital setting. The success of these early efforts prompted Ayllon and colleagues[5] to attempt to analyse more of the symptomatic behaviour of their patients in these terms. To do this, much of the everyday activity of the patients was recorded in order to ascertain what social and other events in the ward environment might generate and maintain the various behaviours exhibited by the patients. In addition, Ayllon set up a 'token economy' on the ward in order to modify these behaviours in desirable ways. Thus personally and socially adaptive behaviours, such as maintaining personal cleanliness and doing useful work on the ward, were rewarded with tokens which could be exchanged for food, clothing, access to entertainment, and the like. Disruptive behaviours, such as shouting, and 'regressive' behaviours such as refusal to eat or hoarding bits of discarded paper, were not reinforced or in some instances 'punished' by the withdrawal of tokens.

The reader who is unfamiliar with this work may wonder how it differs from the many efforts of recent years to treat chronic psychosis with active programmes of social and vocational rehabilitation. The efficacy of these programmes which stress the role of the hospital as a therapeutic milieu probably depends in part on the operation of the same principles of learning. However, the programme described above makes more explicit and systematic use of principles of conditioning. Indeed, the core of Ayllon's programme is the objective measurement and recording of the patient's behaviour as a function of specific reinforcement contingencies. This in turn permits a functional analysis of each patient's behaviour, symptomatic and otherwise, and specification of the environmental events which are maintaining various behaviours. In addition, one can ascertain which behaviours of the patients can be modified by differential reinforcement and which cannot. Thus an efficient programme of treatment can be designed for each patient.

The use of operant-reinforcement procedures to reverse the deterioration in social and personal habits often seen in chronically hospitalized psychotic patients has now been well demonstrated by Ayllon[4] and others[1, 2, 35]. It is likely that these procedures render the patients more amenable to other forms of therapy. Whether these operant-reinforcement procedures by themselves favourably in-fluence the underlying schizophrenic disorder has not been clearly demonstrated at this time. However, there is suggestive evidence that they do[4, 5, 35].

Childhood Schizophrenia and Early Infantile Autism

Operant-reinforcement procedures hold great promise in the treatment of these refractory psychiatric disorders. Early research of Ferster and DeMyer[24] indicated the surprising degree to which the atavistic and socially withdrawn behaviour of markedly autistic children is responsive to reinforcement contingencies. Lovaas and his colleagues[39, 40] extended these procedures in a comprehensive pro-gramme of treatment for autistic children. The general approach is illustrated by their method for helping previously mute or echolalic children to acquire socially useful speech. The core of the procedure is to divide the process of acquiring speech into a series of very small steps. For a totally mute child the first step may simply be shaping the lips in preparation for uttering a single, simple sound. The second step may be actually uttering an approximation to this first sound and so forth. The child is then brought through this series of steps by using food as reinforcement. In this programme virtually all the patient's food is delivered to him in individual spoonfuls contingent upon performance of the next step in his learning-to-speak pro-gramme. With this procedure it has been possible to teach previously very unresponsive, withdrawn and uncommunicative children imitative speech and finally conversational and spontaneous speech. Other deficits in the behavioural repertoire of schizophrenic and autistic children have been similarly treated. In each the child is brought step-by-step through a graduated progression of tasks in which the delivery of positive reinforcement is contingent upon a correct response.

As new behaviours are acquired—speaking, dressing oneself, playing with other children—they may first be performed in a rather mechanical manner without much affective colouring. How-ever, as they become more permanent parts of the patient's be-havioural repertoire, their performance tends to be accompanied by appropriate affects as revealed by gesture, facial expression, and the like. This contrasts with what occurs in the more usual psychothera-peutic approaches to autistic children. In the latter the focus of treatment is usually the child's feelings with the assumption that more adaptive behaviour will follow affective changes. However, in the operant-reinforcement approach altering the child's behaviour is the immediate goal and affective changes are assumed to follow this.

These programmes are still too young and too few to adequately assess their efficacy. However, they appear to be more effective in a much shorter time than the more traditional psychotherapeutic approaches to these very difficult disorders[19, 32, 34, 39, 40].

Neurotic and Other Disorders

Operant-reinforcement principles have been used to fashion effective programmes of treatment for a variety of other disorders. Using procedures similar to those described above, Colman and Baker[18] devised an in-patient programme for the treatment of severe character and behaviour disorders in a military setting. A group of these patients treated within an operant-reinforcement framework did better by the criterion of being successfully returned to active duty than did a control group along more traditional lines. Of particular interest in this study was the observation that the improved behaviours and attitudes acquired by the patients in the course of operant-reinforcement therapy were well maintained when the men returned to active duty and the reinforcement contingencies which prevailed in the treatment setting were no longer operative.

The control of eating behaviour has been the focus of much behaviourally-oriented clinical research. Severe cases of anorexia nervosa have been successfully treated by making rewards such as access to a radio or being permitted to receive company contingent upon a minimal daily weight gain[6]. Blinder and colleagues[10] accomplished the same result by using permission to take exercise off the hospital ward, so rewarding to most anorexia nervosa patients, the reinforcement for a minimal daily weight gain. Stuart[47] devised a programme for the treatment of obesity. The core of this programme consists of a variety of procedures by which the patient gains self-control over his propensity to overeat.

The design of an operant-reinforcement procedure for the treatment of a specific neurotic state issues from a detailed behavioural analysis of the disordered behaviour. In the treatment of hysterical blindness, for example, the patient's use of visual cues to solve problems was differentially reinforced[16]. Patients with persistent, multiple tics were successfuly treated by following tics with aversive consequences and tic-free periods with positive reinforcement[8]. Detailed reports of additional applications of operant-reinforcement procedures to the treatment of neurotic and socially deviant behaviour disorders have been collected by Eysenck[20], Franks[25] and Ullman and Krasner[49].

OTHER PROCEDURES AND APPLICATIONS

Anticipatory Avoidance Learning

Many of the procedures already described involve elements of both Pavlovian and operant conditioning. The present procedure makes explicit use of both. The technique was developed by Feldman and MacCulloch[22] for the treatment of male homosexuality but it is adaptable for the treatment of other disorders as well. A photograph of a male, sexually attractive to the patient, is projected onto a screen. If the projected image is not removed within eight seconds the patient receives an aversive electric shock. The patient is provided with a switch by which he can remove the image at any time before eight seconds have elapsed and thus avoid a shock. However, on some trials which occur at random intervals, the switch is not operative, i.e. operating the switch fails to remove the image and a shock is delivered at the end of the eight-second period. After a number of trials in this situation, the projected image of the male elicits anxiety in the patient since it has been followed on some occasions with an aversive electric shock. This Pavlovian part of the procedure represents conditioned aversion as described earlier. It is expected that looking at and approaching a potential homosexual partner outside the treatment situation will also elicit anxiety (stimulus generalization). An important part of the procedure, however, is the fact that the patient himself is the one who terminates the viewing by operating the switch. This motoric (avoidance) behaviour is reinforced by removal of the image and hence diminution of the anxiety. It is anticipated that this operantly conditioned voluntary behaviour of avoiding homosexual stimuli will also generalize to outside the treatment situation. Feldman and MacCulloch[23] have elaborated their treatment along lines suggested by principles of learning. For example, ten or so different photographs are rank-ordered by the patient in increasing order of sexual attractiveness. The first or least attractive is used first, then the second least attractive and so forth. This is also the order of ease of developing an aversion to each of the photographs. Also, when the patient successfully terminates a male image, and hence experiences removal of anxiety, a photograph of a sexually provocative female is projected in its place. It is anticipated that the pairing of anxiety relief, a positive reinforcement, with female images will increase the patient's willingness to look at and approach previously fearful heterosexual partners outside the treatment sessions. Feldman and MacCulloch[23] report favourable results in 10 of 16 cooperative homosexual patients treated with this procedure.

271

Thought Stoppage

This is a simple procedure by which the patient may gain control over recurrent thoughts of a disturbing nature. The patient simply says 'Stop!' to himself at the moment he perceives the obsessional thought occurring. By persisting in this effort the frequency of occurrence of the thought often rapidly declines. Many variations on this basic procedure have been described[48, 53]. One the author finds especially useful is to equip the patient with a pocket or wrist counter. Then every time he has the obsessional thought he says 'Stop' and advances the counter one. He is instructed further to keep a record of the daily totals. The use of a counter has several advantages. The additional behaviour of advancing the counter seems to further inhibit the obsessional thoughts. The daily tallies allow the patient to follow his own progress. Usually patients are very encouraged by evidence that they are gaining control over their disturbing obsessional habit. This appears to facilitate further self-control. Finally, the daily record made by the patient provides the therapist with a fairly objective record of his patient's progress. Often a rapid change in the daily totals, in either direction, reflects events of emotional significance. The record thus provides the therapist with clues as to experiential variables important in the maintenance or elimination of the obsessional behaviour. Thus the record may aid the therapist in making additional refinements in the behavioural analysis of the patient's disorder.

Treatment of Stuttering

Stuttering offers a special challenge to the behaviourally-oriented therapist. When chronic and severe in an adult, an enduring cure is difficult to achieve by most psychotherapeutic measures. This persistence of the disorder is attributable in part to the self-reinforcing nature of the stutterer's speech problem. The disorder of stuttering consists of two components which interact. There is a dysfluent manner of speaking—the 'stuttering' itself—and the tendency to experience anxiety on approaching a variety of speaking situations. Stuttering is most likely to occur in just those situations in which the patient experiences anxiety, anxiety which is due in part to the experience of having stuttered in similar situations in the past. One would expect an effective programme to be one which takes account of these two components. Thus Brady[15] has developed such a programme in which systematic desensitization is employed to reduce the anxiety associated with speaking situations and operant-reinforcement techniques used to alter faulty habits of speech production. In addition, the programme makes use of a tiny, electronic metronome which resembles a hearing aid of the behind-the-ear type. For reasons which are not clear, most stutterers show an immediate and marked reduction in stuttering if they pace their speech with the rhythmic tick of a metronome. In the treatment programme the patient uses a metronome in a systematic manner. At first he times only one syllable of speech to each tick and uses the device in situations usually associated with minimal difficulty. As he gains experience with the device and confidence in his ability to speak more fluently he gradually speeds up his speech (e.g. by using one tick for two-syllable words) and begins to use the device in more difficult situations. When highly fluent speech is attained with minimal tension and anxiety, the use of the metronome is gradually 'faded out' by systematically reducing the loudness of the tick and gradually discontinuing its use. The total programme has proved to be effective with many patients whose stuttering was both chronic and severe.

CONCLUSIONS

The goal of this chapter has been to convey both the breadth and essence of behaviour therapy. To this end prototypic procedures have been described for the treatment of a variety of disorders. Some of these have strong underpinnings in learning theory. It should be stressed, however, that no procedure should be admitted to the armamentarium of the behaviour therapist merely because it possesses an impressive theoretical visa. Rather, the principal role of theory is to suggest new procedures or innovations in old ones. The decision as to their actual utility must be made on the basis of clinical data. Much carefully controlled clinical investigation still needs to be done to firmly establish the efficacy of many of these procedures.

REFERENCES

1. Agras, W. S. (1967). 'Behavior Therapy in the Management of Chronic Schizophrenia'. *Am. J. Psychiat.* **124,** 240
2. Atthowe, J. M. and Krasner, L. (1968). 'Preliminary Report on the Application of Contingent Reinforcement Procedures (Token Economy) on a "Chronic" Psychiatric Ward'. *J. abnorm. Psychol.* **73,** 37
3. Ayllon, T. and Haughton, E. (1962). 'Control of the Behavior of Schizophrenics by Food'. *J. exp. Analysis Behav.* **5,** 343
4. — and Azrin, N. H. (1965). 'The Measurement and Reinforcement of Behavior of Psychotics'. *J. exp. Analysis Behav.* **8,** 357

5. —— (1968). *The Token Economy: A Motivational System for Therapy and Rehabilitation*. New York: Appleton-Century-Crofts

6. Bachrach, A. J., Erwin, W. J. and Mohr, J. P. (1965). 'The Control of Eating Behavior in an Anorexic by Operant Conditioning Techniques'. In *Case Studies in Behavior Modification*, Chap. 14. Ed. by L. P. Ullmann and L. Krasner. New York: Holt, Rinehart and Winston

7. Bandura, A. (1965). 'Behavior Modification Through Modeling Procedures'. In *Research in Behavior Modification*, p. 310. Ed. by L. Krasner and L. P. Ullmann. New York: Holt, Rinehart and Winston

8. Barrett, B. H. (1962). 'Reduction in Rate of Multiple Tics by Free Operant Conditioning Methods'. *J. nerv. ment. Dis.* **135**, 187

9. Birnbrauer, J. S. and Lawler, J. (1964). 'Token Reinforcement for Learning'. *Ment. Retard.* **2**, 275

10. Blinder, B. J., Stunkard, A. J. and Ringold, A. L. (1968). *Behavior Therapy of Anorexia Nervosa—Effectiveness of Activity as a Reinforcer of Weight Gain*. Paper read at the 124th Annual Meeting of the American Psychiatric Association, Boston, Mass. May 13–17, 1968

11. Brady, J. P. (1966). 'Brevital-relaxation Treatment of Frigidity'. *Behav. Res. Ther.* **4**, 71

12. — (1967). 'Comments on Methohexitone-aided Systematic Desensitization'. *Behav. Res. Ther.* **5**, 259

13. — (1968). 'Drugs in Behavior Therapy'. In *Psychopharmacology: A Reveiw of Progress, 1957–1967*, p. 271. Ed. by D. H. Efron. Public Health Service Publication No. 1836. Washington, D.C.

14. — (1968). 'Psychotherapy by a Combined Behavioral and Dynamic Approach'. *Comprehen. Psychiat.* **9**, 536

15. — (1968). 'A Behavioral Approach to the Treatment of Stuttering. *Am. J. Psychiat.* **125**, 843

16. — and Lind, D. L. (1961). 'Experimental Analysis of Hysterical Blindness'. *Archs gen. Psychiat.* **4**, 331

17. Cautela, J. R. (1966). 'Treatment of Compulsive Behavior by Covert Sensitization'. *Psychol. Rec.* **16**, 33

18. Colman, A. D. and Baker, S. L. (1969). 'Utilization of an Operant Conditioning Model for the Treatment of Character and Behavior Disorders in a Military Setting'. *Am. J. Psychiat.* **125**, 1395

19. Davison, G. C. (1964). 'A Social Learning Therapy Programme with an Autistic Child'. *Behav. Res. Ther.* **2**, 149

20. Eysenck, H. J. (Ed.) (1964). *Experiments in Behavior Therapy* London: Pergamon Press

21. Feldman, M. P. (1966). 'Aversion Therapy for Sexual Deviations: A Critical Review'. *Psychol. Bull.* **65**, 65

22. — and MacCulloch, M. J. (1964). 'A Systematic Approach to the Treatment of Homosexuality by Conditioned Aversion'. *Am. J. Psychiat.* **121**, 167

23. — — (1965). 'The Application of Anticipatory Avoidance Learning to the Treatment of Homosexuality. I. Theory, Technique and Preliminary Results'. *Behav. Res. Ther.* **2**, 165

24. Ferster, C. B. and DeMyer, M. K. (1962). 'A Method for the Experimental Analysis of the Behavior of Autistic Children'. *Am. J. Orthopsychiat.* **32**, 89

25. Franks, C. M. (Ed.) (1963). *Conditioning Techniques in Clinical Practice and Research.* New York: Springer

26. — (1966). 'Conditioning and Conditioned Aversion Therapies in the Treatment of the Alcoholic'. *Int. J. Addictions* **1**, 61

27. Friedman, D. (1966). 'A New Technique for the Systematic Desensitization of Phobic Symptoms'. *Behav. Res. Ther.* **4**, 139

28. Friedman, D. E. I. and Silverstone, J. T. (1967). 'Treatment of Phobic Patients by Systematic Desensitization'. *Lancet* **1**, 470

29. Gelder, M. G. and Marks, I. M. (1966). 'Severe Agoraphobia: A Controlled Prospective Therapeutic Trial'. *Br. J. Psychiat.* **112**, 309

30. — — and Wolff, H. H. (1967). 'Desensitization and Psychotherapy in Phobic States. A Controlled Enquiry'. *Br. J. Psychiat.* **113**, 53

31. Goorney, A. B. (1968). 'Treatment of a Compulsive Horse Race Gambler by Aversion Therapy'. *Br. J. Psychiat.* **114**, 329

32. Hingtgen, J. N., Coulter, S. K. and Churchill, D. W. (1967). 'Intensive Reinforcement of Imitative Behavior in Mute Autistic Children'. *Archs gen. Psychiat.* **17**, 36

33. Jacobson, E. (1938). *Progressive Relaxation.* Chicago, Ill.: University of Chicago Press

34. Jensen, G. D. and Womack, M. G. (1967). 'Operant Conditioning Techniques Applied in the Treatment of an Autistic Child'. *Am. J. Orthopsychiat.* **37**, 30

35. Kennedy, T. (1964). 'Treatment of Chronic Schizophrenia by Behaviour Therapy: Case Reports'. *Behav. Res. Ther.* **2**, 1

36. Lang, P. J., Lazovik, A. D. and Reynolds, D. J. (1965). 'Desensitization, Suggestibility and Pseudotherapy'. *J. abnorm. Psychol.* **70**, 395

37. Lazarus, A. A. (1963). 'The Treatment of Chronic Frigidity by Systematic Desensitization'. *J. nerv. ment. Dis.* **136**, 272

38. — (1964). 'Crucial Procedural Factors in Desensitization Therapy'. *Behav. Res. Ther.* **2**, 65

39. Lovaas, O. I. (1966). 'A Program for the Establishment of Speech in Psychotic Children'. In *Childhood Autism.* Ed. by J. K. Wing. London: Pergamon Press

40. — Freitag, G., Gold, V. J. and Kassorla, I. C. (1965). 'Experimental Studies in Childhood Schizophrenia: Analysis of Self-destructive Behavior'. *J. exp. Child Psychol.* **2**, 67

41. McGuire, R. J. and Vallance, M. (1964). 'Aversion Therapy by Electric Shock: A Simple Technique'. *Br. med. J.* **1,** 151
42. Meyer, V. and Mair, J. M. M. (1963). 'A New Technique to Control Stammering: A Preliminary Report'. *Behav. Res. Ther.* **1,** 251
43. Paul, G. L. (1966). *Insight versus Desensitization in Psychotherapy.* Stanford, Calif.: Stanford University Press
44. — and Shannon, D. T. (1966). 'Treatment of Anxiety through Systematic Desensitization in Therapy Groups'. *J. abnorm. Psychol.* **71,** 124
45. Rachman, S. (1965). 'Aversion Therapy: Chemical or Electrical?' *Behav. Res. Ther.* **2,** 289
46. Salter, A. (1949). *Conditioned Reflex Therapy.* New York: Creative Age Press
47. Stuart, R. B. (1967). 'Behavioral Control of Overeating'. *Behav. Res. Ther.* **5,** 357
48. Taylor, J. G. (1963). 'A Behavioural Interpretation of Obsessive-compulsive Neuroses'. *Behav. Res. Ther.* **1,** 237
49. Ullmann, L. P. and Krasner, L. (Eds) (1965). *Case Studies in Behavior Modification.* New York: Holt, Rinehart and Winston
50. Wolpe, J. (1958). *Psychotherapy by Reciprocal Inhibition.* Stanford, Calif.: Stanford University Press
51. — (1962). 'The Experimental Foundations of Some New Psychotherapeutic Methods'. In *Experimental Foundations of Clinical Psychology.* Ed. by A. J. Bachrach. New York: Basic Books p. 562
52. — (1965). 'Conditioned Inhibition of Craving in Drug Addiction: A Pilot Experiment'. *Behav. Res. Ther.* **2,** 285
53. — and Lazarus, A. A. (1966). *Behavior Therapy Techniques.* London: Pergamon Press

CHAPTER 11

SUPPORTIVE PSYCHOTHERAPY

DAVID STAFFORD-CLARK

INTRODUCTION

At the outset it should be said quite unequivocally, that supportive psychotherapy is not a scientific subject, at least at present. It is an art with a technique, a procedure with various rules which can be learned and which, indeed, can in some degree be passed on, and this must be the object of this contribution. But no work which has as yet been published gives a scientific basis either for its administration or indications, for the selection of any particular technique through which it is given, nor for the results when compared with any other therapeutic technique, by methods such as a double blind trial or indeed any other scientific assessment which can be made.

This is not to say that attempts have not been made, and will not again be made, to fit a procedure which is ultimately so dependent upon individual human relationships into the objective mould of in-animate or predictable living responses: whether through the disciplines of sociology, statistics, or any other biological approach. Nevertheless, it is essential to be clear from the outset that in the author's opinion such attempts as have been made, have been entirely irrelevant to the practice of the subject. The purpose of this chapter will therefore be simply to record a report on experience of a little over a quarter of a century: during which the author has practised this technique with such art as he has learned, and such modest skill as he may have attained, through trial and error: error in particular. Supportive psychotherapy is never easy.

The inevitably individual nature of this contribution and, most of all, its lack of pretention to purely scientific validity is emphasized by the references. The references are to people who have contributed to the subject or made attempts at its evaluation and are, considering the thousands of contributions which have already been made, necessarily highly personal and selective. In view of what has already been said, the student who wishes either to disprove or alternatively to satisfy himself about the scientific respectability of psychotherapy in general, must look elsewhere.

He will certainly discover a whole range of erudite writers on the subject, from Freud[11], at one end to Eysenck[8] at the other. But in the final analysis the merits or demerits of psychotherapy, while arguable in terms of results remain, at least so far, impervious to scientific enquiry. You cannot calibrate the burden of a desolate heart, count the loss of a broken spirit, nor reckon the cost in time and energy of their repair or restoration: yet such are the raw materials of supportive psychotherapy.

This of course does not mean, and should not be taken to imply, that psychotherapy in general, or supportive psychotherapy in particular, are without value. Scientific evaluation demands the validation or refutation of the truth of a hypothesis reached by deductive or inductive reasoning, and experimentally tested. Such truth is indispensable to the totality of human knowledge, and in this respect the rigorousness whereby it is sought, and its worth when obtained, need not be further expounded. But there are other kinds of truth, including emotional and artistic, whose value is essential to man's life, but whose elucidation is not a scientific matter. In this context the words of Sir Charles Sherrington[17] are worth remembering:

> Mind, for anything perception can compass, goes therefore in our spatial world more ghostly than a ghost. Invisible, intangible, it is a thing not even of outline: it is not a 'thing'. It remains without sensual confirmation, and remains without it for ever. All that counts in life, desire, zest, truth, love, knowledge, 'values', and seeking metaphor to eke out expression, hell's depth and heaven's utmost height. . . . Naked mind.

Scope

Psychotherapy is in essence the treatment of the human mind. As a term for a form of activity directed towards that end, it covers all forms of communication between the professional therapist and the patient, including exchange of ideas, discussion, reasoning and emotion: it represents the effort to reach out into the mind and world of a sick person and, by comprehending it, to make it comprehensible to him: even to enable him to see it in a different way, and to modify his behaviour along lines governed by a deeper and wider understanding and by an increased confidence. This is really the basis of psychotherapy.

In practice the term is restricted to those methods which rely for their effect upon the exchange of ideas and understanding between patient and doctor, directed towards relief of the patient's symptoms and distress. This chapter is concerned exclusively with supportive psychotherapy. It therefore has to exclude all other forms of psycho-therapy, from full-scale formal psychoanalysis on the one hand, to any other discreet and self-limiting activity, such as pure decondition-ing by learning therapy, on the other. Just as the scientific endeavours of Freud[11], Jung[13], Adler[1], Wolpe[23] or Eysenck[8] are not really the answer to a purely scientific approach to psychotherapy in general, so their techniques for its administration, while all contributing to the totality of the subject, are not finally the heart of the matter.

The term supportive psychotherapy can sometimes be extended to include marital counselling, or the more professionally expert and specific marital psychotherapy, and certainly one or both partners to a marriage can require and receive supportive psychotherapy as the treatment of choice. So indeed can the marriage itself. But the basic indications, limitations, technique, and prognosis for supportive psychotherapy, while borrowing necessarily from many other aspects of psychotherapy, are not in themselves identical with any of them, and yet by themselves form the greatest single contribution that communication between one human being and another can make, not simply to psychiatric treatment, but throughout the wider range of medicine itself.

The contribution of psychiatry to a fuller understanding of the principles and practice of medicine must ultimately then be to under-line a single fundamental truth: the essential wholeness and dignity of man. For although the technique of psychiatry as part of the training of a medical student is of great importance throughout the entire complicated field of human relationship, and of mental health and sickness, it is in this bridge between what are commonly regarded as essentially medical, surgical, paediatric, gynaecological or obstetric disorders, and their emotional aspects and manifesta-tions, that the whole truth of medicine begins best to be understood.

Confronted by any sick, frightened, disturbed or unhappy person, the doctor can always remember this simple precept: 'Attention must be paid to such a person . . .' Once a patient realizes that you care about how he feels, then you have given him a bridge which he can cross to meet you and which you can cross to meet him. Good doctors have always recognized the necessity for such a bridge and the best have discovered something of the way to build it for them-selves and their patients. In this sense the better the doctor, the fuller will be his recognition of his own need for psychiatric know-ledge and skill and the more complete his attainment of these objectives, the better doctor will he yet become.

No good doctor can afford to be totally ignorant of supportive psychotherapy. Many good doctors believe that they practise it, but lack perhaps a precision in recognizing its indications and a clear grasp of some of those techniques upon which it rests and with this preamble we can now go forward to examine just those aspects of the subject.

Our goal must be to reach a concept of supportive psychotherapy which will include the potential use of relaxation under light hypnosis, of deconditioning to specific noxious stimuli, of long-term support, and equally long-term relationship therapy directed towards modification of the personality, including some knowledge of transactional analysis[5], but underlying each and every aspect of it must be the concept of bridge building, whereby the patient can pass from isolation to a more fruitful and less unhappy involvement with the rest of the world, and particularly with the other people in it, than was previously possible.

IMPLICATIONS

Before examining indications, techniques, and outlook, it seems reasonable at this point to attempt to give the reader some opportunity both to reflect upon, and to question, the concept under consideration. One way of doing this by a Socratic dialogue, compiled from questions asked by interested and critical students, both undergraduate and postgraduate, and answers aimed at meeting them, based on the author's experience which, as the earlier part of this chapter will already have warned the reader, is ultimately his sole justification for its appearance, as well as the foundations of the material it supplies.

Q. Well, I still don't feel that I really know what supportive psychotherapy is. How would you define it, if you like, in purely laymen's terms?

A. I think it can best be defined as a holding action, to preserve an individual's contact with life and with other people at the best possible level for that individual, for as long as may be necessary.

Q. Well, how long may this be?

A. It depends on the situation: the shortest period over which supportive psychotherapy is likely to make a significant difference could be as little as one or two interviews of half an hour to an hour each. The longest period could be a lifetime.

Q. Do you really mean that? That supportive therapy can last that long?

A. Yes.

Q. Well, in that case, how do you do it?

A. There will be something about this in the concluding section of this chapter which is devoted to indications, technique, and outlook: but bearing in mind that this may be a holding operation needing to last indefinitely, in most cases the doctor will usually have started out by seeing the patient once a week for a limited period, which may be as much as several months, after which the interviews will be progressively spaced out until they reach a point at which the patient is coming only when some crisis makes it necessary or, if at reasonably regular but longer intervals, as frequently as once every three or four months up to once or twice a year.

Q. But how can this possibly help anybody?

A. Because the relationship combines two essential qualities which are unlikely to be found in any other relationship which the patient has. The first is a purely objective kindness and perspicacity in understanding the patient's personality and life situation; the second, a willingness and a capacity to reflect that understanding in discussion with the patient, without becoming personally involved in resolving any of his or her life problems.

Q. Does that mean that the doctor never does anything practical to help the patient except either listening or talking to him or her?

A. Often it means exactly that. Very rarely the doctor may put the patient in touch with some other agency, from his psychiatric social service to more general agencies dealing with employment, legal aid, housing authorities, or other sources of help in critical life situation: and by providing this type of introduction may lead the patient into an ongoing possibility of practical help from people trained and dedicated towards its special provision.

Q. Apart from interviews is there anything else that the doctor may do?

A. Again, only exceptionally. But he may sometimes write a letter himself to an employer, a spouse, or other member of the family, or to somebody else or some other organization directly connected with the patient's difficulties and life situation or even offer to see other people on the patient's behalf, if they are prepared to come, always, however, with the aim of clarifying the problem for the patient, and thereby enabling the patient to reach a more realistic solution. If he can do this through interviews with other people which partially resolve the problem itself, such as postponing the patient's being sacked from a job, while the patient himself modifies his attitude towards it, so much the better.

Q. But the essence of supportive psychotherapy is the professional interview between the psychotherapist who is a doctor, and the patient who comes to see him by appointment?

A. Yes.

Q. Cannot this sometimes be done by lay people: Freud, for example, set great store by the hope of trained lay analysts?

A. That is perfectly true. But the purpose of this chapter is to give some information which doctors can use, and which they can safely use within our total arena of professional knowledge so that, for example, if the patient's response to supportive psychotherapy is to produce a string of hypochondriacal complaints, the therapist neither rejects him on this account, nor always feels bound to refer him to somebody else for their elucidation, nor indeed need the doctor be in any way inhibited from examining such patients to discover whether or not their complaints have any other structural or biologically functional foundation. This a doctor can do, but even the best lay therapists cannot. That is why this chapter, in what is essentially a medical book, is itself essentially a chapter for doctors.

Q. Bearing in mind that you have yet to describe technique, indications, and outcome, could you still not say something at this point about how this is done?

A. I could say this: that the essence of supportive psychotherapy is the relationship between the two people, and that therefore in one sense it would be described by analysts of all kinds as a transference.

Q. Do you mean by the transference what Freud[11] meant, or what Jung[13], Adler[1], or more recently Melanie Klein[14] or Michael Balint[3] have meant?

A. A good supportive psychotherapist is bound to acknowledge the inspiration of each and all of those whom you have mentioned. But he means both more and less than that. He means the relationship which develops when one person has confided as fully as he can in another, and because of this comes to have a special relationship with his confidante, and to assume more and more that the doctor will be as concerned with what the patient has told him as the patient is bound to be himself, without however being comparably involved in or overwhelmed by it.

Q. May not this make the patient too dependent upon the doctor?

A. Not if the doctor chooses his patients correctly, and particularly if he realizes that they need the kind of help which supportive psychotherapy essentially supplies, in that they are already too dependent, without having necessarily anyone to depend upon.

Q. So that one of the objects of supportive psychotherapy is to increase their independence?

A. Put simply, yes. But in fact we are all interdependent upon one another and, when we talk about independence, what we really mean is our ability to make our own contribution to the total situation of human interdependence in such a way that, in our journey through life, we are neither utterly passive passengers, nor always fighting for the exclusive right to drive the bus.

Q. Given then that this special relationship develops, and granted that this is not the part of the chapter dealing with techniques, can you still say how this relationship can be used to help the patient?

A. By enabling the patient to recognize something of the nature of personality: his own personality first, and then the reality of the personalities of other people. He can then begin to perceive the inevitability of difference involving potential clashes between personalities in their ordinary everyday transactions[5]; most of all and most inevitably in the transactions which occur between people who are closely bound to each other by family life, by marriage, by work or by any other kind of association which calls for an acknowledged interdependence, although neither of them may have realized that this will make the demands upon them which inescapably it does.

Q. Well perhaps this dialogue could go on for ever, but the chapter certainly can't so may I content myself with one last and perhaps impossible double question? Do you really think that supportive psychotherapy is worth the time and effort it costs, and does it really do much good? Wouldn't an ordinary good friend do just as well, and isn't supportive psychotherapy really a name for befriending someone in the hope that this friendship will cure them—and anyway does supportive psychotherapy ever cure anybody?

A. To answer the last and hardest question first, supportive psycho-therapy is sometimes followed by what amounts to a cure. But I would ask you to remember that medicine itself is concerned

primarily with attendance upon the sick and with relief of suffering; when possible with prevention; rather less often with what
may be regarded as total cure. When somebody is ill or injured,
complete recovery is naturally the goal of the doctor. But this
goal, and the role which the doctor can fulfil, are only identical in
about 20 per cent of all the cases with which the doctor has to deal.
Inevitably in the long run, for example, he fights a losing battle
with death. But while he is caring for a patient, his aim can be
well summed up in Trudeau's words 'To cure sometimes, to relieve
often, to comfort always'[21]. Supportive psychotherapy is more
than ordinary friendship because it brings professional detach-
ment: and with it the increased perception which the long view,
and the lack of involvement in any other way in the patient's life,
can always afford. But the way in which the doctor translates this
additional gain into the special professional service which supportive psychotherapy involves will, I hope, gain some clarification from the last part of the chapter which follows now.

TECHNIQUES

Supportive psychotherapy of any kind can always be combined with
appropriate medicinal symptomatic treatment, which it is not the
object of this contribution to specify. The first step is essentially a
comprehensive medical and psychiatric history: of the kind which
must indeed form the foundation of the psychiatric approach to any
human problem. Although the history can, for purposes of con-
venience, be recorded by the therapist under the various headings as
set out in textbooks, it is almost always wise to let the patient begin
by telling his own story, or putting his own complaint, in his own
words. Not infrequently the first 20 minutes of the first interview will
consist in a torrent of mingled information and emotional release,
in the form of a bewildered monologue, to which literally no one in
the patient's life has ever found the time to listen before.

Whenever an outburst of this kind may be imminent or necessary,
it is part of the art of supportive therapy to allow it to take place. For
in the first interview, above all, it is likely to be what the patient
tells the doctor, rather than what the doctor tells the patient, which
may well determine the subsequent course, and with it success or
failure, of treatment of this kind.

While the doctor is eliciting the history in this informal but un-
obtrusively skilful fashion, he should also be cataloguing, in his own
mind, potential goals for future exploration and clarification. To
some extent his recognition and his identification of these goals will

be conditioned by his own training. The analytically trained psychotherapist will be on the alert for, and will readily recognize, evidence
of repressed complexes: from the classical oedipal situation, through
other all too familiar human experiences so often productive of
human woe such as early sibling rivalry, parental rejection, penis
envy in girls, castration fears and complexes in men, and indeed the
whole range of human unconscious psychodynamic patterns, whose
recognition forms part of our inheritance from Freud[11] and those who
came after him. Jungian[13] or Adlerian[1] psychotherapists may find
comparable evidence respectively of hitherto unrecognized arche-
types, or life plans aimed at compensating for unconscious inferiority, in these revelations: while the therapist trained principally
along behavioural[23] lines is likely to discover evidence of conditioning, repeated stimulus responses, and ultimate stimulus generalization.

It is important to remember that all these things are likely to be
present, and therefore all of them can be found, in the life history of
every human being. In a chapter on composite methods in modern
psychotherapy, part of a book which has received perhaps less
attention than it deserved, Dr. Leslie Weatherhead[22] illustrates this
with an apt example. He starts from the imagined dream of a crippled
married woman, and shows how a characteristic interpretation along
Freudian, Adlerian, Jungian, and behavioural lines, each illuminating one aspect of her total predicament, could be derived. Clearly,
the wider the basic training of the therapist, the greater will be his
potential insight into the raw material produced by the patient in the
course of the history. But once the initial goals have been selected,
and the assessment of the patient's basic personality made, the next
stage in the task of supportive psychotherapy is to embark on treatment itself.

TREATMENT

The basic starting framework has already been defined as weekly
interviews, which must later be reduced in frequency if a reasonable
number of patients are to be treated simultaneously. The goals themselves can be listed in the therapist's treatment plan and, once the
initial history is completed, can be tackled in whatever order proves
most appropriate in the light of the patient's presentation of his
difficulties. Often a good starting point is the initial complaint. This
is unlikely to be purely somatic, since by the time the patient is
referred for supportive psychotherapy, or recognizes his need for it,
much water will have flowed under many investigational bridges:

and persistent distress will almost certainly have emphasized a need for recognition of the role of life situation, personality, and immediately exacerbating emotional factors, in the total clinical picture. Given the opportunity to elaborate the initial complaint, a patient will often tell the doctor a great deal more about his life, its frustrations, fulfilments, hopes and fears, than he may previously have been able to see for himself.

Included amongst the goals must be every combination of circumstances which strike the therapist as being of recurrent importance in the patient's life. The late Dr Jacob Finesinger[9] devised a simple technique for undertaking what he called insight therapy which is based on goal selection along analytical lines, followed by a limited number of goal-directed interviews. These can at times form a useful part of supportive psychotherapy, although the amount of insight which a patient can achieve or tolerate will always form an important part of the therapist's overall assessment of the case.

Interpretations come later in the course of treatment and they should always be based on the material which the patient has already provided, rather than upon any hypothetical constructions of the therapist's own training, no matter how accurate or reliable these may have proved to be. For example, it is least likely to cause avoidable complication or difficulty in the course of treatment if an interpretation is always put to the patient in a deliberately open-ended or speculative way along the lines of 'Do you think it's possible that you feel X and Y now, because when you first experienced them they were always associated with A and B in your life . . .?' The X and Y can be, for example, a sense of personal shame, connected with blushing, bronchospasm, or symptoms of acute headache or urgency of micturition whilst A and B can relate to childhood situations involving siblings, parents or school. Somatic symptoms and their sexual setting can also be related in the same way. People who would argue angrily and defiantly about an interpretation based on a psychodynamic formulation will as often eagerly accept and find relief in it when it is conveyed indirectly, as a possibility put up for their consideration by a therapist who recalls what they have themselves told him, and perceives the link between that and what is happening to them now.

Part of Finesinger's original technique was to insist that the record kept by the therapist, whether on tape or in any kind of shorthand or manuscript of which he might be capable, was as detailed as possible and included his own as well as the patient's contributions, while specifically avoiding any suggestion of what he expected, or sought to find.

He taught what amounted to a simple course in professional acting whereby the therapist could assume at will the role of an interested, neutral or even occasionally deliberately remote (although never unobservant) listener. The technique perfected by Finesinger therefore assists the doctor to appreciate the differing degree to which he is implicated in each patient's situation. Doctors trained under him also learned to extract from their patients a continuous stream of information, often by essentially nonverbal communications, such as nods, smiles, or sometimes a remote or distant look although where it was necessary to stimulate the patient to further revelation, without suggesting what form it should take, a repetition of key words from the patient's last sentence was preferred.

This latter technique can be tested in practice in many otherwise routine social situations, provided obvious rudeness or exploitation is scrupulously avoided, when for any reason the observer is not feeling particularly inclined to exhibit his own social parlour tricks. (In the following fictional example O is the observer and R the respondent, that is, the person addressing him.)

R. It must be fascinating to be a psychologist—I mean, being able to read people's minds and all that . . .

O. *Fascinating?*

R. Well yes, I mean to know all our darkest thoughts.

O. *Ours?*

R. No, not necessarily mine, I don't *think* I have any, I mean, for all I know, you can tell *what I'm thinking now*, but anybody else's you know, people who come to see you.

O. *What you're thinking now?*

R. Well that's just it, I mean if it was something I couldn't tell you here.

O. *Where could you tell me?*

R. Well I suppose in your consulting room—not that I'd ever go there.

O. *Not ever?* (smiling enquiry: no trace of hostility)

R. Well, you know what I mean.

O. Tell me *what you mean.*

The combination of the repetition of selected words and occasional deliberate encouragement by saying 'tell me about that . . . . . .' (whatever it happens to be) or, alternatively, the interested look followed by what Max Beerbohm once described as 'plying the weapon of silence' can be extremely effective.

287

RESULTS

Whether the goals be few or many, and the plan for treatment brief, perhaps a few weeks, several months, or in selected cases longer but at less frequent intervals, two things will inevitably occur. One is that a relationship will have been created between the doctor and the patient, in which the patient has learnt to accept the doctor's interest as dependable and sustained, without being conditional upon the patient's own moods: and the doctor will have formed an increasingly clear overall appreciation of the patient's predicament and life situation: using the term 'appreciation' here in its military sense.

Indeed a competent psychiatrist can often see in essence the core of a patient's problems by the time he has completed the preliminary study of the patient's life. Sometimes patients, sensing something of the purpose of this study, will demand an exposition of what is in the doctor's mind, in the belief or hope that this will offer them an immediate key to recovery. But in this sense unfortunately no one can learn from another's experience of his life, no matter how expert or accurate the impression formed by the doctor may prove to be.

We build up our patterns of thought and feeling slowly and often painfully, and the emotional experiences which have gone into them have to be relived rather than retold before we are liberated from their influence upon us. There is all the difference in the world between the intellectual formulation of a man's problems and personality, and that change of heart which alone can bring him release from the chains in which they have bound him. Whether we call the link which the doctor can establish between the one and the other the transference situation or the patient–doctor relationship, we are really dealing with an emotional bond which acts as a catalyst for all the chaotic feeling and experience of the sick or unhappy person.

On the patient's side much of this emotional bond springs, as we have seen, from the reservoirs of stifled and forgotten passions: on the doctor's side from the detached but absolutely sincere and dedicated concern to help, however humbly, another human being. Behind them both there must be that greatest gift of all, a capacity for unselfish love: and for all the wisdom, skill and technical accomplishment which ought to go into it, psychotherapy is fundamentally but another way of using the creative power of love towards the restoration of human happiness and peace of mind.

There is another and perhaps equally illuminating sense in which the concept of love can usefully be employed to help the doctor delineate his task. Part of it must necessarily involve a plan for the limitation, or, if the reality situation demands it, the ultimate termination of the therapeutic relationship: for example if the doctor or patient are only going to be in the same country for a limited period of time. This situation can arise either because the patient has travelled to seek treatment, or because the doctor who is giving it is himself available for only a limited period, either because of training requirements, or because of his own life plans.

Neither of these considerations preclude recognition that ideally the needs of the situation may be infinite—and therefore impractical: they simply impose inescapably realistic limitations, which also have to be acknowledged. There is a sense in which a psychotherapeutic relationship can be likened to a love affair although in practice this is just what it must never become. But just as an inexperienced psychotherapist tends to think principally in terms of gaining rapport and creating the relationship, so an ardent young adventurer may be constantly preoccupied in looking for a new love affair. An experienced psychotherapist, like an experienced lover, knows that the difficulty will be not to begin it, but to end it. So a part of his efforts are always directed towards seeing how and when it has to be ended: and how it can be ended with the least distress for the most vulnerable person, usually the patient.

CONCLUSIONS

In summary, some supportive psychotherapy can in fact be quite brief. It can include direct, simple and sympathetic advice, sometimes sheer reassurance and encouragement; it may be combined with practical intervention into the social circumstances of the patient whereby emotional complications of the family life or employment are constructively modified through contact with family or employer, often by a trained psychiatric social worker attached to the out-patient clinic and under the supervision of the psychotherapist concerned.

Even so, it is important in even the briefest supportive psychotherapy that such advice or explanation that the doctor has to offer should be based not upon his own personal feelings about the desirability of any particular solution and still less upon the projection on his part of what he would do if he were in the patient's shoes. These are the two shortcomings from which so much well-intentioned lay advice so often suffers. By contrast, the doctor's advice and explanation will be based upon his objective assessment of the patient's individual needs and possibilities, gained from his knowledge of the patient acquired in the way described, and accepted without prejudice of any kind.

He may also consider that the patient will require periodic advice and supervision for some time, in order that the readjustment which is desirable may be followed and consolidated. From the patient's point of view, the knowledge that there exists somebody who not only understands him and his symptoms, but who is able to accept him without hostility and distress, to explain to him the nature of his difficulties and their connection with symptoms which he has developed, and to help and support him through the stresses which underlie these symptoms, is in itself a very great help and comfort. It may enable such a patient to resume work and domestic responsibility which have formerly proved impossible, and to take his place once again as an active member of the community. Treatment of this kind represents the first line of defence against mental illness which the medical profession has to offer and much of the avoidable unhappiness caused by fear, anxiety, tension or guilt in daily life, is often successfully relieved or prevented in this way. Often it is quite unnecessary to acquaint the patient with more than a fraction of the underlying implications which the detailed study of his life has revealed: but as a basis for any kind of advice, explanation or reassurance, insight on the part of the doctor, as accurate and complete as his skill and training can render it, is indispensable.

In practise a useful framework for such brief psychotherapy may be constructed by planning eight to a dozen interviews at weekly intervals, each of 30 to 45 minutes duration, for which the following targets are set:

(1) Establishment of rapport; effective doctor–patient relationship; adequate history (for two interviews). This can lead to an appreciation of the situation—here again using the word appreciation in its military sense.

(2) Selection of goals; formulation of overall plan of treatments; exploration of goals (subsequent three to four interviews).

(3) Interpretation of material (begun at appropriate stages of exploratory interviews, but completed within context of overall treatment); integration of these interpretations with the patient's own concept of his life situation and implications; recognition and acceptance by the patient, support and reassurance by doctor (final three to four interviews).

The methods, mechanisms, and special techniques involved are indicated on p. 291 (J. J. Fleminger, personal communication).

As a general rule, it is reasonable to regard the ratio of the three contributions of ventilation, exploration and guidance, in the total course of treatment, as being 7:2:1. It is sometimes possible to complete the process within a dozen or so interviews, but whether or not this is so, it is always practicable at about this stage to lengthen the intervals between the interviews, and to settle the basis of supportive psychotherapy onto a practical and effective relationship

Percentage of time	Methods		Mechanisms	Special techniques
	Patient	Doctor		
Ventilation 70	Describes symptoms Discharges emotions	Listens Accepts Encourages	Internal and Passive (Stress reaction dissolves)	Abreactive
Exploration 20	Recalls trauma Discovers connections	Questions Interprets	Internal and Active (Stress reaction resolved by patient)	Analytic
Guidance 10	Listens Comments Questions	Reassurance Explanation Advice	External and Passive (Stress or reaction reduced by doctor)	Counselling Suggestion Social aid

which can accompany the emotional maturation of the patient in all aspects of his or her personality.

Special Techniques

Apart from the overall technique of supportive psychotherapy already indicated, group therapy, and deconditioning techniques using relaxation under light hypnosis (and thereafter following the pattern of behaviour therapy especially indicated in phobic anxiety states, as described by Wolpe[23]) all have their place. The special techniques of hypnosis, and ways in which group therapy can be used for support, would require entirely separate consideration for their adequate description[19]. There remain for consideration the principle indications for supportive psychotherapy, and their reasonable expectation in terms of outlook and prognosis for the patient who learns to accept and benefit from such treatment.

Indications

The most important single indication is that the patient is aware of

subjective emotional disability, capable of some degree of communication, and willing to spend the time and the effort necessary to
make it effective. Patients with personality disorders are often among
the most importunate in appealing for this kind of help, and may
indeed include some whose need is greatest. But selection is always
inseparable from elimination of those unsuitable. In general, the more
grossly immature the patient's personality, the longer and more
arduous will be the course of any kind of psychotherapy. At the
emotionally infantile level of psychopathic personality, the choice
may lie between complete analysis if the patient is capable of it, or
interminable failure if he is not.

Supportive psychotherapy is far more valuable for patients whose
emotional maturity has reached adolescence but, in varying degrees,
has failed to transcend it. Chronic anxiety states, phobic anxiety
states, sometimes obsessive compulsive disorders, and often chronic
psychotic or chronic hysterical disorders may all lend themselves to
supportive psychotherapy in combination with other specific
medicinal or therapeutic measures. The common denominator of all
the indications for supportive psychotherapy is that a human being
in dire distress can neither recognize its origins, nor discover any way
of dealing with it, in the absence of effectively sustained communication. Such a human being can usually be helped by a form of psychotherapy as flexible, professional, and as realistically compassionate,
as supportive psychotherapy needs to be.

Prognosis

In the author's experience, between 20 and 30 per cent of all
patients attending for supportive psychotherapy eventually recover and no longer require it, within a relatively limited period. But
they may still require, after the 3, 6 or 12 months during which
they may have been seen regularly, an occasional lifeline to the
therapist; in practice an opportunity to come back if the need
arises. Often the mere knowledge that such an opportunity exists provides a specific prophylactic against its being required. In the remaining 70 per cent of cases, the therapist and the patient learn to think
not so much in terms of complete recovery, as of re-establishment of
equilibrium: sometimes simply a less vicious and self-destructive
circle of repetitive failure than the patient has originally contrived
for himself.

While an abandonment of commitments or a jettisoning of responsibilities prove sometimes to be part of the inevitable price which
a crippled personality may have to pay for any kind of stable
equilibrium, the wise supportive psychotherapist will not urge or

advise these measures, particularly when they involve other people to whom the patient is under some obligation. Every kind of human retreat from difficulty including divorce, separation, or desertion in marriage, resigning from a post or accepting dismissal, a general lowering of the sights which had previously been inseparable from a patient's self esteem, can form part of the material which comes up for discussion in the course of supportive psychotherapy, but none of the decisions ultimately implicit in them need or should be taken solely on the psychotherapist's personal advice or responsibility. As indicated in the dialogue in the central section of this chapter, supportive psychotherapy is essentially a kind of holding action, and if the holding lasts until recovery or relief comes about so much the better. But even if it does not, neither on therapist's nor on the patient's part can abandonment of responsibility, rejection of someone else's need, or betrayal of their trust, ever form part of the treatment plan.

Two final observations will perhaps exemplify the essence of the outlook which should become the aim of both patient and therapist in supportive psychotherapy. The first is that the mere payment of attention to stress can be a significant step towards its alleviation; the second that, whenever the physician is confronted by an acutely unhappy, distracted, or suffering patient, he must never withhold acceptance, compassion, or understanding, but he must take care how he shows it. To place a comforting hand on the shoulder of a depressed, schizophrenic, or otherwise psychotic patient may be an act of simple kindness—or occasionally of inspired communication. To do the same to someone in the anguish of neurosis, particularly to someone with hysterical personality, may be to invite misunderstanding and perhaps to court disaster.

The key to this is simple. Psychotic patients are often like children in a nightmare whereas neurotic patients are more like disturbed and accusing adolescents, and require a different kind of attention—and respect.

All patients can benefit from supportive psychotherapy at some stage in their lives, whatever the nature of their illness. There will never be enough of it to go round. But it is as much a part of the armoury of the competent physician as is manual dexterity or gentleness in handling tender or painful tissues and patients are entitled to expect this level of expertness from those who offer them treatment.

Psychotherapy of this limited but invaluable kind should be within the capacity of every practising doctor. The expenditure of a limited amount of time in this way is not only humane, but economical, for by the skilled use of a few hours spread out over weeks or months, the physician may not only avert the chronic invalidism and demoralization of the neurotic patient, but may also spare himself the bitterness and frustration which inevitably assail a practitioner continually confronted with this aspect of human suffering and who has never acquired the interest or understanding necessary to deal with it effectively.

REFERENCES

1. Adler, A. (1924). 'The Practice and Theory of Individual Psychology'. Translated by P. Radin. London: Kegan Paul
2. Atkin, I. (1962). *Aspects of Psychotherapy*. London, Edinburgh: Livingstone
3. Balint, Michael (1964). *The Doctor, his Patient and the Illness*, 2nd edn. London: Pitman
4. — and Balint, Enid (1961). *Psychotherapeutic Techniques in Medicine*. London: Tavistock Publications
5. Berne, Eric (1966). *Games People Play*. London: Andre Deutsch
6. Carkhaff, Robert R. and Berenson, Bernard (1967). *Beyond Counselling and Therapy*. New York: Holt, Rinehart and Winston
7. Courtenay, Michael (1968). *Sexual Discord in Marriage*. London: Tavistock Publications
8. Eysenck, Hans J. (1967). *The Effects of Psychotherapy*. New York: International Science Press
9. Finesinger, Jacob E. (1959). *Interviewing Techniques*. Film sponsored by the Veterans Administration, U.S.A.
10. Frank, Jerome D. (1962). *Persuasion and Healing*. Baltimore: Johns Hopkins Press
11. Freud, S. (1933). *New Introductory Lectures on Psychoanalysis*. Translated by James Strachey, Anna Freud, Alix Strachey and Alan Tyson. Standard Edition. London: Hogarth Press
12. Gaylin, Willard (1958). *The Meaning of Despair*. New York: Science House.
13. Jung, C. (1962). Collected papers on *Analytical Psychology*. London: Bailliere, Tindall and Cox
14. Klein, Melanie (1948). *Contributions to Psychoanalysis*. London: Hogarth Press
15. Malan, D. H. (1963). *A Study of Brief Psychotherapy*. London: Social Science Paperbacks
16. Ross, T. A. (1937). *The Common Neuroses*, 2nd edn. London: Edward Arnold
17. Sherrington, Sir Charles (1955). *Man on his Nature*. The Gifford Lectures, Edinburgh, 1937–8. Harmondsworth, Middlesex: Penguin

18. Stafford-Clark, David (1952). *Psychiatry Today*. Harmondsworth, Middlesex: Penguin
19. — (1964). *Psychiatry for Students*. 1st edn, p. 162 and appendix II. London: Allen and Unwin
20. Storr, Anthony (1960). *Integrity of the Personality*. London: Heinmann
21. Trudeau, Edward Livingstone (1916). *Autobiography*. New York
22. Weatherhead, Leslie D. (1951). *Psychology, Religion and Healing*. London: Hodder and Stoughton
23. Wolpe, J. (1963). 'Pychotherapy: The Nonscientific Heritage and the New Science'. *Behav. Res. Ther.* **1,** 23

CHAPTER 12

THE PATHOLOGICAL ANATOMY OF THE TEMPORAL LOBE WITH SPECIAL REFERENCE TO THE LIMBIC AREAS

J. A. N. CORSELLIS

The temporal lobe is susceptible in general to the same pathological processes that may affect other parts of the brain. There are, however, some conditions in which the damage tends to be concentrated in the anterior and medial parts. When this happens certain forms of mental disorder are prone to occur.

The areas which now seem to be most relevant in this connection (*Figures 1* and *2*) are the uncus and the parahippocampal (or hippo-campal) gyrus on the surface of the brain; the deeper structures include the amygdaloid nucleus in the roof of the inferior horn and the hippocampus (or Ammon's horn) which lies inferomedial to the ventricle and projects through the fornix to the diencephalon, and, in particular, to the mamillary bodies and the septal region. These areas together make up the inferior half of the ring of grey matter which, with the cingular gyrus dorsally, encircles the medial wall of each cerebral hemisphere. The entire ring, with its deeper connections and perhaps with extension into the posterior orbital and insular cortex, is now often referred to as the limbic lobe, limbic areas, or, more tendentiously, as the limbic system.

The functions of these areas have been debated for many years and are still far from clear. What little is known has been the result of progress in clinical, anatomical and physiological knowledge as much as in the field of pathology.

A short incursion into the way ideas have developed about the nature of the limbic system, and in particular about its temporal component, may therefore be helpful if the pathological aspects are to be seen in perspective.

HISTORICAL BACKGROUND

Willis had already in the seventeenth century made use of the term 'limbic' to describe the anatomy of the brain around the corpus callosum. It was not, however, until the early part of the nineteenth

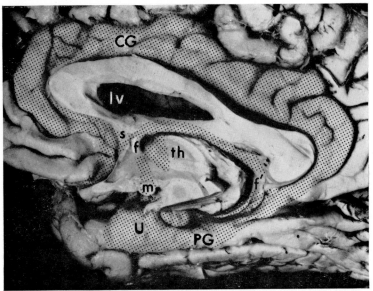

Figure 1. Sagittal view of the medial surface of a human hemisphere. The shading illustrates the general disposition of the limbic areas. CG—cingular gyrus; PG—parahippocampal gyrus; f—anterior column of fornix; f'—posterior column of fornix; lv—lateral ventricle; m—mamillary body; s—septal area; th—thalamus; U—uncus

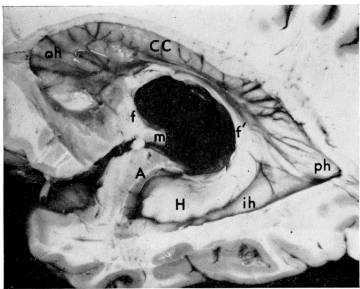

Figure 2. Dissection of hemisphere with the convexity and the thalamus removed to expose the lateral ventricle (CC—corpus callosum; ah—anterior horn; ih—inferior horn; ph—posterior horn). The hippocampus (H) is seen lying in the floor of the inferior horn and connecting through the fornix with the mamillary body. The amygdaloid nucleus (A) lies deep in the uncus in the roof of the inferior horn

century that this area began to be studied in such a way that the limbic lobe emerged as an entity.

Two French anatomists, Gerdy[34] and Foville[29], were concerned with this development. The former described, in 1838, an annular convolution on the medial side of each hemisphere. In the following year Foville named this ring of grey matter the 'convolution of the hem' since he envisaged it as running, like the edge of a bonnet, round the inner margin of each hemisphere. He laid great importance on this convolution but he gave no reasons why he done had so.

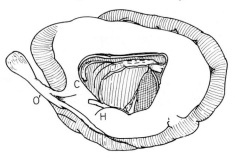

(Reproduced from Atom Broca (1878) by courtesy of the Editor of the *Revue anthropologique*)

Figure 3. The drawing of an otter's brain which Broca used to illustrate the extent of the 'great limbic lobe'. O'—olfactory tract; C— cingular gyrus; H—hippocampal (now known as parahippocampal) gyrus. The peripheral shaded area represents the extralimbic mass of the hemisphere

Some 40 years later Foville's observations were resurrected by Broca[14] in his extensive study on the comparative anatomy of the cerebral mantle.

Broca introduced the term 'the great limbic lobe' and compared its shape to a tennis racquet. He described how the handle was formed by the olfactory lobe, the dorsal part of the frame by the cingular gyrus and the ventral part by the medial grey matter of the temporal lobe (*Figure 3*).

Broca considered that these parts together constituted a separate and fundamental division of the cerebral mantle which, since it was more than a mere lobe of the brain, should be distinguished as the 'great limbic lobe'. Broca often returned to the special nature of this lobe, contrasting it with the 'extra-limbic' mass. In doing so, he foreshadowed in a most remarkable way ideas about cerebral localization that only began to reappear in the last 30 years. He wrote '. . . these two parts of the hemisphere, so different in their structure, differ also in their functions . . . one comes to recognize that the first is the seat of the lower faculties which predominate in the beast, and the second is the seat of those superior faculties which predominate in the intelligent animal . . .' and again '. . . the cerebral hemisphere is composed of two parts, the one *brutish* represented by the great limbic lobe, the other *intelligent* represented by the rest of the mantle. . . .'

Broca did not elaborate these ideas and the term 'brutal' was left ill-defined. The way, however, in which he described the sense of smell as a brutal sense indicated that the olfactory pathways formed, in his opinion, an important part of the great limbic lobe. It is wrong, however, to think, as Ferrier suggested, that Broca held the great limbic lobe to be concerned only with the sense of smell.

Schwalbe[86] accepted Broca's delineation of the great limbic lobe, but preferred to call it the falciform, or sickle-shaped, lobe. Schwalbe took more account than Broca of its deeper connections and he therefore divided this falciform lobe into an outer and an inner component, a division which is still of practical use today. The outer part was the cortex seen on the surface and consisted of the fornicate gyrus, which is a joint name for the cingular and parahippocampal gyri. The inner, deeper, part was formed by the hippocampus (which Broca probably included in his great limbic lobe), the fornix and the septum pellucidum, neither of which was mentioned by Broca.

Ferrier[28] considered that his own experimental work, as well as that of Horsley and Schäfer[48], confirmed the identity of Broca's great limbic lobe, which he preferred, like Schwalbe, to call the falciform lobe. Ferrier maintained that only a small anterior part of this lobe was concerned with smell and that 'all the facts receive the most satisfactory explanation if we regard the falciform lobe as a whole and in each and every part the centre of tactile sensation . . .'.

Such views, however, were not without their critics. Zuckerkandl[110] disagreed with Ferrier's experimental work, claiming that his own contributions had clearly demonstrated that the Ammon's horn belonged to the olfactory system.

The reintroduction of the term rhinencephalon at this time by Turner[100] gave further support to Zuckerkandl's view, not because of anything Turner wrote but because the word 'rhinencephalon' satisfied an anatomical need and it soon came to be used, or misused, as a replacement for the term 'limbic lobe'. Such a substitute was readily taken up, for Broca's theories had proved unacceptable to many anatomists. Elliot Smith[26], for example, remarked in 1901 on the 'strange fascination' which the theory of the limbic lobe still exercised over the minds of many writers.

As the years passed, however, this fascination seems to have weakened, and as neurohistological techniques developed the interest seemed more in establishing with greater precision the architecture and the connections of these areas than in investigating their possible role. It is, for instance, noticeable that in Rose's exhaustive study[80] of the 'so-called olfactory cortex in men and monkeys', function was mentioned only in the last paragraph and, interestingly enough, the suggestion was then made that this was not restricted to the sense of smell.

The modern reawakening of interest in the human limbic areas was the result of an article published by Papez[72]. Papez's aim was to integrate the work of Cannon[16] and others, who had been investigating the functions of the hypothalamus, with advances in neuroanatomical knowledge which had emphasized the importance of the direct pathways linking the medial wall of the cerebral hemisphere to the diencephalon. Papez summarized his views in the proposition that 'the hypothalamus, the anterior thalamic nuclei, the cingular gyrus, the hippocampus and their interconnections, constitute a harmonious mechanism which may elaborate the functions of central emotion as well as participate in emotional expression'. Papez culled from the literature a body of information which helped to support this idea but, as he pointed out, he did not present negative or contradictory evidence. Once again, it was emphasized that there was no good reason to connect these areas simply with the sense of smell, a view which was later strongly supported, in so far as the hippocampus was concerned, by Brodal[15].

At about the same time that Papez published his hypothesis, Klüver and Bucy[54, 55] reported gross behavioural and affective disturbances in monkeys after the removal of both temporal lobes and therefore of a major part of both limbic areas. Experimental work on the effects of ablation or disturbances of one or other parts of these areas increased and in 1949 MacLean[58] developed his concept of the visceral brain—a term which is at least reminiscent of the 'brutal brain' of Broca. MacLean's argument is separated from that of Broca by 70 years, but the following sentences by MacLean could almost have been written by Broca:

Although in the ascension to higher forms, the rhinencephalon yields more and more control over the animal's movements to the neocortex, its persistent strong connections with lower autonomic centres suggest that it continues to dominate in the section of visceral activity. Hence the rhinencephalon might be justifiably considered a visceral brain and will be so referred to . . . to distinguish it from the neo-cortex which holds sway over the body musculature and subserves the function of the intellect.

MacLean called on a wide range of clinical and experimental data to support his concept of the visceral brain. Shortly afterwards Fulton[30] attempted to link the visceral brain to various forms of leucotomy. He showed how the study of the clinical and the neuro-anatomical effects of leucotomy (e.g. Meyer and Beck[62]) had led to the trend for the operation to become more precisely localized and to move away from the neocortex of the prefrontal areas into the regions of the limbic grey matter, such as the cingular gyrus and the posterior orbital cortex.

Scoville then extended the field of 'psycho-surgery' beyond the prefrontal areas into the temporal lobes. In so doing, he discovered that the removal of the medial, or limbic, parts of both temporal lobes was followed by the development of a severe disorder of recent memory[87, 88].

Interest in these same areas was further stimulated by the results of the operation of temporal lobectomy which had been introduced for the treatment of psychomotor and allied forms of epilepsy[74].

During the subsequent 15 years the limits and the functions of the limbic system have been extensively investigated. Comprehensive reviews with references include those by Green[37], Hassler[44], Poeck[78], Stephan[95], Lowell White[107], and most recently there is the stimulating monograph of Smythies[90] which is concerned with 'the mechanisms of emotion, memory, learning and the organisation of behaviour, with particular regard to the limbic system'.

Apart from that by Hassler, however, none has been primarily concerned with the neuropathological aspects. This is no doubt partly due to the way in which nearly all pathological processes or lesions involving the human limbic areas fail to respect anatomical boundaries. It is, therefore, peculiarly difficult to assess the significance of an apparent link between pathological and clinical observations, particularly when both are always complex and often ill-defined. The two main exceptions to this are the rôle of the temporal component in epilepsy and in memory disorder and these will now be discussed.

EPILEPSY

Study of the pathology of the temporal lobes in epilepsy has tended to concentrate on two main areas within the lobe. One of these is the anteromedial grey matter of the uncus and the underlying amygdaloid nucleus; the other is the more posteriorly situated hippocampus or, as it is also known, the Ammon's horn.

301

Although a link between the anteromedial part of the temporal lobe and epilepsy had been hinted at in several earlier case reports[3, 43, 82] it was firmly established by Hughlings Jackson[49] in a series of papers dated from 1888 onwards. He and his colleagues described the occurrence of a peculiar form of epilepsy characterized by a 'dreamy state' in several patients who were later found to have a focal abnormality in the region of the uncus.

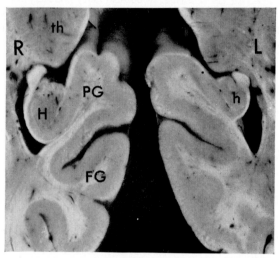

Figure 4. The medial temporal gyri from both hemispheres of an epileptic patient. These have been cut coronally and laid side by side. The right side appears normal. H— hippocampus or Ammon's horn; PG—parahippocampal gyrus; FG—fusiform gyrus; th—thalamus. On the left side the hippocampus (h) is greatly shrunken; the parahippocampal gyrus is considerably less affected. The atrophy of the hippocampus usually increases the size and alters the shape of the inferior horn

Jackson, however, scarcely mentioned the hippocampus and the original investigation of a possible connection between this area and epilepsy was largely confined to France and Germany. As early as 1825, two of Esquirol's assistants, Bouchet and Cazauvieilh[10], had noticed the exceptional hardness or sclerosis of the Ammon's horn in the brains of some epileptic, and other, patients that they had examined (*Figure 4*). They made no further comment on this observation at the time although 28 years later Bouchet expressed the view that, in spite of the frequency of the sclerosis in epilepsy, it was not the cause of the fits.

The histological examination of the area seems first to have been undertaken in Germany when Sommer[91] described the microscopic appearances of hippocampal or Ammon's horn sclerosis and showed how in many, but not all, cases of epilepsy this area of cortex, and possibly that adjacent to it, loses many of its nerve cells, becomes heavily gliosed and eventually may shrink to a small scar. Since the normal human hippocampus is three to four centimetres long and a centimetre or more in cross section, the extent of the scarring may be greater than generally realized[108].

The abnormalities in the different regions were also different in nature. Those in the uncinate area were tumours or infarcts; the hippocampal lesion, although at one time thought to be a malformation, was seen generally as the result of some unidentified pathological process leading to atrophy.

It has always been easy to accept Jackson's view that the type of epileptic attack he described was related to the uncinate lesion; the relevance of the hippocampal sclerosis to epilepsy has proved a more intractable problem.

Firstly, although indisputable sclerosis of the Ammon's horn can be found on one or other side of the brain, and occasionally on both sides, in about 50 per cent of patients with long-standing epilepsy, similar areas of neuronal loss, gliosis and atrophy are often present in other parts of the brain, such as the cerebellum (32 per cent of cases), the thalamus (19 per cent), and the cerebral cortex (31 per cent)[73]. Similar figures were found by Margerison and Corsellis[61].

With damage so often disseminated throughout the brain it has seemed to many invidious to incriminate as an epileptogenic lesion only that in the hippocampus, particularly as 40–50 per cent of chronic epileptic patients do not show any hippocampal damage.

Secondly, the origin of this type of brain damage has always been obscure. The generally accepted view, at least until recent years, was that put forward in general terms by Turner[99], more firmly established by Spielmeyer[93] and later elaborated by Scholz[84, 85]. According to this, the nerve cells die as the result of a disturbance in their blood and oxygen supply occurring during an epileptic attack. The glia proliferate as a reaction to the dying neurons and in the course of time scar tissue develops. Such an interpretation implies that the damage, which is now often but loosely called hypoxic, occurs as the sequel to the epileptic attack. It does not adequately explain why certain areas such as the hippocampus or the cerebellum are exceptionally vulnerable nor does the hypothesis of itself account for the initial epileptic episode.

All these points, coupled with the knowledge that some kind of hippocampal abnormality is often seen in patients who were not epileptic, led to the conclusion that a scarred hippocampus was of no clinical significance, and interest in this aspect of the pathology of epilepsy waned.

The position was changed by the introduction of electroencephalography and the identification of paroxysmal electrical activity centred over one or both temporal lobes of many patients with what had come to be called psychomotor epilepsy[35, 51]. The next step was the surgical removal of the apparently disordered temporal lobe, followed by its pathological examination[5, 39, 52, 69, 74].

The results of the pathological study of the resected specimens and particularly the reports of Earle, Baldwin and Penfield[24] and Meyer, Falconer and Beck[64] brought to life again the old controversies about the pathology of epilepsy.

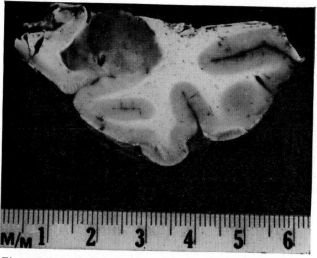

Figure 5. Coronal cut through a temporal lobe which had been removed surgically for the treatment of epilepsy. Most of the hippocampus is represented on the left of the picture and a small glioma can be seen in the region of the parahippocampal and the fusiform gyri

Not surprisingly, the kinds of abnormality found in the lobectomy specimens were comparable to those recorded in the earlier postmortem studies on the brains of epileptic patients. Thus, in some of the specimens, a tumour, malformation or well-defined circumscribed abnormality was identified (*Figure 5*). These tended to lie anteromedially in the region of the uncus, the amygdaloid nucleus and the tip of the inferior horn of the lateral ventricle. These abnormalities were, therefore, of the same order as those described by Hughlings Jackson and were also, although smaller, in roughly the same anatomical area.

Meyer, Falconer and Beck[64] gave a figure of 25 per cent for such abnormality, and a more recent survey[27] agreed with this. Other figures, however, have not been so high and some of the reasons for this discrepancy should be discussed briefly. Different criteria used in the selection of patients for operation may be important, but another possible factor is the way in which the lesions tend to lie deep in the limbic grey matter rather than in the more superficial parts of the temporal cortex. The operation of temporal lobectomy can range from the removal of part of a single gyrus on the convexity to the resection in one piece of the full coronal extent of the lobe and some 5·0 cm back from the temporal pole. It is only in the latter case, and when the deeply-placed tissue is available to the pathologist, that abnormalities lying in the periamygdaloid, and particularly in the hippocampal, regions are likely to be identified.

There is then the further problem that a fully-resected lobe measures several centimetres in all three planes. Since some tumour-like masses and some focal neuronal or glial anomalies may be remarkably circumscribed (Cavanagh, 1958. Personal observation) the more extensively the tissue is sampled for microscopy, the more likely it is that any anomaly present will be detected.

When the abnormality is definite, focal and probably visible to the naked eye, it is reasonable to assume that the epilepsy is related to it. Even here, however, there are problems. Although some of the tumours found are classifiable as gliomata (such as an astrocytoma or an oligodendroglioma), or more rarely as meningiomata, other small glial and possibly vascular masses[25] are also not infrequently found. These appear to be indolent in growth, if indeed they do continue to grow, and are better looked on as malformation or as hamartoma than as neoplasm. Circumscribed cellular aggregations of this kind, which measure little more than a centimetre across, are occasionally encountered in the temporal lobes of patients who have been epileptic for many years. Recently, a young man with a history of 'temporal lobe attacks' for four years was found after operation to have had a small grossly abnormal mass of cells which was only visible under the microscope and which was virtually restricted to one part of the hippocampus. Janz and Neimanis[50] have reported several cases in which they believe such masses to have lain almost dormant for years and only later to have become transformed into rapidly growing gliomata.

In other patients frankly abnormal neurons and glial cells, disseminated or in clusters, have been found. Sometimes the pathological condition has been recognized as tuberous sclerosis[75]. Occasionally, the only finding has been of an alien population of large nerve cells in some part of the temporal cortex, but not necessarily limited to the limbic grey matter. These relatively subtle and rare anomalies may easily be overlooked. When they are suspected they have to be assessed with particular care since the dividing line between normal and abnormal may at times be difficult, or even impossible, to draw. Once its presence has been verified, the possible significance of such an anomaly in relation to the epilepsy should not be lightly dismissed for it at least indicates that the anatomical organization of the lobe in question is disturbed.

The significance of lesions in the temporal lobes of epileptic patients becomes particularly crucial when the old problem of damage to the hippocampus and the adjacent grey matter, including at times the amygdaloid nucleus[63], is reconsidered. This is because Ammon's horn or hippocampal sclerosis has been found in 50 to 65 per cent of the temporal lobes removed from patients with temporal lobe epilepsy[27, 38].

This sclerosis of the medial temporal areas, therefore, constitutes by far the commonest abnormality in lobectomy specimens just as it is the commonest lesion to be found after death in the brains of chronic epileptic patients.

Whereas, however, the surgically treated patients have, without exception, been diagnosed on clinical and on electrical grounds as suffering from temporal lobe epilepsy, the earlier post-mortem observations were made on people who had spent much of their lives in hospital and who had been classified for the most part as suffering from idiopathic or cryptogenic epilepsy. The fact that the same lesion occurs so often in the two different groups of epileptic patients suggests either that the clinical and EEG findings in patients who have undergone a temporal lobectomy are unrelated to the presence of the hippocampal scar or that evidence of a temporal lobe disturbance would be found, if looked for, in many patients with cryptogenic epilepsy.

The latter possibility had already been anticipated by Stauder's clinico-pathological study[94]. He had demonstrated a remarkably close association between the occurrence of clinical signs of a temporal lobe disorder (which he defined in great detail) and the presence of an Ammon's horn sclerosis after the patient had died.

Sano and Malamud[83] came to a similar conclusion and showed in a series of epileptic patients studied post mortem that the pattern of the fits, and in a few cases the occurrence of an anterior temporal spike or sharp wave focus in the EEG, were related to the presence of an Ammon's horn sclerosis. More recently Liddell[57] and Margerison and Liddell[60] analysed the clinical and the EEG findings in a large series of epileptic patients living in hospital and found that more than half of them showed evidence of a temporal lobe disorder. Margerison and Corsellis[61] later found in the 55 cases who had subsequently died a close association between the presence or absence of the clinical and EEG features of temporal lobe epilepsy and the presence or absence of hippocampal sclerosis. No similar association was found with any of the other areas of the brain that had also been examined.

Such evidence would seem to confirm the view that those epileptic patients in whom the medial parts of the temporal lobe are sclerosed will be particularly liable to suffer from the temporal lobe type of epilepsy. This assertion, however, is not without its critics. As already mentioned, it has long been known that damage to the hippocampus can occur in many different conditions without the development of any epileptic phenomena[68]. For example, patients with severe cerebrovascular disease are often found to have microinfarcts in one or both hippocampi; less often the entire hippocampus is destroyed by the occlusion of a posterior cerebral artery. Moreover, severe neuronal loss, gliosis and other evidence of degeneration are commonly seen in the Ammon's horn in Alzheimer's disease, senile dementia, and in kernicterus. Although sporadic epileptic attacks may occur in these conditions, it seems to be immaterial whether the hippocampus is damaged or not[20, 45].

However, both the appearances and the pathogenesis of such hippocampal damage are radically different from the hippocampal sclerosis found in epilepsy. It is, therefore, important to make the distinction that indiscriminate hippocampal abnormality is not manifestly associated with epilepsy; the link is only between hippocampal sclerosis and epilepsy. In order to establish the nature of this link the pathogenesis of the sclerosis has to be considered, particularly as this has been the subject of considerable controversy. Although, as already mentioned, the precise origin of the sclerosis in the epileptic brain is still far from clear, it is generally agreed to result from a disturbance of the blood and oxygen supply to the brain. It is how and when this disturbance comes about that is unclear. The controversy started when Earle, Baldwin and Penfield[24] reversed the traditional view already outlined which stated that the damage occurred as a result of hypoxia developing during an epileptic attack. They proposed that the damage antedated the epilepsy, having been caused by deformation of the skull at the time of birth. The distortion led to the herniation of the brain through the tentorial opening with compression of the adjacent branches of the posterior cerebral artery by the free tentorial edge.

There are, however, several difficulties inherent in this proposal. Firstly, Norman[70, 71] has pointed out that the distribution of the damage, with the emphasis on the hippocampus and the almost constant sparing of the calcarine cortex, does not follow the pattern which usually results from obstruction to the flow in a posterior cerebral artery. The hypothesis also fails to explain satisfactorily the origin of the damage so often seen in other parts of the epileptic brain. Secondly, Veith[103], in a study of the brains of a large series of neonatal deaths, found remarkably little evidence of temporal lobe herniation or of neuronal damage in the hippocampus. Thirdly, a history of difficult birth is not elicited any more often from epileptic patients found to have a hippocampal sclerosis than from those without it.

Another possible explanation of the damage was put forward by Gastaut and his colleagues[32, 33] who attributed the hippocampal damage, or pararhinal sclerosis as they called it, to an episode of brain-swelling that might follow any one of the various insults that can occur to the brain in infancy or early childhood. These include head injury and infection. Most of the objections just outlined could, however, still apply to what is a comparable mechanism to that proposed by Penfield and his colleagues, except that the interference to the blood supply is seen as the result of brain-swelling in the early years of life rather than of distortion of the head at birth.

Nevertheless, since cerebral trauma is often followed by epilepsy it might well be an important factor in the origin of the hippocampal sclerosis, the more so as it is the temporal lobes which tend to be the the most bruised parts of the brain in closed head injury. It is also well known that the temporal lobes are not infrequently scarred in chronic epileptic patients[83] and that similar cortical scars are found at times in the temporal lobe specimens removed from epileptic patients. As Courville[22] has pointed out, however, this scarring, both in cases of head injury and in chronic epilepsy, damages the temporal pole and the more laterally placed gyri rather than the inferomedial, or limbic, areas. The hippocampus itself is usually unaffected. It also seems probable, and at times it is obvious, that the cortical scarring in chronic epilepsy does not antedate the onset of fits but derives from a fall as a consequence of one. Although this is still a controversial issue, it seems doubtful whether trauma plays a major rôle in the causation of hippocampal sclerosis. Certainly head injury does not figure more prominently in the early history of patients with a sclerosed hippocampus than in those without one[27].

One factor that does appear to be linked to the development of hippocampal sclerosis is the occurrence of severe convulsions, sometimes amounting to status epilepticus, in the early years of life[19]. These convulsive attacks may in some cases be the result, as Gastaut emphasized, of an acute infection or other illness, but more often their cause is not known. This is similar to the pathogenetic situation that Spielmeyer and his followers described. In other words, the destruction of the hippocampal neurons, as well as that of neurons in other sensitive areas of the brain (cerebellum, thalamus, etc), usually results from an inadequate blood and oxygen supply which develops after the onset of epileptic attacks particularly in early life.

Thus hippocampal sclerosis may be regarded as part of a post-hypoxic scarring process which preferentially, but not exclusively, affects the medial temporal areas. Contrary to earlier views such a scar is not necessarily inert but may in due course, like scarring elsewhere in the brain, so disrupt normal cerebral activity that the incidence and the pattern of epileptic attacks are influenced by its presence. This interpretation does not require that this should inevitably happen or that such damage should be the only determining factor. There is, for example, evidence that a genetic factor may also be important. The interpretation would, however, help to explain why there is so close an association between the presence or absence of hippocampal sclerosis and the presence or absence of the clinical and EEG manifestations of temporal lobe epilepsy, both in patients selected for lobectomy operation and in those in hospital with long-standing epilepsy.

It now seems justifiable, therefore, to add this atrophy and sclerosis of the medial temporal areas to the list of abnormalities which are liable to result in temporal lobe epilepsy. It is as well to emphasize again, however, that damage of this type is rarely confined to a single temporal lobe or even to both. It is possible that concomitant damage in other parts, such as the thalamus and the cerebellum, may also influence the clinical picture or the electroencephalographic findings.

Finally, it should be stressed that even when all the various abnormalities are taken together, there are still some 20 per cent of cases left in which no definite abnormality in the temporal lobes can be found. The elucidation of this, and of many other problems, still offers plenty of scope for further investigation, particularly in collaboration with other disciplines.

MEMORY DISORDER

Some disturbance of memory is a feature of many conditions in which there is widespread degeneration of brain tissue. There are, however, two relatively circumscribed areas of the brain which appear to be particularly important. One is the mamillary body, possibly with the nearby medial parts of the thalamus; the other is the inferomedial part of the temporal lobe and in particular the hippocampus. These two areas are closely related through the connecting link of the fornix and together they make up a major part of the limbic areas.

Two reports[6, 56], appearing towards the end of the nineteenth century, led the way. Korsakow described the illness, now named after him, in which 'together with the confusion, nearly always a profound disorder of memory is observed, although at times the disorder of memory occurs in pure form . . . this manifests itself in an extraordinarily peculiar amnesia in which the memory of recent events is chiefly disturbed, whereas the remote past was remembered fairly well.' Korsakow said little about the pathological basis of the condition apart from attributing it to a toxaemia resulting from many different causes, including alcohol.

Wernicke[106] had already established that a severe tissue reaction occurred at times in the periventricular grey matter of patients dying from alcoholism and from other causes. Gudden[42] noticed that this process was particularly severe in the mamillary bodies. He was followed by Bonhoeffer[9] who suggested that there might be a connection between the damage in this area and the Korsakow state.

It was not until 1928 that Gamper[31] produced substantial evidence to support this hypothesis. He found that although the damage was scattered along the length of grey matter around the aqueduct and the third and fourth ventricles, it was nevertheless most severe and most constant in the mamillary bodies (*Figure 6*). Gamper postulated that this lesion, by interfering with the pathways connecting the mamillary bodies with the mid-brain, the thalamus and eventually the cortex, was responsible for the memory disorder in the Korsakow state.

This hypothesis was not at first accepted in this country. Carmichael and Stern[17], as others had done some years before, emphasized the importance of diffuse, but unremarkable, changes in the cerebral cortex while failing to examine the periventricular grey matter. Many subsequent studies, however, have confirmed Gamper's observations, and the illness described by Korsakow is now generally recognized in most cases to be the result of the brain damage caused by an attack of Wernicke's encephalopathy, whether due to the effects of alcoholism or of any other disorder leading to thiamine deficiency[59].

This and many other investigations have repeatedly shown the damage to be concentrated in the periventricular grey matter, as first outlined by Gamper. The mamillary bodies have nearly always been found to be more vulnerable than other parts and occasional cases have been reported in which they are the only areas affected[12].

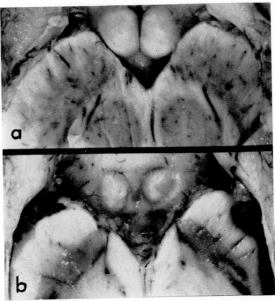

Figure 6. A surface view of (a) normal mamillary bodies, for comparison with (b) the atrophied and discoloured mamillary bodies of a "Korsakovian" patient

There is, nevertheless, a particularly marked tendency for the medial parts of the thalamus also to be affected, and Adams, Collins and Victor[2] have argued that it is the disorganization of the dorso-medial nucleus of the thalamus that is the more important factor. Part of this nucleus, however, usually degenerates as the result of a leucotomy operation, while attempts have been made to destroy it stereotactically[92]. In neither instance has a lasting disorder of memory been attributed to such damage. It seems doubtful whether enough is known at present to justify the incrimination of one part of the deep grey matter rather than another. The crucial points are that the damage is always bilateral and that it lies somewhere along the di-encephalic sector of the limbic pathways.

The possible effect on memory of damage to the temporal lobes in man was first considered in a brief clinico-pathological report by von Bechterew[6]. This does not appear to have been followed up and the next step was in 1954 when Scoville removed the inferomedial parts of both temporal lobes from several psychotic patients as a form of treatment for their illness. He found, unexpectedly, that some of them had developed a severe defect in recent memory. Scoville and Milner[88] analysed the results further and came to the conclusion that the effect on recent memory was not produced by resecting the uncus and amygdala alone but only when the operation included bilateral removal of the hippocampus and the parahippocampal gyrus. They considered that the more extensively these latter areas were removed, the worse was the memory defect.

Petit-Dutaillis and colleagues[76] had in 1954 removed the anterior part of both temporal lobes from an epileptic patient but the operation did not include the hippocampus on either side. In this case there was only a transient disorder of recent memory although the patient was left with a permanent retrograde amnesia covering a period of several months. In contrast, Terzian and Ore[98] removed the entire anterior portions of both temporal lobes but went back far enough to include most of the hippocampus. Although they listed 'a serious deficiency in memory' as one of the effects, the main emphasis was on the resemblance of the postoperative clinical picture to the Klüver-Bucy Syndrome.

The only other sources of further information on this problem are the reports on the effects of unilateral temporal lobectomy and the study of those rare pathological conditions in which the limbic, and particularly the medial temporal, areas are selectively involved.

A disturbance of recent memory usually occurs only when the temporal lobe damage is bilateral, but a unilateral resection of the medial structures is not always without effect. Milner and Penfield[67] reported on two patients out of a total of 90, in whom a defect in recent memory developed after the removal of the lobe on the dominant side. In both cases, however, there was reason to believe that the opposite hippocampus was abnormal.

Several studies by Falconer and colleagues are also relevant. Meyer and Yates[66] and Meyer[65] found that the ability to learn new verbal and auditory material could be seriously impaired by removal of the lobe on the dominant side, although a longer follow-up of the cases by Blakemore and Falconer indicated that the defect in auditory learning tended ultimately to disappear. Serafetinides and

Falconer[89] found that the removal of the non-dominant hemisphere was occasionally (seven out of 34 patients) followed by an inconvenient rather than incapacitating impairment of recent memory. In six of the cases, however, there was electrical evidence of medial temporal abnormality on the opposite side and it was therefore argued that bilateral temporal lobe disturbance was responsible for the memory defect.

Stepien and Sierpinski[96] have discussed the impairment of recent memory after temporal lobe lesions. They described several epileptic patients in whom the memory disorder was associated with electrical abnormalities in both temporal lobes. Following the removal of one lobe, however, both the contralateral discharges and the memory disturbance cleared up. They explained this by postulating that unilateral lesions may interfere with the normal activity of the opposite side and their excision would remove the source of irritation.

There are several pathological conditions in which the medial parts of the temporal lobes tend to be more severely affected than the rest of the brain. These include certain forms of encephalitis, some forms of vascular disease, and some cases of organic dementia.

ENCEPHALITIS

Van Bogaert, Radermecker and Devos[8] drew attention to a severe form of acute encephalitis in which the brunt of the damage was borne by the temporal lobes. Many cases have now been reported. The entire lobe of each hemisphere may be affected, but the damage usually shows a marked tendency to concentrate on the inferomedial temporal gyri and the insular, the posterior orbital and the cingular cortex. The inflammatory reaction is severe and there is usually massive necrosis with destruction of cortex and white matter obvious to the naked eye. The damage is sometimes asymmetrical[1]. Viral, serological and histological studies strongly suggest that the illness is usually due to an infection with the herpes simplex virus, which has often been isolated from the brain tissue of affected patients. Furthermore type A intranuclear inclusion bodies in nerve or glial cells may be found either in biopsy or in post-mortem material and electron microscope studies have shown the presence of herpes-like particles in areas of brain tissue containing inclusion bodies[102]. Serological tests may also be positive. There have, however, been several reports of cases in which no positive evidence of a herpes simplex infection has been found and in one case Coxsackie B5 virus was isolated from the cerebrospinal fluid during life[46]. In another patient, known to the present writer, the illness developed following the treatment of a snake-bite with antivenom serum.

The encephalitis, whether evidence of a herpes infection has been demonstrated or not, is usually fatal within two weeks. According to Adams and Jennett[1] it presents in childhood as well as in adult and late adult life as an acute pyrexial attack with headache, confusion and possibly a hemiparesis or convulsions. The cerebrospinal fluid shows an increase in protein and in cells. Partial, or very rarely complete, recovery has been recorded; there are several clinico-pathological reports of patients who have died after an illness lasting months or even years. These longer-surviving patients suffer from the effects of extensive damage to both temporal lobes and this may bring them to the attention of the psychiatrist. A severe disorder of recent memory was described[23] in two patients who had survived an attack. Similarly, Rose and Symonds[79] reported on several patients in whom a severe defect in recent memory and retrograde amnesia had followed an attack of acute encephalitis which was considered on clinical grounds to have been the type under discussion. The more usual sequel, however, would seem to be the development of dementia and not merely a disturbance of recent memory, but there is remarkably little definite known about this. Aszkanazy, Tom and Zeldowicz[4] described a patient who had survived, demented, for seven months, and Adams and Jennett mentioned another. The present writer has twice seen this. One patient, a man of 40, lived for three years with a moderate degree of dementia but with a particularly severe disorder of recent memory. The limbic grey matter, including therefore both hippocampi, was found to have been destroyed in a remarkably selective way by a severe sub-acute necrotizing encephalitis (*Figure* 7). In the second case, scarcely any remnant of either temporal lobe was found after death while the immediately adjacent cortex and to a lesser extent the white matter showed a severe inflammatory reaction with necrosis. The patient had lived for two years after the fulminating onset of his illness. Following partial recovery after several days of coma he was found to be demented. In addition, he showed remarkably clear evidence of the 'oral tendencies' described by Klüver and Bucy[55] as being one of the effects of total bilateral temporal lobectomy in monkeys.

Not all cases of encephalitis of the limbic areas are of the necrotizing type. Brierley and colleagues[13] reported several patients who became demented in their fifties over a period lasting from a few months to a year. No cause for the dementia (or for the marked memory loss noted in two of the three patients) was established during life although the possibility of a viral encephalitis had been considered. In two of the three cases the cerebrospinal fluid showed an increase in lymphocytes and in the protein content; in one, the colloidal gold curve was strongly paretic in type.

The common neurohistological feature was a marked inflammatory reaction which was focused on the limbic grey matter.

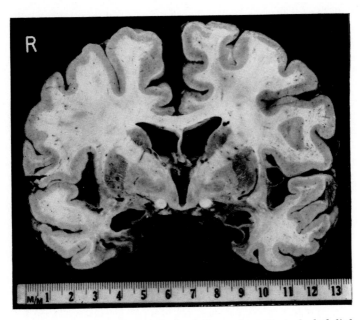

*Figure 7. Coronal cut through the hemispheres of a patient who had died three years after the onset of a necrotizing encephalitis in which the brunt of the damage had been borne by the medial temporal areas and the insula.
(The cingular gyrus is often similarly affected)*

Intranuclear inclusion bodies were absent and the limited investigation that was carried out produced no positive evidence of infection by a particular virus. The cause of the encephalitis in these cases is therefore unknown but a finding in one of them has introduced a further problem. In this case a secondary deposit from an unsuspected bronchial carcinoma had been found. This was thought at the time to have been a coincidence, but a number of similar observations have since been reported and, taken together, these suggest that there may be a connection.

315

Limbic Encephalitis and Carcinoma

It has long been known that a variety of neurological disorders may develop in patients with carcinoma. Usually in such patients there is clinical evidence of damage to the cerebellum, to the brain stem or to the spinal cord which consists of degeneration and loss of nerve cells, some gliosis and possibly tract degeneration. In some instances, however, there is also an appreciable inflammatory-like reaction in the degenerating areas. This was at first thought to be a reaction to the break-down of tissue, but Russell[81] and others have pointed out that the inflammatory component can be too marked for such an explanation to be acceptable and that it may at times be so severe as to be indistinguishable from that seen in a viral encephalitis. Both the degenerative changes and the inflammatory-like reaction had until recently been identified only at levels caudal to the basal ganglia but it is now clear that a similar tissue reaction may occur in the cerebral hemispheres with particular emphasis on the limbic grey matter. Examples have been reported by Verhaart[104], Störring, Hauss and Ule[97], Yahr, Duvoisin and Cowen[109] and by Ulrich, Spiess and Huber[101]. Corsellis, Goldberg and Norton[21] have recently reviewed these reports and added three further cases.

Clinically, the patients have all been over 50 years old. A marked disturbance of affect has been an early and constant feature, several patients have been hallucinated and several have had epileptic attacks. The cerebrospinal fluid was usually abnormal, the commonest abnormality being a raised lymphocyte count and a raised level of protein. A paretic type of colloidal gold curve has occasionally been recorded.

The carcinoma in nearly all the patients has been bronchial in origin, but in several instances no primary growth had been found although the intrathoracic lymph nodes contained secondary deposits. No evidence of direct spread of the tumour to the central nervous system has been found.

In all but one of the patients in whom there was marked bilateral hippocampal damage, a disturbance of recent memory had been a major feature. Indeed, Störring, Hauss and Ule[97] had reported their case because of the striking association between the disorder of recent memory, without intellectual deterioration, and the localized hippocampal abnormality.

Some of the patients also became demented. The exceptions were the cases described by Henson, Hoffman and Urich[47] who were unable to attribute any definite symptoms to the involvement of the limbic areas. This apparent anomaly, however, is probably related to the fact that in all their cases the pathological changes were mild and nerve cell loss was slight or absent. In all the other reported cases the damage has been severe and often visible to the naked eye.

It seems unlikely that the occurrence of this limbic 'encephalitis' in association with carcinoma is coincidental but why it should happen is unknown. It has been attributed to a viral infection, and even to the herpes simplex virus, but there is little to support this view. Metabolic and immune factors have also been invoked but they too remain unidentified.

Even though the condition is rare and its causes obscure, it should be kept in mind if a patient is encountered with evidence of malignant disease and of an organic psychotic disorder with a defect in recent memory.

There are several other conditions in which the medial temporal areas are prone to damage, although when the damage occurs it is usually as part of a more generalized process.

VASCULAR DEGENERATION

Occlusion of the posterior cerebral artery is probably the commonest cause of infarction of the medial temporal gyri (*Figure 8*). Most or all of the hippocampus and the parahippocampal gyrus is then likely to be destroyed, together with part of the inferomedial surface of the occipital cortex. This is not uncommonly found in the brains of elderly patients with marked cerebral atherosclerosis. In most instances, however, the occlusion is unilateral and the patients are likely to be demented. Much more rarely the arteries on both sides may be occluded. Von Bechterew[6] may have recorded the first example when he described a patient with a gross memory disorder and apathy, in whose brain there was softening of the medial parts of both temporal lobes. A remarkable instance of this was recorded by Victor and colleagues[105]. They made a careful study over five years of a man of 59 with bilateral visual defects, who suffered from a profound defect of recent memory, an inability to learn and an incomplete retrograde amnesia for the two years before his illness. His memory for recent events was virtually unaffected. His intelligence remained good, but he became inactive and apathetic. In the brain, much of the hippocampus, the fornix and the mamillary body on both sides was severely degenerated while the unci and the amygdaloid nuclei were spared. Although other damage was present, the authors argued effectively that it was the relatively small lesions in the medial temporal areas that had led to the defects in memory and learning.

317

It is also conceivable that disease of the small cerebral vessels can play an important part in memory disorder in old age, for even though no gross lesions may be found, microinfarcts are remarkably common in the hippocampi of elderly patients. They are moreover not infrequently bilateral. Since, however, other parts of the brain are also liable to be affected it would be unwise to emphasize too strongly the possible significance of localized damage.

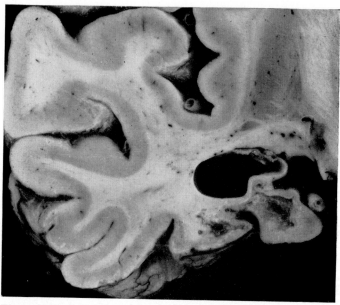

Figure 8. The medial temporal gyri have been almost completely destroyed following the occlusion by atheroma of the posterior cerebral artery. (The occluded vessel can be seen to the right of the infarcted parahippocampal gyrus)

DEMENTIA

This comment applies even more to the problem of memory disorder in senile dementia. The 'senile' type of cerebral degeneration, which consists mainly of loss of nerve cells and gliosis, together with the formation of senile plaques and neurofibrillary change, is a diffuse process affecting the cerebral grey matter. Once again, however, the hippocampus appears to be more vulnerable than other parts of the cerebral cortex, and the way the memory tends to fail in later years may be related to this local susceptibility.

It has also been suggested from time to time that bilateral

damage to the medial temporal areas may result not only in the disorganization of recent memory, but may play an important part in the development of dementia[36, 40, 41]. Others have attributed one or more of the features of the Klüver-Bucy Syndrome to the concentration of damage in the temporal lobes and particularly in the limbic part[53, 77]. These ideas are supported to a limited extent by the various observations, including those already quoted, in which dementia or bizarre behavioural abnormalities have followed either an encephalitis of the limbic areas, or the surgical removal of the temporal lobes.

The extreme variability from case to case, however, not only in the clinical picture, but also in the distribution of the brain damage, makes it difficult to draw any firmer conclusions at the present time. It may not be irrelevant that the neuropathologist Bratz[11] could remark in 1923 that psychiatry had even then been trying to understand the Ammon's horn for over 150 years. Judged on this time scale, perhaps some recent progress has been made.

REFERENCES

1. Adams, J. H. and Jennett, W. B. (1967). 'Acute Necrotizing Encephalitis: A Problem in Diagnosis'. *J. Neurol. Neurosurg. Psychiat.* **30**, 248

2. Adams, R. D., Collins, G. H. and Victor, M. (1962). 'Troubles de la Mémoire et de l'Apprentissage chez l'Homme; leurs Relations avec des Lésions des Lobes Temporaux et du Diencéphale'. In *Physiologie de l'Hippocampe*, p. 273. Paris: Centre National de la Recherche Scientifique

3. Anderson, J. (1886). 'On Sensory Epilepsy'. *Brain* **9**, 385

4. Aszkanazy, F. L., Tom, M. I. and Zeldowicz, L. R. (1958). 'Encephalitis Presumably of Viral Origin Associated with Massive Necrosis of the Temporal Lobe'. *J. Neuropath. exp. Neurol.* **17**, 565

5. Bailey, P. and Gibbs, F. A. (1951). 'Surgical Treatment of Psychomotor Epilepsy'. *J. Am. med. Ass.* **145**, 365

6. Bechterew, W. V. von (1900). 'Demonstration eines Gehirns mit Zerstörung der vorderen und inneren Theile der Hirnrinde beider Schläfenlappen'. *Neurol. Zentbl.* **19**, 990

7. Blakemore, C. B. and Falconer, M. A. (1967). 'Long-term Effects of Anterior Temporal Lobectomy on Certain Cognitive Functions'. *J. Neurol. Neurosurg. Psychiat.* **30**, 364

8. Bogaert, L. van, Radermecker, J. and Devos, J. (1955). 'Sur une Observation Mortelle d'Encéphalite Aigue Nécrosante'. *Revue. neurol.* **92**, 329

9. Bonhoeffer, K. (1897). 'Klinische und anatomische Beiträge zur Kenntnis der Alkoholdelirien'. *Mschr. Psychiat. Neurol.* **1**, 229

10. Bouchet and Cazauvieilh (1825). 'De l'épilepsie considerée dans ses rapports avec l'aliénation mentale'. *Archs gén. Méd.* **9**, 510

11. Bratz, E. and Grossmann, W. (1923). 'Über Ammonshornsklerose'. *Z. ges. Neurol. Psychiat.* **81**, 45

12. Brierley, J. B. (1966). 'The Neuropathology of Amnesic States'. In *Amnesia*, p. 150. Ed. by C. W. M. Whitty and O. L. Zangwill. London: Butterworths

13. — Corsellis, J. A. N., Hierons, R. and Nevin, S. (1960). 'Subacute Encephalitis of Later Adult Life, Mainly Affecting the Limbic Areas'. *Brain* **83**, 357

14. Broca, P. (1878). 'Anatomie Comparée des Circonvolutions Cérébrales'. *Rev. anthropol.* Series 3, **1**, 385

15. Brodal, A. (1947). 'The Hippocampus and the Sense of Smell'. *Brain* **70**, 179

16. Cannon, W. B. (1927). 'The James-Lange Theory of Emotion: A Critical Examination and an Alternative Theory'. *Am. J. Psychol.* **39**, 10

17. Carmichael, E. A. and Stern, R. D. (1931). 'Korsakow's Syndrome: Its Histopathology'. *Brain* **54**, 189

18. Cavanagh, J. B. (1958). 'On Certain Small Tumours Encountered in the Temporal Lobe. *Brain* **81**, 389

19. — and Meyer, A. (1956). 'Aetiological Aspects of Ammon's Horn Sclerosis associated with Temporal Lobe Epilepsy'. *Br. med. J.* **2**, 1403

20. Corsellis, J. A. N. (1957). 'The Incidence of Ammon's Horn Sclerosis'. *Brain* **80**, 193

21. — Goldberg, G. J. and Norton, A. R. (1968). ' "Limbic Encephalitis" and its Association with Carcinoma'. *Brain* **91**, 481

22. Courville, C. B. (1958). 'Traumatic Lesions of the Temporal Lobe as the Essential Cause of Psychomotor Epilepsy'. In *Temporal Lobe Epilepsy*, p. 220. Ed. by M. Baldwin and P. Bailey. Springfield, Ill.: Charles C. Thomas

23. Drachman, D. A. and Adams, R. D. (1962). 'Herpes Simplex and Acute Inclusion-body Encephalitis'. *Archs Neurol., Chicago* **7**, 45

24. Earle, K. M., Baldwin, M. and Penfield, W. (1953). 'Incisural Sclerosis and Temporal Lobe Seizures produced by Hippocampal Herniation at Birth'. *A.M.A. Archs Neurol. Psychiat.* **69**, 27

25. Edgar, R. and Baldwin, M. (1960). 'Vascular Malformation associated with Temporal Lobe Epilepsy'. *J. Neurosurg.* **17**, 638

26. Elliot Smith, G. (1901). 'Notes upon the Natural Subdivision of the Cerebral Hemisphere'. *J. Anat. Physiol., Lond.* **35**, 431

27. Falconer, M. A., Serafetinides, E. A. and Corsellis, J. A. N. (1964). 'Etiology and Pathogenesis of Temporal Lobe Epilepsy'. *Archs Neurol., Chicago* **10**, 233

28. Ferrier, D. (1886). *Functions of the Brain*, 2nd edn. London: Smith, Elder

29. Foville, M. (1844). *Anatomie, Physiologie et Pathologie du Système Nerveux*, Vol. 1, p. 193. Paris

30. Fulton, J. F. (1951). *Frontal Lobotomy and Affective Behaviour*. London: Chapman and Hall

31. Gamper, E. (1928). 'Zur Frage der Polioencephalitis der chronischen Alcoholiker. Anatomische Befunde bei alcoholischen Korsakow und ihre Beziehungen zum klinischen Bild'. *Dt. Z. Nerv-Heilk.* **102**, 122

32. Gastaut, H. (1957). 'Étiologie, Pathologie et Pathogénie des Épilepsies du Lobe Temporal'. *Revue. fr. Étude clin. biol.* **2**, 667

33. — Toga, M., Roger, J. and Gibson, W. C. (1959). 'A Correlation of Clinical, Electroencephalographic and Anatomical Findings in Nine Autopsied Cases of "Temporal Lobe Epilepsy" '. *Epilepsia* **1**, 56

34. Gerdy (1838). Quoted by Broca (1878)

35. Gibbs, E. L., Gibbs, F. A. and Fuster, B. (1948). 'Psychomotor Epilepsy'. *Archs Neurol. Psychiat., Chicago* **60**, 331

36. Glees, P. and Griffith, H. B. (1952). 'Bilateral Destruction of the Hippocampus (Cornu Ammonis) in a Case of Dementia'. *Mschr. Psychiat. Neurol.* **123**, 193

37. Green, J. D. (1964). 'The Hippocampus'. *Physiol. Rev.* **44**, 561

38. Green, J. R. and Scheetz, D. G. (1964). 'Surgery of Epileptogenic Lesions of the Temporal Lobe'. *Archs Neurol., Chicago* **10**, 135

39. — Duisberg, R. E. H. and McGrath, W. B. (1951). 'Focal Epilepsy of Psychomotor Type. A Preliminary Report of Observations on Effects of Surgical Therapy'. *J. Neurosurg.* **8**, 157

40. Grünthal, E. (1947). 'Über das klinische Bild nach umschriebenen beiderseitigen Ausfall der Ammonshornrinde. Ein Beitrag zur Kenntnis der Funktion des Ammonshorns'. *Mschr. Psychiat. Neurol.* **113**, 1

41. — (1959). 'Über den derzeitigen Stand der Frage nach den klinischen Erscheinungen bei Ausfall des Ammonshorns'. *Psychiatria Neurol.* **138**, 145

42. Gudden, H. (1896). 'Klinische und anatomische Beiträge zur Kenntnis der multiplen Alkoholneuritis'. *Arch. Psychiat. Nerv-Krankh.* **28**, 643

43. Hamilton, A. M. (1882). 'On Cortical Sensory Discharging Lesions (Sensory Epilepsy)'. *N.Y. med. J.* **35**, 575

44. Hassler, R. (1964). 'Zur funktionellen Anatomie des limbischen Systems'. *Nervenarzt* **35**, 386

45. Haymaker, W., Pentschew, A., Margoles, C. and Bingham, W. G. (1958). 'Occurrence of Lesions in the Temporal Lobe in the Absence of Convulsive Seizures'. In *Temporal Lobe Epilepsy*, p. 166. Ed. by M. Baldwin and P. Bailey. Springfield, Ill.: Charles C. Thomas

46. Heathfield, K. W. G., Pilsworth, R., Wall, B. J. and Corsellis, J. A. N. (1967). 'Coxsackie B5 Infections in Essex, 1965, with Particular Reference to the Nervous System'. *Q. Jl Med.* **36,** 579

47. Henson, R. A., Hoffman, H. L. and Urich, H. (1965). 'Encephalomyelitis with Carcinoma'. *Brain* **88,** 449

48. Horsley, V. and Schäfer, E. A. Quoted by Ferrier (1886)

49. Jackson, Hughlings (1888). 'On a Particular Variety of Epilepsy ("Intellectual Aura"), One Case with Symptoms of Organic Brain Disease'. *Brain* **11,** 179

50. Janz, D. and Neimanis, G. (1966). 'Clinical Aspects and Morphology of Diffuse Blastomas of the Temporal Lobe, the so-called Spongioblastomas of the Rhinencephalon'. *Dt. Z. NervHeilk.* **188,** 92

51. Jasper, H. H. and Kershman, J. (1941). 'Electroencephalographic Classification of the Epilepsies'. *Archs Neurol. Psychiat., Chicago* **45,** 903

52. —— Pertuisset, B. and Flanigin, H. (1951). 'EEG and Cortical Electrograms in Patients with Temporal Lobe Seizures'. *A.M.A. Archs Neurol. Psychiat.* **65,** 272

53. Jelgersma, H. G. (1964). 'Ein Fall von juveniler hereditärer Demenz vom Alzheimer Typ mit Parkinsonismus und Klüver-Bucy-Syndrom'. *Arch. Psychiat. NervKrankh.* **205,** 262

54. Klüver, H. and Bucy, P. C. (1937). ' "Psychic Blindness" and Other Symptoms Following Bilateral Temporal Lobectomy in Rhesus Monkeys'. *Am. J. Physiol.* **119,** 352

55. —— —— (1938). 'An Analysis of Certain Effects of Bilateral Temporal Lobectomy in the Rhesus Monkey, With Special Reference to "Psychic Blindness" '. *J. Psychol. Neurol., Lpz* **5,** 33

56. Korsakow, S. S. (1890). 'Über eine besondere Form psychischer Störung combinirt mit multipler Neuritis'. *Arch. Psychiat. NervKrankh.* **21,** 669

57. Liddell, D. W. (1953). 'Observations on Epileptic Automatism in a Mental Hospital Population'. *J. ment. Sci.* **99,** 732

58. MacLean, P. D. (1949). 'Psychosomatic Disease and the "Visceral Brain"—Recent Developments Bearing on the Papez Theory of Emotion'. *Psychosom. Med.* **11,** 338

59. Malamud, N. and Skillicorn, S. A. (1956). 'Relationship between the Wernicke and the Korsakow Syndrome'. *A.M.A. Archs Neurol. Psychiat.* **76,** 585

60. Margerison, J. M. and Liddell, D. W. (1961). 'The Incidence of Temporal Lobe Epilepsy among a Hospital Population of Long-stay Female Epileptics'. *J. ment. Sci.* **107,** 909

61. —— and Corsellis, J. A. N. (1966). 'Epilepsy and the Temporla Lobes'. *Brain* **89,** 499

62. Meyer, A. and Beck, E. (1954). *Prefrontal Leucotomy and Related Operations: Anatomical Aspects of Success and Failure.* Edinburgh, London: Oliver and Boyd

63. —— (1955). 'The Hippocampal Formation in Temporal Lobe Epilepsy'. *Proc. R. Soc. Med.* **48,** 457

64. — Falconer, M. A. and Beck, E. (1954). 'Pathological Findings in Temporal Lobe Epilepsy'. *J. Neurol. Neurosurg. Psychiat.* **17,** 276

65. Meyer, V. (1959). 'Cognitive Changes following Temporal Lobectomy for Relief of Temporal Lobe Epilepsy'. *A.M.A. Archs. Neurol. Psychiat.* **81,** 299

66. — and Yates, A. (1955). 'Intellectual Changes following Temporal Lobectomy for Psychomotor Epilepsy'. *J. Neurol. Neurosurg. Psychiat.* **18,** 44

67. Milner, B. and Penfield, W. (1955). 'The Effect of Hippocampal Lesions on Recent Memory'. *Trans. Am. neurol. Ass.* **80,** 42

68. Morel, F. and Wildi, E. (1956). 'Sclérose Ammonienne et Épilepsies'. *Acta neurol. belg.* **56,** 61

69. Morris, A. A. (1950). 'The Surgical Treatment of Psychomotor Epilepsy'. *Med. Ann. Distr. Columbia* **19,** 121

70. Norman, R. M. (1962). In *Acute Hemiplegia in Childhood,* p. 37 Little Club Clinics in Developmental Medicine No. 6. London: Heinemann

71. — (1966). In *Biological Factors in Temporal Lobe Epilepsy.* By F. Ounsted, J. Lindsay and R. Norman. Clinics in Developmental Medicine, No. 22

72. Papez, J. W. (1937). 'A Proposed Mechanism of Emotion'. *Archs Neurol. Psychiat., Chicago* **38,** 725

73. Peiffer, J. (1963). *Morphologische Aspekte der Epilepsien.* Berlin: Springer-Verlag

74. Penfield, W. and Flanigin, H. (1950). 'Surgical Therapy of Temporal Lobe Seizures'. *Archs Neurol. Psychiat., Chicago* **64,** 491

75. Perot, P., Weir, B. and Rasmussen, T. (1966). 'Tuberous Sclerosis. Surgical Therapy for Seizures'. *Archs Neurol., Chicago* **15,** 498

76. Petit-Dutaillis, D., Christophe, J., Pertuisset, B., Dreyfus-Brisac, C. and Blane, C. (1954). 'Lobectomie Temporale Bilaterale pour Epilepsie. Evolution des Perturbations Fonctionelles Postopératives'. *Revue neurol.* **91,** 129

77. Pilleri, G. (1961). 'Orale Einstellung nach Art des Klüver-Bucy-Syndroms bei hirnatrophischen Prozessen'. *Schweiz. Arch. Neurol. Neurochir. Psychiat.* **87,** 286

78. Poeck, K. (1964). 'Die Klinische Bedeutung des Limbischen Systems'. *Nervenarzt* **35,** 152

79. Rose, F. C. and Symonds, C. P. (1960). 'Persistent Memory Defect following Encephalitis'. *Brain* **83,** 195

80. Rose, M. (1927). 'Die sogenannte Riechrinde beim Menschen und beim Affen. II Teil des "Allocortex bei Tier und Mensch"'. *J. Psychol. Neurol., Lpz.* **34,** 261

81. Russell, D. S. (1961). 'Encephalomyelitis and "Carcinomatous Neuropathy"'. In *Encephalitides*, p. 131. Ed. by L. van Bogaert, J. Radermecker, J. Hozay and A. Lowenthal. Amsterdam: Elsevier

82. Sander, W. (1874). 'Epileptische Anfälle mit subjektiven Geruchsempfindungen bei Zerstörung des linken Tractus Olfactorius durch einen Tumor'. *Arch. Psychiat. NervKrankh.* **4,** 234

83. Sano, K. and Malamud, N. (1953). 'Clinical Significance of Sclerosis of the Cornu Ammonis'. *A.M.A. Archs Neurol. Psychiat.* **70,** 40

84. Scholz, W. (1951). *Die Krampfschädigungen des Gehirns,* Heft 75. Berlin: Springer-Verlag

85. — (1959). 'The Contribution of Patho-anatomical Research to the Problem of Epilepsy'. *Epilepsia* **1,** 36

86. Schwalbe, G. (1878). 'Der Lobus Falciformis, Sichellappen'. In *Hoffman's Lehrbuch der Anatomie des Menschen,* II

87. Scoville, W. B. (1954). 'The Limbic Lobe in Man'. *J. Neurosurg.* **11,** 64

88. — and Milner, B. (1957). 'Loss of Recent Memory after Bilateral Hippocampal Lesions'. *J. Neurol. Neurosurg. Psychiat.* **20,** 11

89. Serafetinides, E. A. and Falconer, M. A. (1962). 'Some Observations on Memory Impairment after Temporal Lobectomy for Epilepsy'. *J. Neurol. Neurosurg. Psychiat.* **25,** 251

90. Smythies, J. R. (1966). *The Neurological Foundations of Psychiatry.* Oxford: Blackwell

91. Sommer, W. (1880). 'Erkrankung des Ammonshornes als aetiologisches Moment der Epilepsie'. *Arch. Psychiat. NervKrankh.* **10,** 631

92. Spiegel, E. A., Wycis, H. T., Orchinik, C. W. and Freed, H. (1955). 'The Thalamus and Temporal Orientation'. *Science* **121,** 771

93. Spielmeyer, W. (1927). 'Die Pathogenese des epileptischen Krampfes'. *Z. Neurol.* **109,** 501

94. Stauder, K. H. (1935/6). 'Epilepsie und Schläfenlappen'. *Arch. Psychiat. NervKrankh.* **104,** 181

95. Stephan, H. (1964). 'Die kortikalen Anteile des limbischen Systems'. *Nervenarzt* **35,** 396

96. Stepien, L. and Sierpinski, S. (1964). 'Impairment of Recent Memory after Temporal Lesions in Man'. *Neuropsychologia* **2,** 291

97. Störring, G. E., Hauss, K. and Ule, G. (1962). 'Zur topischen Diagnostik des amnestischen Symptomenkomplexes'. *Psychiatria Neurol.* **143,** 161

98. Terzian, H. and Ore, G. D. (1955). 'Syndrome of Klüver and Bucy reproduced in Man by Bilateral Removal of the Temporal Lobes'. *Neurology, Minneap.* **5,** 373

99. Turner, J. (1907). 'The Pathological Anatomy and Pathology of Epilepsy'. *J. ment. Sci.* **53,** 1

100. Turner, W. (1891). 'The Convolutions of the Brain'. *J. Anat. Physiol.* **25,** 105

101. Ulrich, J., Spiess, H. and Huber, R. (1967). 'Neurologische Syndrome als Fernwirkung Maligner Tumoren'. *Schweiz. Arch. Neurol. Neurochir. Psychiat.* **99,** 83

102. Vanderhaeghen, J. J., Périer, O. and Bossaert, Y. (1966). 'Acute Necrotizing Encephalitis'. *Path. europ.* **1,** 29

103. Veith, G. (1960). 'Über die Pathogenese des perinatalen Hirnschadens'. *Geburtsh. Frauenheilk.* **20,** 905

104. Verhaart, W. J. C. (1961). 'Grey Matter Degeneration of the C.N.S. in Carcinosis'. *Acta neuropath.* **1,** 107

105. Victor, M., Angevine, J. B., Mancall, E. L. and Fisher, M. (1961). 'Memory Loss with Lesion of the Hippocampal Formation'. *Archs Neurol., Chicago* **5,** 244

106. Wernicke, C. (1881). *Lehrbuch der Gehirnkrankheiten für Ärzte und Studierende.* Kassel, Berlin: Fischer

107. White, L. E. (1965). 'A Morphologic Concept of the Limbic Lobe'. *Neurobiol. Int. Rev.* **8,** 1

108. Williams, D. (1968). 'Man's Temporal Lobe'. *Brain* **91,** 639

109. Yahr, M. D., Duvoisin, R. C. and Cowen, D. (1965). 'Encephaolpathy Associated with Carcinoma'. *Trans. Am. Neurol. Ass.* **90,** 80

110. Zuckerkandl, E. (1887). *Uber das Riechcentrum.* Stuggart: Enke

CHAPTER 13

ELECTROENCEPHALOGRAPHY AND THE
DIAGNOSIS OF TEMPORAL LOBE DISEASE

M. V. DRIVER

THE NORMAL EEG OF THE TEMPORAL REGIONS

In the scalp EEG of the healthy adult it is difficult to distinguish any activity that relates exclusively to the temporal lobe. The only rhythms that are prominent (alpha, occasionally beta) are recordable also over the sylvian-central, parietal and occipital regions. Though there may be subtle differences in frequency or amplitude from one area to another the variability is so great from person to person that allocation of any 'specific' feature to the temporal lobe is impossible. The alpha rhythm as usually recorded can be shown by automatic analysis to be made up of a number of different frequencies which presumably—and this can sometimes be demonstrated by recording from the exposed brain during a neurosurgical operation—have different loci of origin within the cortex, and some of these are probably temporal, or at least posterior temporal. Differences in the readiness with which the various alpha components attenuate when the subject's eyes open (at one time called the 'blocking' reaction) may be made out according to location but, again, in the healthy person it is generally difficult to determine the changes in purely temporal activity.

Similar considerations apply with the most prominent EEG features of normal sleep. Thus the high voltage slow arousal phenomena ('K complexes'), the sigma rhythm ('sleep spindles'), the vertex sharp waves (V waves, biparietal humps) as well as the various 'slowing' phenomena which precede them can be recorded over the temporal lobes but they do not appear to contain any components which can be said to arise specifically in them (*see* van Leeuwen[38] for a Glossary of terms used in EEG).

The physiological basis of the EEG is still only imperfectly understood, though it is believed that what is recorded from the scalp or from the exposed cortex represents a modification, perhaps a 'driving', of the inherent slow potential changes recordable in the vicinity of cells by influences which have their immediate origin in the thalamus. There is now a vast literature on this subject, but one can refer to the early animal experiments of Morison and Dempsey[25], more recently confirmed in human beings by Housepian and Purpura[17] to the effect that under conditions in which rhythmic EEG activity no longer appears spontaneously (e.g. in a state of moderately deep anaesthesia) it can be restored in the form of the 'recruiting response' by suitable electrical stimulation of the mesial and intra-laminar areas of the thalamus.

However, there is now evidence that regions of the thalamus other than those situated mesially may play a similar role and the latter need not necessarily and in all circumstances act as the central pace-maker system controlling rhythmic electrocortical activity. Andersen and colleagues[3] have shown that under certain conditions of light anaesthesia rhythmic activity may remain localized to one thalamic region and its restricted cortical projection only, whereas at other times such activity may spread throughout the thalamus and give rise to spindle formations involving large areas of the cerebral cortex. The rate of spindle recurrence may be higher in lateral than in mesial thalamic nuclei, with a tendency for a more generalized spindle to 'lead' in the lateral nuclei. It can be assumed then that the normal rhythmical EEG activity, as recorded from the cortex of the temporal lobes and elsewhere, is a reflection of normal function of the thalamus as a whole and of all those systems which use the thalamo-cortical projections as a final common path. To what extent it also depends on the interhemispheric commissures is a matter of some doubt, though much has been made of such connections in relation to the abnormalities of epilepsy.

The EEG of the healthy adolescent child contains slower rhythmical components than are seen in the adult. These include waves which appear to have an origin in the posterior temporal regions and which have properties similar to those of the alpha rhythm. They range in frequency from the low alpha limit of 8 c/sec to 3 c/sec or so and frequently appear to have a sub-harmonic relationship with the alpha. The slowest of these waves may stand out as a 'focal' phenomenon against a background of more usual alpha activity and can be misinterpreted as a sign of cerebral disease. The more distinctly rhythmic slow waves may, on occasion, be the most prominent or 'dominant' activity of the EEG and difficulty may then be experienced in their interpretation too since similar waves may be seen in children with petit mal and other disorders. These various phenomena will be discussed more fully later.

The other typical childhood EEG activity is the theta rhythm, which commonly appears more prominently in the frontotemporal regions than elsewhere. It does not react to 'alerting' stimuli as obviously as does the alpha rhythm, but it has been said in some circumstances to respond to emotional changes and in particular to appear with frustration and disappointment. Its actual physiological meaning is, like that of the alpha rhythm, obscure and in clinical electroencephalography it is rarely regarded as having any importance unless it is grossly asymmetrical or unusually persistent into late adolescence and early adulthood.

Alpha, beta and theta rhythms are to some extent artificial abstractions resulting from attempts to simplify and order, and it may well be considered preferable to describe these forms of cerebral activity purely in terms of location, frequency and reactivity. However described, though, they are the only prominent and more or less continuous features of the normal EEG in adolescence and adult life and subtle variations from person to person can be said to have no very well-established relation to psychological or psychiatric factors.

Several phenomena of irregular or paroxysmal occurrence have been described in the temporal regions of the EEG and are important in that they have some properties similar to those of features seen in temporal lobe epilepsy. The most important are *rhythmic positive spikes*, *'background' temporal spikes* and *posterior temporal sharp waves*.

Rhythmic Positive Spikes

These were first reported in 1951[10] as the '14 and 6 per second positive spike phenomenon'. The pattern is more variable than this description might suggest, any frequency between six and eight for the slower and 12 to 16 for the faster rhythm being common. The waves characteristically occur in brief bursts, up to a second or so in duration, the frequency of repetition within the burst being constant though the occurrence of the bursts themselves is without obvious rhythmicity. The waveform shows a very fast positive going spike alternating with a much slower negative phase and the amplitude is commonly about 50 μV. In many subjects these phenomena stand out more clearly from the 'background' activity of the EEG with unipolar rather than a bipolar recording, and it is recommended that a nose or joined ear reference (A_1–A_2 in the 10–20 system[18]) or a common average reference lead is used. With such a system the positive spikes are seen most clearly in the midtemporal, midsylvian and posterior temporal areas (*Figure 1*). There has been considerable controversy over the incidence and physiological and psychiatric significance of this phenomenon and a very large literature now exists, much of it of no great value. The spikes rarely

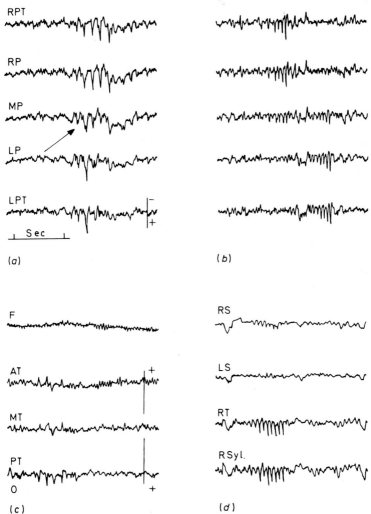

Figure 1. Rhythmic positive spikes. (a) 6/sec 80–100 μV positive spikes recorded against a reference electrode from both posterior temporal-parietal regions, but asynchronously (double spike at arrow gives time interval, right leading left by about 40 m sec); (b) 14–15/sec 50–70 μV positive spikes, same subject and recording conditions as (a). This shows a greater time interval between the phenomena of the two sides. On other occasions intervals of several seconds were observed; (c) 6/sec positive spikes, but using a bipolar recording technique (compare with (a)); (d) 13–14/sec 50–80 μV positive spikes recorded against a reference electrode fiom midtemporal and sylvian scalp electrodes but at low voltage only from a sphenoidal electrode (R—right; L—left; F—frontal; AT—anterior temporal; MT—midtemporal; PT—posterior temporal; P—parietal; MP—midparietal; O—occipital; S—sphenoidal; Syl—sylvian)

appear in alert subjects, but do so in states of drowsiness and light sleep. They are seen frequently in the EEG of adolescents and young adults and much less frequently at the extremes of life. Their actual incidence in health at various ages is very difficult to assess, however, but it is high enough in most age groups to make its 'abnormality' a matter of painstaking statistics rather than mere subjective impression.

The physiology of the phenomenon is also obscure. The form and occurrence of the bursts is rather reminiscent of sigma waves (sleep spindles) though the apparent cortical location is different. One would expect that such phenomena would have a thalamic basis (as did Gibbs when he introduced the name 'thalamic epilepsy' for the combination of certain paroxysmal clinical features with an EEG showing positive spikes), though as yet none appears to have been demonstrated adequately.

The greatest controversy has arisen over the clinical importance of this EEG feature. The 'thalamic or hypothalamic epilepsy' as described by Gibbs was said to have a less specific, generally milder and less incapacitating symptomatology than the classical forms of epilepsy previously recognized, and included various sensory, visceral and emotional symptoms. The important features of the '14 and 6 per second syndrome', which is now perhaps a more commonly used term than the original, have recently been summarized from the literature[12]. They include organized and not necessarily aggressive but socially inappropriate acts which cannot be stopped. The patient's affect is said usually to be blunted and he will have ruminated before the act was committed and shown no remorse or concern afterwards. Numerous publications have supported the view that the positive spike phenomenon is significantly associated with such or similar phenomena, details of which are available in review articles[13] but a number of investigators have been less impressed[32].

A recent publication by Lombroso and colleagues[23] was critical of early work for failure to give exact criteria for the selection of 'control' and 'normal' subjects and for paying insufficient attention to the duration of sleep as a factor of possible importance. They analysed their results in a large group of 13–15 year old boys judged to be neurosurgically and mentally healthy and found that of 155 who became drowsy or fell asleep during the course of the EEG recording 90 (58 per cent) showed positive spikes ('ctenoids'). Their experience led them to the conclusion that almost every healthy child, in this age group at least, would show positive spikes if the sleep EEG continued long enough. One feels that a critical appraisal of all published work is likely to lead to a judgement of not proven and it would be unwise to accept that in any given patient the presence of these positive spikes in the EEG had any neurological or psychiatric significance.

'Background' Temporal Spikes

As temporal lobe epilepsy is so commonly associated with an EEG finding of anterior and midtemporal spikes or sharp waves (no distinction of clinical importance can usually be made between these phenomena and none will be made in the remainder of this account) it is important to know whether such spikes can occur in non-epileptic psychiatric patients and in normal subjects. As mentioned in the introductory paragraphs, the usual EEG pattern recorded from the temporal regions in the healthy adult consists of rhythmic waveforms. However, the description of these waveforms as 'sinusoidal' does not allow for the fact that they may display certain irregularities even in health, the commonest being an occasional extreme elevation above the general amplitude and the interspersion of a single wave or brief group of waves of lesser or greater frequency than is habitual (*Figure 2*). When such elevations and interspersions occur frequently the EEG may assume a very irregular or 'dysrhythmic' appearance but their occasional occurrence may produce a waveform that can only be described as a 'spike'. Such waveforms appear to comprise the phenomena reported by Kooi and colleagues[21] and are probably the basis for some statements to the effect that the identification of spikes in the EEG of the temporal regions is not necessarily confirmatory of the diagnosis of temporal lobe epilepsy.

Distinction on neurophysiological grounds between spikes with and without epileptic significance is difficult, though it is a problem which merits attention in view of the increasing use of automatic analysis and computer techniques in electroencephalography. In another publication, Kooi[20] studied several properties of rapid EEG transients, including the amplitude and duration of waves, rise and descent times and the peak angle, and came to the conclusion that the 'segmental velocity' (i.e. rate of change of voltage) was the most useful. He showed that the segmental velocity in both naturally occurring and simulated spikes generally exceeded $2 \mu V/msec$ whereas that found in normal EEG patterns was largely below 1·5. No reference was made to the relative placing of the 'spikes' reported in the previous study. Until these and similar studies are validated in practice and until suitable analysing devices become available it will be necessary to continue to use such empirical criteria as enable, in the majority of cases, a reasonably clear distinction to be made. These are, firstly, that the focal spikes of epilepsy commonly appear

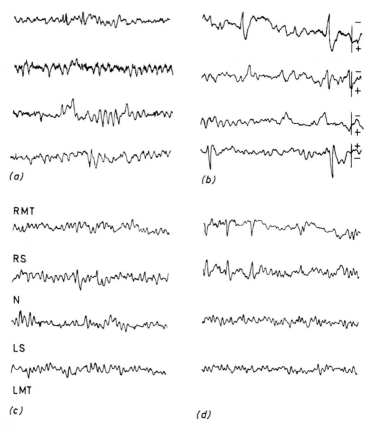

Figure 2. Midtemporal and anterior temporal spikes. (a) Irregular sharp and spike activity recorded from the midtemporal region of four alert psychiatric patients, none of whom had histories suggestive of epilepsy or organic cerebral disease; (b) the upper two tracings were taken simultaneously from the anterior temporal and midtemporal regions of a patient with psychomotor epilepsy. The first is more readily distinguished from those in (a) than is the second. None of those in (a) showed spikes in the anterior temporal region. The third sample of, (b) a midtemporal record from a patient with temporal lobe epilepsy, shows long duration sharp waves appearing after the alpha rhythm has attenuated with drowsiness (compare with the third one of (a)). The fourth tracing is of midtemporal spikes from a behaviourally disturbed, but apparently non-epileptic, child of 10. A sphenoidal recording failed to disclose anterior temporal spikes; (c) mixed fast rhythms recorded during thiopentone induced sleep in a patient with temporal lobe epilepsy. No spikes had occurred for several minutes; (d) thiopentone recording several seconds later than. (c). Focal spikes appear at the right sphenoidal electrode, at which time the fast activity in the sphenoidal-ear (RMT) channel, though not the sphenoidal-frontal (nose) channel, becomes considerably attenuated (All bipolar recordings. R—right; L—left; N—electrode on tip of nose; MT—midtemporal; S—sphenoidal)

to be unassociated with the 'background' rhythms (e.g. alpha) whereas the spikes of the non-epileptic subject appear, in a sense, to arise out of these rhythms and, secondly, the focal spikes of epilepsy may be preceded or more commonly followed by a definite attenuation in the background activity, whereas the non-epileptic spikes are not (*Figure 2*). Two other points of distinction are crucial: first, the spikes seen in non-epileptic subjects tend to be prominent when the background EEG is prominent and to be less obvious when it changes character as in light or moderately deep sleep, whereas the spikes of epilepsy are unaffected by the background and they tend to appear much more frequently in drowsiness and sleep than when the subject is awake. Secondly, a spike focus at a 'sphenoidal' electrode in light sleep is almost invariable in temporal lobe epilepsy. Though such a focus may also appear in subjects with intracranial disease without epilepsy (e.g. with some large pituitary lesions) it is not seen in healthy subjects. It is, therefore, important to record during sleep—and preferably with sphenoidal electrodes—if there are some doubts about the diagnosis of temporal lobe epilepsy and unequivocal EEG evidence is required.

Posterior Temporal Sharp Waves

The slow posterior temporal phenomena of childhood and adolescence usually assume a rounded or sinusoidal form, but other waveforms may be seen especially when occurring singly rather than in runs. Waves of saw tooth and sharp outline occasionally appear very clearly, in which case description without qualification may lead to a mistaken impression that the 'focus' represents a pathological disturbance of function and, therefore, a cerebral lesion. Quite commonly these waves show similar characteristics to the alpha rhythm, not only in relation to apparent origin but also in their tending to be more prominent in the right side, their behaviour to alerting stimuli (attenuation) and their disappearance with drowsiness and light sleep. It is, in fact, doubtful whether such waves have any significance different to that of the more usual rounded waves of this region, whether in their presence in childhood or their unusual persistence into adult life. Certainly, if they are the only unusual feature in an otherwise 'normal' EEG it would be unwise to look upon them as in any way confirmatory of organic cerebral disease (*Figure 3*).

ABNORMALITIES OF THE EEG IN TEMPORAL LOBE DISEASE

Epilepsy

The typical and sometimes the only prominent EEG abnormality

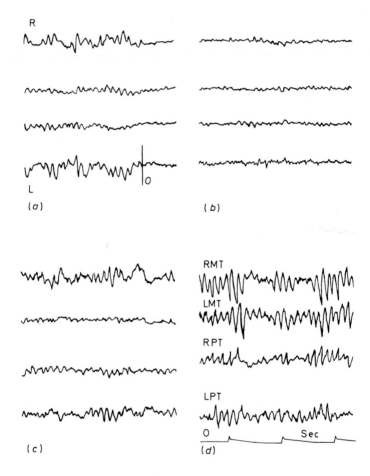

Figure 3. Posterior temporal slow and sharp waves. (a) Recording is from a 19 year old female patient who suffered from temper tantrums and emotional instability since age of 11. The bilateral posterior temporal slow waves disappear when the eyes open (O); (b) as (a) 6 sec later, the eyes are still open. The slow waves are absent but the alpha rhythm is returning. The slow waves indicate a lesser level of arousal than does the alpha rhythm; (c) Recording is from a 24 year old male patient diagnosed as a schizophrenic with no history of violence; (d) recording from a 37 year old male patient with a history of episodic violent behaviour but without clinical evidence of epilepsy (All bipolar recordings. (a), (b) and (c) are transverse right to left posterior temporal-parietal regions; (d) anteroposterior, alternately right, left. R—right; L—left; MT—midtemporal; PT— posterior temporal; O—occipital)

in temporal lobe epilepsy in adults is the anterior temporal spike focus. Its exact location on the scalp may vary from patient to patient and, not uncommonly, from time to time in the same patient, but generally it appears as a 'phase reversal' (in bipolar recording) at an anterior temporal convexity electrode or at a sphenoidal electrode and often at both together. It is frequently observed to have a wide distribution over the antero-inferior temporal regions, perhaps wider, so that channels connected to electrodes in the frontal, sylvian, midtemporal and posterior temporal regions also register it. This does not necessarily mean that the whole cortex of these areas is functioning abnormally but usually only that the properties of the skull and scalp are such as to spread out or perhaps smooth out the potential fields from one or more relatively restricted zones of cortical dysfunction to a wide area of scalp. The properties of non-homogeneous volume conductors are of relevance here[4]. Whether in a given case such a 'widespread' focus is to be explained on these lines or is to be considered as a sign of synchronous involvement of a large area of lateral temporal cortex is usually impossible to determine. One can say though that such synchrony (particularly if no resolution is obtainable by a cathode ray oscilloscope) is most unusual and also that a much more punctate spike focus is almost always demonstrable when the cortex is exposed in the operating theatre.

Two or more spike foci may be recordable in the temporal area, the most common finding being apparently independent spikes in the anterior temporal-sphenoidal and midtemporal-sylvian regions.

The form of the spike is much more varied than its apparent location, very rapid spikes, longer duration sharp waves and mixed forms such as spike-slow, polyspike or spike-sharp complexes being common. It is doubtful whether the variation of form has any importance from a practical point of view, though with the more complex waves it is important to establish that the phenomena are, in fact, anterior temporal foci and not discharges of more general and possibly extratemporal cortical distribution.

The exact location and morphology of the spike focus in temporal lobe epilepsy are of far less importance than whether it appears at all, and every effort should be made in doubtful cases to record the EEG under the most favourable circumstances. A brief EEG recorded in an out-patient department may well be quite normal whereas one recorded from a relaxed patient in a quiet room may show a very active spike focus. Drowsiness and sleep, whether natural or drug induced, are conducive to the appearance of spikes. Before thinking of 'excluding' the possibility of temporal lobe epilepsy on EEG grounds one should be prepared to take at least three sleep records, for which purpose the ordinary scalp electrodes may well suffice (preferably applied as described by Pampiglione[28], though the 10–20 system[18] is often adequate). Sphenoidal electrodes are of greatest value when the question of lateralization of the actual epileptogenic lesion arises in a case with bilateral spikes or when there is some apparent disagreement between the clinical, radiological, psychological and electroencephalographic evidence.

A relative reduction in the amount of barbiturate-induced fast activity on one side, and in particular in those channels connected to one of the sphenoidal electrodes, may provide confirmatory lateralizing evidence in cases of mesial temporal sclerosis[19]. However, this finding needs some care in interpretation, both in relation to prediction of responsible pathology, since it may be found also with small focal lesions, and in regard to lateralization. Margerison and Corsellis[24] found in their group of institutionalized epileptics that, though such a reduction was significantly associated with mesial temporal sclerosis, the presumed EEG lateralization only coincided with that of the lesion disclosed at autopsy in about half the cases. It seems certain that factors other than the presence of an underlying tumour or sclerosis can lead to a reduction in amplitude of fast activity, though the original observation may be used as a lateralizing sign—of a lesion or of the epileptogenic process—except in cases where the reduction is accompanied by a very rapidly repeating EEG spike focus, when confirmation that the apparent reduction persists in the absence of such spikes should be sought on another occasion (*see Figure 2*). Slow activity also, particularly if of mixed or irregular form, may occasionally be of lateralizing value whether it relates directly to the presence of a cortical lesion or to a localized postictal dysfunction.

The use of sphenoidal electrodes may be combined not only with the injection of barbiturates (e.g. thiopentone and methohexital) but also with that of such drugs as chlorpromazine, amitriptyline and procyclidine[39] or convulsant drugs such as leptazol ('metrazol') and bemegride. In the more difficult cases electroencephalographic recordings have been taken from electrodes placed within the brain, though this has not emerged from the trial period as a really successful or practical technique. These, and more recent procedures, including the injection of amylobarbitone and leptazol into the internal carotid arteries, are discussed more fully elsewhere[6].

That there is such a number of techniques available for use in the investigation of patients with bilateral EEG spike abnormalities reflects the belief that not every such case, nor even every patient with probable bilateral pathology, is necessarily a case of independent bilateral epilepsy. A great deal of attention has been paid to this problem in experimental epilepsy and in particular addressed to the phenomenon of the 'mirror focus'. The basic observation[26, 27] was that the production in a suitable laboratory animal, e.g. a cat, of a single and clearly lateralized cortical epileptic lesion would lead after some lapse of time to the appearance of a 'mirror' spike focus in the EEG of the homotopic contralateral cortex. Initially, this focus would show a clear time relationship with that related to the lesion, but given sufficient time this relationship would disappear and the mirror focus would behave as though independent. Callosal section or removal of the lesion before the contralateral spikes became independent would be followed by the disappearance of the mirror focus, but not so after independence had been achieved. If these observations could be related directly to EEG foci in human temporal lobe epilepsy they would suggest that resection of the 'leading' temporal lobe in cases showing bilateral time-related spikes would be likely to result in a relief from seizures, whereas resection of one lobe after independence had been established would not. Such time-related bilateral focal spikes are rarely met with in practice, but many patients with apparently independent bilateral foci become seizure free or nearly so following a unilateral resection.

The probability is that the 'mirror' phenomenon is not so simple as it originally appeared and it can develop in different circumstances in different experiments. For example, Holubář[16] found with penicillin-induced foci in the rat that the mirror focus developed even in animals which had had the corpus callosum sectioned beforehand, presumably via the deeper subcortical structures. Species differences as well as lesion differences are obviously of great importance in applying the results of animal experiments to the study of human epilepsy, and the reaction of the monkey to an alumina cream lesion may well be as different from the reaction of the rat cortex to penicillin as from the reaction of the human brain to a small temporal lobe astrocytoma. Another source of difficulty is in exactly what is implied by the term 'epileptic' or 'epileptogenic': the primary lesion may lead not only to a local spike focus but also to observed contralateral motor seizure activity, though it appears to be very unusual for the mirror focus to do the same and if it does not it cannot be regarded as an 'epileptogenic focus'.

Though the precise relevance of the mirror focus to human epilepsy is obscure the anatomical relationships between the area of a cerebral lesion and distant parts of the brain may be of importance clinically and detectable by EEG. For example, Falconer, Driver and

Serafetinides[9] described two cases with posterior temporoparietal lesions which themselves appeared to be 'silent' but which appeared to provoke seizures via activation of the mesial temporal structures. Schneider, Crosby and Farhat[31] noted the importance of the apparent two-way anatomical relationship of the frontal and temporal lobes via the uncinate fasciculus, a relationship which can lead to symptoms of both temporal and frontal dysfunction with lesions limited to the temporal lobe. These reports also indicate a possible reason for failure of resection to bring relief in some cases of temporal lobe epilepsy with unilateral temporal spikes. Being small, without 'local' signs and unobserved by radiology, the responsible lesion may escape notice. If part of the projection area is left behind, the seizures may well continue.

One of the most interesting points about the spike focus is that though it would obviously appear to have a meaning in the disease or syndrome of temporal lobe epilepsy it seems to play little or no part in the actual seizure itself. The typical EEG phenomena of the latter are rhythmic slow waves that may or may not show the same location as the interictal spike (*Figure 4*). Whether or not the spike focus itself has any concomittants of psychological or psychiatric importance is impossible to say with certainty on the basis of present knowledge. The methods of investigating perceptive and other deficits in patients with brief spike-wave bursts in the EEG[35] are not easily applied to the study of the effects of 'focal' spiking, but the problem deserves more attention. In rhesus monkeys epileptogenic lesions and non-epileptogenic ablations of the parietal cortex do not appear to differ significantly in their effects on certain aspects of learning[7], but the degree to which such a finding can apply to temporal lobe lesions and the associated spiking is not certain.

Whatever the effect of the anteromesial temporal spike focus in the symptomatology of the patient, it is an extremely useful sign in diagnosis and the level of agreement between independent assessments of the patient as a temporal lobe epileptic and the EEG spike focus as an indicator of temporal lobe epilepsy is high. For example, Margerison and Corsellis[24] reported, amongst other interesting findings, agreement in 85 per cent of 39 cases, a comparable agreement to that found between clinical versus neuropathological, and EEG versus neuropathological assessments.

Foci confined to the midtemporal region of the scalp are, however, by no means reliable indicators of temporal lobe epilepsy or pathology, particularly in children. Such foci have been reported as the result of a migration from a more posterior situation, sometimes as the end result, in which case the prognosis is stated to be very good, and

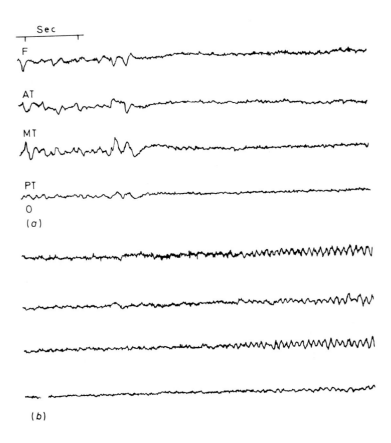

Figure 4. Development of a temporal lobe seizure. (a) The interictal pattern of sharp waves is seen on the left. Their disappearance marks the beginning of the electroencephalographic seizure, characterized by low amplitude activity without obvious focal phenomena; (b) record follows directly from the end of (a) and shows the developing rhythmic slow activity characteristic of the seizure. Sharp waves and spikes do not usually return until the postictal period (Bipolar recording. F—frontal; AT—anterior temporal; MT—midtemporal; PT—posterior temporal; O—occipital)

sometimes as a stage on the way to the development of an anterior temporal focus, the prognosis of which is serious[11]. It appears doubtful whether such a migration occurs in practice and it seems much more likely that the posterior and anterior foci represent the responses of the relatively immature and the relatively mature brain respectively to the dysfunction brought about by the basic lesion. The work of Trojaborg[36, 37] on spike foci in brain-damaged children can be interpreted in a similar way. As noted earlier, posterior temporal spike forms are not uncommon in children in the absence of actual cerebral disease. Lombroso[22] described the midtemporal spike focus in childhood as the EEG correlate of lingual epilepsy, that is, of a type of sensory seizure involving the tongue, gums and the inside of the cheeks. Other features of the seizure might include non-dysphasic speech arrest, excessive salivation and motor involvement of the face, pointing to a low Rolandic rather than a temporal lobe origin (though Gibbs felt that it was in fact temporal, the symptomatology relating to the spread of seizure discharge rather than to its origin). As the prognosis with this type of seizure was good (50 per cent becoming seizure free with a normal EEG within 4–5 years), Lombroso felt that differentiation from true temporal lobe epilepsy was very important. Such differentiation must be done mainly on the basis of an accurate analysis of the seizure since the apparent temporal location of the spike and its tendency to appear more frequently in sleep might well be considered in rather doubtful cases as indicative of primarily anterior temporal lobe dysfunction. Some assistance could probably be obtained from recordings using sphenoidal electrodes, and especially if an EEG were obtained during the course of an actual seizure, but, as with other varieties of epilepsy in childhood, precise diagnosis can be extremely difficult.

Temporal Lobe Phenomena in Behaviour Disturbances

One of the earliest comprehensive accounts of the types of EEG activity to be found in patients with episodic psychotic disorders and psychopathic behaviour was that of Hill[14]. He differentiated between slow but normal variants of the alpha rhythm and the 'posterior temporal slow wave focus' which was one of the EEG phenomena of the temporal lobes apparently related in some way to aggressive traits within the psychopathic population. However, as Hill pointed out, the study failed to show any EEG characters which could be related specifically to patients of the types investigated: a variety of patterns appeared, all of which could be recognized in a proportion of the normal population. In a later presentation[15] he noted that posterior temporal slow waves might be regarded as a physiological phenomenon in early childhood but their persistence into adult life, as part of a defect of cerebral maturation, could be associated with serious psychiatric disabilities. Such disabilities, including psychopathic aggressive behaviour, were more commonly met with, and more serious, posterior temporal foci more than the anterior temporal spike focus. The various points introduced in this work; the definition of posterior temporal focus, its incidence in the normal population, its relationship with deviant behaviour and its importance relative to the anterior temporal spike (and thus to temporal lobe epilepsy) have been the subjects of much discussion since.

An analysis of unusual—and especially slow—activity to be found in the posterior temporal and occipital regions was made by Aird and Gastaut[1]. They described four types of such activity, including a class of slow posterior waves often associated with high voltage sharp waves of negative polarity, all of which blocked with the alpha rhythm when the eyes opened. These were common in their patient population—especially in the 6 to 25 year group—but were also found as a distinct and developed phenomenon in 10 per cent of a presumed normal population of 500 young men of 19 to 22 years of age.

There are many difficulties in the way of a reliable assessment of the frequency with which this phenomenon is to be expected in the various psychiatric disorders with which it has been associated. The manifestations of 'behaviour disorder' are many and varied and findings in a group described as 'young adult psychiatric patients' cannot realistically be compared and contrasted with those in a second such group from a different hospital and perhaps a different country. No limitation of the imprecision is possible by other investigations, for example pathological or radiological studies, and EEG assessment has not yet reached that degree of precision which would enable one investigator adequately to compare his recordings with those made use of by another. The study by Wiener, Delano and Klass[40] appears to have as few imponderables as possible, being of a limited age group (13–18 years) of male subjects without signs, symptoms or history of organic brain disease or mental retardation—80 were classified as 'delinquent', having been so judged in a court of law, and 70 as 'normal'. Each had a lengthy EEG recording, including periods of overbreathing and sleep, which was analysed without prior knowledge of individual classification. No very great differences were found between the groups in relation to slow activity though there were differences within each group between the 13 to 14 year olds and those of 17 to 18, i.e. 'maturation' proceeded about equally in both delinquents and non-delinquents. The group of 100 behaviourally disordered children studied by Aird and Yamamoto[2] was different in age group ($1\frac{1}{2}$ to 16 years) and in neurological status (11 had positive signs of CNS disorder and others had a past history of intracranial disease). Almost one half (49) of these children had definite EEG abnormalities of which 27 were mainly temporal, seven having spikes or sharp waves 'suggestive of focal epileptic discharge' even though none of the 100 was said to be epileptic. In another group of patients with temporal EEG foci reported by the same authors 39 per cent had a behaviour disturbance.

These represent two widely different approaches to the deviant behaviour population, one relating to such slight departures from normal that the difference between 'subjects' and 'controls' may be largely accidental, and the other to a group of mixed neuro-psychiatric symptomatology such as is much more commonly met within hospital practice. Experience with EEG studies in children in the latter category suggests that whether the EEG is abnormal or not is related far more definitely to positive neurological signs, or a suggestive history, than to the type or severity of the behaviour disorder.

The question of the exact relationship between psychopathic aggressive behaviour and the posterior temporal EEG features so often found associated with it remains unanswered. Possibly they do in fact represent nothing more than a sign of one or more defects in cerebral maturation, but experience with EEG teaches that few if any of its phenomena have one single distinct and specific meaning. Slow posterior temporal waves in the EEG of a normal 11 year old boy may not signify that similar waves in a 20 year old psychopath relate to an 11 year old 'rest' in his brain. The EEG of the temporal lobe reflects thalamic function, which relates to the function of the middle and lower brain stem and this, as Zivin and Marsan[42] point out, serves the organism's need to make adjustments to environmental changes. At this level slight defects of development or very limited disease processes can result in profound disturbances of sensory integration and modify response to any aspect of the environment which is capable of evoking an emotional reaction.

Williams[41] approaches the problem of EEG and aggressive anti-social behaviour on a broad front, putting the anterior temporal region ahead of the posterior in importance, and including the orbital and lateral frontal areas also. It is possible that the postulated brain stem-thalamic dysfunction responsible for the disturbed behaviour acts at a non-cortical level, or if at a cortical level then without EEG signs, and at the same time results in slow or sharp wave disturbances which can appear in any or all of its projection areas. As de Jong[5] points out, the behaviour disorder should not be considered too closely related to the site of EEG disturbance. The problem is, however, very complicated as is confirmed, if confirmation were needed, by the beneficial effects on behaviour that can follow a temporal lobectomy for the relief of epilepsy[8] and by reports such as those of Small, Small and Hayden[33] and Stevens[34] to the effect that psychiatric evaluation of temporal lobe and non-temporal lobe epileptics does not confirm that there is anything distinctive about the personalities of the former.

REFERENCES

1. Aird, R. B. and Gastaut, Y. (1959). 'Occipital and Posterior Electro-encephalographic Rhythms'. *Electroenceph. clin. Neurophysiol.* **11,** 637

2. — and Yamamoto, T. (1966). 'Behaviour Disorders of Childhood'. *Electroenceph. clin. Neurophysiol.* **21,** 148

3. Andersen, P., Andersson, S. A. and Lømo, T. (1966). 'Patterns of Spontaneous Rhythmic Activity within Various Thalamic Nuclei'. *Nature, Lond.* **211,** 888

4. Brazier, M. A. B. (1968). *The Electrical Activity of the Nervous System*, Chap. 7. London: Pitman

5. De Jong, R. N. (1957). ' "Psychomotor" or "Temporal Lobe" Epilepsy. A Review of the Development of Our Present Concept'. *Neurology, Minneap.* **7,** 1

6. Driver, M. V. (1969). 'Electroencephalography in the Study of Epilepsy'. In *Recent Advances in Neurology and Neuropsychiatry,* 8th edn. Ed. by Lord Brain and M. Wilkinson. London: Churchill

7. — Ettlinger, G., Moffett, A. M. and St. John-Loe, P. (1968). 'Epileptogenic Lesions in the Monkey'. *J. Physiol.* **196,** 93

8. Falconer, M. A. and Serafetinides, E. A. (1963). 'A Follow-up Study of Surgery in Temporal Lobe Epilepsy'. *J. Neurol. Neurosurg. Psychiat.* **26,** 154

9. — Driver, M. V. and Serafetinides, E. A. (1962). 'Temporal Lobe Epilepsy due to Distant Lesions: Two Cases Relieved by Operation'. *Brain* **85,** 521

10. Gibbs, E. L. and Gibbs, F. A. (1951). 'Electroencephalographic Evidence of Thalamic and Hypothalamic Epilepsy'. *Neurology, Minneap.* **1,** 136

11. Gibbs, F. A. and Gibbs, E. L. (1960). 'Good Prognosis of Mid-temporal Epilepsy'. *Epilepsia* **1,** 448

12. Greenberg, I. M. and Rosenberg, G. (1966). 'Familial Correlates of 14 and 6 cps EEG Positive Spike Pattern'. *Psychiat. Res. Rep.* **20,** 121

13. Henry, C. E. (1963). 'Positive Spike Discharges in the EEG and Behavior Abnormality'. In *E.E.G. and Behaviour*, Chap. 13. Ed. by G. H. Glaser. New York: Basic Books

14. Hill, D. (1952). 'EEG in Episodic Psychotic and Psychopathic Behaviour'. *Electroenceph. clin. Neurophysiol.* **4,** 419

15. — (1953). 'Clinical Associations of Electroencephalographic Foci in the Temporal Lobe'. *A.M.A. Archs Neurol. Psychiat.* **69,** 379

16. Holubář, J. (1965). 'Mode of Activation of the Mirror Focus Initiated by Local Penicillin Application to the Contralateral Cerebral Cortex in Rats'. *Physiologia bohemoslov.* **14,** 509

17. Housepian, E. M. and Purpura, D. P. (1963). 'Electrophysiological Studies of Subcortical-cortical Relations in Man'. *Electroenceph. clin. Neurophysiol.* **15,** 20

18. Jasper, H. H. (1958). 'The Ten Twenty Electrode System of the International Federation'. *Electroenceph. clin. Neurophysiol.* **10,** 371

19. Kennedy, W. A. and Hill, D. (1958). 'The Surgical Prognostic Significance of the Electroencephalographic Prediction of Ammon's Horn Sclerosis in Epileptics'. *J. Neurol. Neurosurg. Psychiat.* **21,** 24

20. Kooi, K. A. (1966). 'Voltage-time Characteristics of Spikes and Other Rapid EEG Transients: Semantic and Morphological Considerations'. *Neurology, Minneap.* **16,** 59

21. — Güvener, A. M., Tupper, C. J. and Bagchi, B. K. (1964). 'Electroencephalographic Patterns of the Temporal Region in Normal Adults'. *Neurology, Minneap.* **14,** 1029

22. Lombroso, C. T. (1965), 'Lingual Seizures and Midtemporal Spike Foci in Children. *Sixth Int. Congr. Electro enceph., Vienna*, p. 19

23. — Schwartz, I. H., Clark, D. M., Muench, H. and Barry, J. (1966). 'Ctenoids in Healthy Youths: Controlled Study of 14- and 6- per-second Positive Spiking'. *Neurology, Minneap.* **16,** 1152

24. Margerison, J. H. and Corsellis, J. A. N. (1966). 'Epilepsy and the Temporal Lobes. A Clinical, EEG and Neuropathological Study of the Brain in Epilepsy, with Particular Reference to the Temporal Lobes'. *Brain.* **89,** 499

25. Morison, R. S. and Dempsey, E. W. (1942). 'A Study of Thalamocortical Relations' *Am. J. Physiol.* **135,** 281

26. Morrell, F. (1959). 'Experimental Focal Epilepsy in Animals'. *Archs Neurol. ,Chicago* **1,** 141

27. — (1960). 'Secondary Epileptogenic Lesions'. *Epilepsia* **1,** 538

28. Pampiglione, G. (1966). 'Some Anatomical Considerations upon Electrode Placement in Routine EEG'. *Proc. electro-physiol. Technol. Ass.* **13,** 166

29. — and Kerridge, J. (1956). 'EEG Abnormalities from the Temporal Lobe Studied with Sphenoidal Electrodes'. *J. Neurol. Neurosurg. Psychiat.* **19,** 117

30. Rovit, R. L., Gloor, P. and Rasmussen, T. (1961). 'Sphenoidal Electrodes in the Electrographic Study of Patients with Temporal Lobe Epilepsy'. *J. Neurosurg.* **18,** 151

31. Schneider, R. C., Crosby, E. C. and Farhat, S. M. (1965). 'Extra-temporal Lesions Triggering the Temporal Lobe Syndrome'. *J. Neurosurg.* **23,** 246

32. Small, J. G. and Small, I. F. (1964). 'Fourteen and Six per second Positive Spikes'. *Archs gen. Psychiat.* **11,** 645

33. — Small, I. F. and Hayden, M. P. (1966). 'Further Psychiatric Investigation of Patients with Temporal and Nontemporal Epilepsy'. *Am. J. Psychiat.* **123,** 303

34. Stevens, J. R. (1966). 'Psychiatric Implications of Psychomotor Epilepsy'. *Archs gen. Psychiat.* **14,** 461

35. Tizard, B. and Margerison, J. H. (1963). 'Psychological Function during Wave-spike Discharge'. *Br. J. Soc. clin. Psychol.* **3,** 6

36. Trojaborg, W. (1965). 'Serial EEG Investigation of Children with Focal Spike Discharges'. *Electroenceph. clin. Neurophysiol.* **19,** 613

37. — 'Spike Foci in Children'. *Sixth Int. Congr. Electro enceph., Vienna,* p. 31

38. Van Leeuwen, W. S. (1966). 'Proposal for an EEG Terminology by the Terminology Committee of the International Federation for Electroencephalography and Clinical Neurophysiology. *Electroenceph. clin. Neurophysiol.* **20,** 306.

39. Vas, C. J., Exley, K. A. and Parsonage, M. J. (1967). 'Activation of the EEG by Procyclidine Hydrochloride in Temporal Lobe Epilepsy'. *Epilepsia* **8,** 241

40. Wiener, J. M., Delano, J. G. and Klass, D. W. (1966). An EEG Study of Delinquent and Non-delinquent Adolescents'. *Archs gen. Psychiat.* **15,** 144

41. Williams, D. (1968). 'Man's Temporal Lobe'. *Brain* **91,** 639

42. Zivin, L. and Marsan, C. A. (1968). 'Incidence and Prognostic Significance of "Epileptiform" Activity in the EEG of Non-epileptic Subjects'. *Brain* **91,** 751

CHAPTER 14

TEMPORAL LOBE EPILEPSY:
CLINICAL FEATURES, PATHOLOGY, DIAGNOSIS, AND
TREATMENT

MURRAY A. FALCONER and DAVID C. TAYLOR

Before leaving this part of my subject, I remark, by way of recapitula-
tion, that he who neglects the 'dreamy state' because it is indefinite
and 'merely curious' and such symptoms as chewing, etc., movements,
and apparent alterations in the size and distance of external objects,
because they seem trifling things, may not even surmise that his
patient has the serious disease of epilepsy in a rudimentary form, until
a severe fit comes to tell him so. Even then it may be said that the
slight paroxysms 'developed into' epilepsy; but I insist that such slight
paroxysms are themselves epileptic.

J. Hughlings Jackson, 1888

INTRODUCTION

Although modern methods of treatment have probably reduced the
number of epileptic patients who require long-term mental hospital
management, there remain many whose incapacity is such as to lead
them frequently into the care of psychiatrists. It is now generally
agreed that temporal lobe epilepsy is disproportionately over-
represented among such patients. Therefore it falls frequently to the
psychiatrist to distinguish temporal lobe epilepsy from other
epilepsies and from a variety of functional states which it closely
resembles or which are frequently superimposed upon it. The
therapeutic implications and the prognosis demand that an accurate
diagnosis should be made.

There is still some semantic dispute over the wisest terminology
to use for this condition, largely stemming from the fact that not all
psychomotor seizures are derived from the temporal lobe and not all
temporal lobe epilepsies are of psychomotor type. The term 'temporal lobe epilepsy' has a practical value, at least from a neurosurgical standpoint, and means a group of epilepsies which originate
within one or both temporal lobes[17, 89]. Psychomotor seizures, how-

346

ever, have been described under various rubrics since the time of Hippocrates before they were renamed as such by Gibbs, Gibbs, and Lennox[36]. For these authors the term was descriptive of a variety of seizures frequently found by them in association with flat-topped, relatively slow-wave discharges seen in the EEG. Such an EEG pattern was, as it happened, a product of the particular technique used at that period and is no longer seen in modern EEGs. None the less it remains true that the most characteristic type of temporal lobe epilepsy has a psychomotor component which, on careful enquiry, makes the diagnosis possible clinically. The clinical diagnosis may then be pursued with investigations to an extent proportional to the seriousness of the disorder. In children, particularly, it may be many years before clinically obvious psychomotor epilepsy declares itself in the EEG with a clear-cut temporal lobe focus[23, 65]. The development of our concepts of temporal lobe epilepsy have been well summarized[11, 32, 53]. Among the terms used for temporal lobe epilepsy in the past are 'uncinate epilepsy', 'grand mal intellectuel', 'psychic variants', and 'psychic equivalents'[11, 53].

Anatomy and Physiology

Part of the semantic difficulties have stemmed from differing definitions of what constitutes the temporal lobe. The anatomist may limit the structure to an area of cortex anterior to the vein of Labbé and inferior to the sylvian fissure, although the clinician may include the uncus, the hippocampus (Ammon's horn) with the dentate gyrus, the hippocampal gyrus (parahippocampal gyrus) as well as the amygdala. The only other structures outside these regions which commonly have the potentiality for producing psychomotor attacks are the insula, the inferior orbital cortex, and other parts of the limbic system including the cingulate gyrus, and even these structures are closely related anatomically to the temporal structures proper. However, lesions affecting them are less common.

Knowledge of the functions subserved by these structures makes the nature of temporal lobe seizures more comprehensible[17, 19, 20]. According to Penfield[68, 69] the neocortical mantle of the lobe has an interpretive and perceptual function. Part of the superior temporal gyrus is concerned with hearing and equilibration. Olfactory and gustatory functions are subserved in the uncus and amygdala while all the mesial structures are intimately concerned with the regulation of the autonomic nervous system. Memory recording mechanisms are also present in the temporal lobe. Thus disturbed temporal function can affect a wide variety of fundamental activities, the emphasis of which may vary from individual to individual.

CLINICAL FEATURES

Incidence and Prevalence

The true prevalence of the epilepsies is still arguable because of serious problems in the interpretation of the epidemiological data. The problem is that many people and many parents will not declare the fact of their own or of their children's epilepsy. Furthermore, all studies choose an idiosyncratic definition of what constitutes 'epilepsy'. Thus many people with a history of seizures in the past, or with only occasional seizures, are excluded. Prevalence varies with the age group under consideration. Published figures therefore constitute a minimal estimate. Even so the College of General Practitioners[9] survey gave an estimate of four persons per 1,000, thus suggesting a quarter of a million epileptics in Great Britain. The recent Isle of Wight survey[39] gave a prevalence figure of 0·72 per cent of children between the ages of five and 15; extrapolating from this figure there would be some 50,000 schoolchildren with epilepsy in the country. In Pond's studies of general practices the overall prevalence was 6·2 per 1,000, of whom 7 per cent had been in a mental hospital[75, 76]. Half the mental hospital group suffered from temporal lobe epilepsy. De Jong[11] drawing on statistics from various sources indicated 'that anywhere from 30 to 80 per cent of epileptic patients have temporal lobe manifestations even though their attacks may not in all cases be of the pure psychomotor type'. Though the prevalence of temporal lobe epilepsy will vary with the population under study, it largely depends upon the clinical skill of the examiner and the extent of the investigations backing up the enquiry.

Seizure Patterns

A patient with temporal lobe epilepsy may exhibit more than one type of seizure pattern:
  (1) Auras only
  (2) Absences
  (3) Psychomotor attacks
  (4) Falling attacks
  (5) Grand mal attacks

The diagnosis is fundamentally a matter of clinical enquiry and interpretation. Absences may be overlooked while psychomotor attacks not followed by a generalized seizure are liable to misinterpretation as functional or hysterical manifestations. Abnormalities of mood or behaviour or of consciousness are more likely to be epileptic when they are sudden, out of character, brief and irregularly recurrent. Temporal lobe attacks, however, may be precipitated by emotion or fatigue. Where there are obvious major or minor seizures their psychomotor character will be apparent if five questions are asked. What evidence is there that an attack is 'in the air'? How does the patient describe his experience? What do observers see at the onset of the attack? What happens during the attack? And what happens after the attack?

The salient clinical features of psychomotor attacks are in Table 1.

TABLE 1

Features of Psychomotor Attacks

---

(1) Objective Concomitants
    Impaired consciousness—dazedness to unconsciousness
    Motor activity—confusional behaviour to reorientating reactions
    Autonomic reactions—mastication, pallor, flushing, etc.
    Speech disturbances—dysphasia and ictal speech automatisms.

(2) Subjective Concomitants
    Crude somatic sensations   Epigastric → throat
                          Cephalic
                          Tinnitus and vertigo
                          Taste and smell
    Emotional   Fear
                          Pleasure
    Perceptual illusions   Strangeness and familiarity
                          Micropsia and macropsia
                          Micrusia and macrusia
                          Déjà vu and déjà entendu
    Memory hallucinations   Reminiscence
                          Panoramic memory

(3) Automatisms

Changes in mood, irritability, and bad dreams may at times precede the attack by several hours or days, but such prodromes are not confined to temporal lobe epilepsy. The most common auras, particularly when the onset of seizures has been early in life, are crude visceral sensations. The commonest is a feeling perceived in the epigastrium which sometimes rises up into the throat. Patients may describe them as 'a turning of the stomach', as 'fear in the stomach', or even pain. Next in frequency come inexplicable 'odd feelings in the head'. Sometimes the visceral sensations are referred to the penis, vagina, or rectum. Tinnitus and vertigo also occur and are frequently accompanied by changes in auditory perception. All these crude phenomena are common when the lesion is mesial temporal sclerosis[26]. Fear, or more properly anxiety, is the most common premonitory emotional experience[105], but sometimes, as was noted by Jackson and described by Dostoiewsky[13, 14], the attacks may cause

349

pleasure of considerable intensity. Indeed, after the relief of epilepsy, some of our patients have complained that this pleasure is now denied them. The more intelligent adult patients may describe auras of depersonalization or of derealization, or that objects, sounds or events suddenly acquire a peculiar vivid significance for them. At times perceptual anomalies may lead to apparent variations in size or distance, and sounds may seem remote or unbearably loud. Among the disorders of memory are various phenomena which seem like a record of some remote event being replayed in the mind visually or auditorially. Some of these hallucinations have a musical quality. More than one aura may occur simultaneously and their content be so rich and strange that the patient has not the vocabulary to describe them. Olfactory and gustatory auras, once said by Gowers to be diagnostic of temporal lobe seizures, are in fact rare, and when they do occur, suggest the presence not of mesial temporal sclerosis but of a tumour or a hamartoma[11, 22].

With the onset of the aura the attack may be apparent to a perceptive witness. Minimally there is blankness or dazedness, the patient may blanch or blush, or he may move out of company into a quieter situation. The intensity of the attack in any patient will vary from time to time, depending on the extent of the spread of abnormal neuronal activity. Occasionally the attack may cease with the onset of the aura and there may be only the briefest period of dazedness. Alternatively, disturbed motor activity in the form of falling or slumping, confused psychomotor behaviour, or even a grand mal convulsion, may follow. We prefer to limit the term 'automatism' to the Jacksonian ideophone of snatches of apparently purposeful behaviour such as searching, drinking, smoking, or undressing, rather than to describe the lip-smacking, pursing, and trivial motor movements which some authors include but which we prefer to call 'psychomotor confusion' or 'reactively compelled behaviour'[18, 19]. Such automatic behaviour generally follows the attack proper, but at times may represent the only observable evidence that a fit has occurred.

One of our patients, for example, would rise after the aura in an amnesic phase and void urine into any handy container. This was all that his friends had noted. Following a psychomotor attack most patients are confused and have little recollection of the events subsequent to the aura. Occasionally a patient can recall observing events during the psychomotor attack but being unable to speak at the time. This is ictal dysphasia which may persist after the seizure has apparently stopped. Infrequently an adult patient with a psychomotor attack of temporal lobe origin cannot recall his aura.

We agree with De Jong[11] that psychomotor seizures, although usually of temporal lobe origin, can sometimes arise in other parts of the brain, probably in connection with the limbic system. The Montreal school appear to regard seizures having certain auras as definitely arising within the temporal lobe[3, 37]. These auras include 'experiential illusions, such as déjà vu and feelings of strangeness or unreality; perceptual illusions or hallucinations (auditory or organized or both, complex visual hallucinations); olfactory phenomena; ictal automatism; ictal fear or other emotions; mastication, licking and swallowing movements; and epigastric sensation'[3]. One of us (Falconer. 1969. Unpublished observations), however, has occasionally seen patients, usually with neoplasms or angiomas affecting the inferior frontal region or the cingulate gyrus, who have presented with psychomotor attacks with one or more of these various features, but without detectable spike discharges in the temporal lobes on EEG examination. Schneider and colleagues[83] have made similar observations. We therefore do not regard these auras as pathognomic of temporal lobe epilepsy, although they usually do indicate it, as temporal lobe lesions are much more common.

Having established the nature of the current attacks it is imperative to determine the circumstances and timing of the first attack ever, as well as their subsequent progression. Often many years separate the initial attack from the onset of habitual seizures. We have found that when the first attack was status epilepticus in early childhood, or where there was a history of febrile convulsions, the pathology is usually mesial temporal sclerosis.

The age of onset of the habitual seizures is important, both in understanding the likely nature of the associated handicaps, as well as in indicating the aetiology of the epilepsy. In a recent series of 100 cases of temporal lobe epilepsy[96] 32 out of 47 cases who proved to have mesial temporal sclerosis had established their habitual seizures before the age of 10 years. Cases in which no specific pathological lesion was found tended to have a later onset (11 out of 25 cases developed habitual seizures between 10 and 20 years). Hamartomas, scars, and infarcts were more prevalent in the older age groups. In general, the earlier the onset of epilepsy the greater the degree of intellectual and social damage. Thus the I.Q. scores in the Wechsler tests tended to be lower in patients whose habitual seizures began in the first decade (only nine out of 29 patients with a verbal I.Q. of over 110 started having seizures in the first decade compared with 17 out of 23 with scores below 90). Where epilepsy started early, schooling was more disturbed and 55 per cent of the early onset group had required institutional care compared with 35 per cent of the remainder. Early onset epilepsy and poor ratings on all items of social adjustment were found to be correlated together. Thus in obtaining the nature and timing of the onset of the epilepsy data of considerable significance are often established.

Mental State

There are, broadly speaking, three groups of mental abnormalities in epilepsy which have been used as a basis for their classification since the time of Falret[27]. These were fully reviewed by Pond[72]. They are peri-ictal disorders, inter-ictal disorders, and long-term psychoses. The peri-ictal disorders present as acute problems whenever the abnormal behaviour observed during a psychomotor attack or the resulting automatism gives rise to concern. Among these disorders can be included outbursts of violence (usually provoked by interfering with a patient during an attack), relatively brief fugue-like wanderings, and occasional sexual misdemeanours. Marked prodromal changes of mood or behaviour sometimes warn relatives or attendants of an attack, and such changes of mood usually disappear after the attack. Following a seizure or series of seizures, changes of mood, usually towards depression, are common and may be severe. At times a confusional psychosis, often coloured with ecstatic religious feelings and vivid hallucinations, occurs in the post-ictal period, though such twilight states may occur without a clear relationship to observed attacks.

The majority of temporal lobe epileptics requiring psychiatric help suffer from long-term inter-ictal personality disorder. Most people dealing regularly with chronic epileptic patients are aware of the frequency of slow pedantic 'stickiness' and shallow religiosity in their personalities, but the term 'epileptic personality' is so all-embracing that it serves little nosological function at least within the epileptic population[91, 98]. A more useful concept is that of maturity: 'they are children in their EEGs and their personalities', wrote Rey, Pond, and Evans[79]. Aggressiveness and immaturity have been the main personality features in our population especially in those with early onset epilepsy[43, 47, 85, 93]. The sudden, inexplicable, extreme, and remorseless nature of their tantrums attests to their infantile quality.

Since maturity is difficult to define in purely psychological terms and usually extends into social function, we measured the social adjustment in order to assess the degree of incapacity of our patients before operation and to record the changes wrought by surgery[26, 96]. The measurement included ratings of the extent of institutionalization, interpersonal relationships within and beyond the family, the use made of leisure, sexual adjustment, and working capacity. The intercorrelation of these scales was high and a sum of scores was used as an estimate of the total adjustment. Preoperative adjustment was reduced with a family history of mental illness, with early onset of epilepsy, with the need for special schooling, and with low I.Q. Adjustment was reduced with increasing frequency of grand mal seizures, or attacks involving falling and slumping (i.e. those obvious to observers) and not with the frequency of psychomotor attacks. Adjustment within the family was the item least influenced by seizure frequency. There was a clear relationship between social adjustment and psychiatric diagnosis, being worst for psychotic and psychopathic patients and best for normal or neurotic patients.

Esquirol believed that all manner of abnormal reactions may follow in the wake of epilepsy. Most modern studies confirm this view in relation to disturbance of temporal lobe function[29, 31, 32, 50, 77, 101]. Falret[27] suggested that the epilepsy may merely make the individual more vulnerable to mental disorder, the precise form of which would depend on the patient's age, milieu, and genetic endowment. While concurring with this view we recently attempted to correlate mental state with a wide range of variables in the life history and in the epileptic process[91]. In the series of 100 patients referred to only 13 were considered normal before operation, 30 were diagnosed neurotic, 48 psychopathic, 16 psychotic, and 5 of epileptic personality. Thus in 12 cases two diagnoses were made. In the neurotic group depressive reactions, anxiety and phobic states were the most common. Of the psychopathic group 27 were aggressive and 15 immature or inadequate. Eight of the 16 psychotic cases suffered long-term schizophrenic psychoses of the type described by Hill[42], by Pond[72], and more fully by Slater, Beard, and Glitheroe[87].

Patients who were normal, or who became normal after operation, tended to have good interpersonal relationships and work records before operation. The neurotic patients were more intelligent than average, had better schooling, and were operated on later in life (20 out of 24 diagnosed neurotic alone were operated on after the age of 25 years). Psychopathy was associated with a younger age of onset, lower intelligence, male sex, low social class, poor work adjustment, and poor interpersonal relationships. Psychotic patients had poor social adjustment on all scales, and tended to have hamartomas or non-specific lesions in the resected specimens and not to have mesial temporal sclerosis.

Although 40 per cent had a family history of mental illness and a third were permanently separated from at least one parent before the age of 15 years, these factors did not correlate with the development of any particular mental state. About two-thirds of the neurotic patients had a right temporal focus for their seizures, whereas nearly two-thirds of the psychopathic patients had a left-sided focus. These interhemispheric differences are supported by the finding of Lishman[54] that damage to the left hemisphere leads to more psychiatric disability than does damage to the right. Further, Flor-Henry[30] showed that epileptic disturbance of the left temporal lobe is more likely to be associated with schizophrenic reactions, and right-sided epilepsy more with depressive reactions.

Thus, long-term personality disorder is the most frequent finding in patients with temporal lobe epilepsy, although affective changes are often seen. Our experience supports that of Slater, Beard, and Glitheroe[87] that schizophrenia-like psychoses occur more frequently than chance association will allow, although these particular psychoses are chronic and relatively benign (only four of our 19 patients considered psychotic at follow up were chronically hospitalized).

Two aspects of temporal lobe epilepsy which have received attention recently are sexual behaviour and criminality. Abnormal sexual behaviour associated with temporal lobe epilepsy has frequently been described in man and in experimental animals[33, 51, 84]. Classically, the disorder in man is hyposexuality, but instances of hypersexuality and perversity have been reported. The extent to which patients complain of absence of libido seems dependent on the age of acquisition of epilepsy[6, 92] since series largely made up of patients who developed temporal lobe epilepsy in adult life complain of their loss[40, 48] whereas those who developed early onset epilepsy rarely do and when questioned express indifference or disdain. Thus in our own experience the commonest abnormality has been low sexual drive rather than failure of erection or ejaculation. Perverse sexuality, usually compulsive excessive masturbation, was evident in 15 per cent of our sample[92]. Improved intensity of libido and relief of complex bizarre perversions have occurred with relief of epilepsy by surgery[45, 60]. In man the complete Klüver-Bucy syndrome has never followed bilateral temporal lobectomy, and heterosexual hypersexuality has not been reported[97]. In fact, true heterosexual hypersexuality in temporal lobe epilepsy is extremely rare. The view of Maeder[55] that the sexuality of epileptics is polymorphous 'like a normal child' is not only vindicated by recent research, but also reinforces the view held by many psychiatrists that the essential psychological defects of epileptics are immaturity and low motivation[74].

The cases reported by Walker[103] and by Fenton and Udwin[28] again raise the question, which so preoccupied psychiatrists at one time, of criminal responsibility and crimes of violence during epileptic seizures. One of us (M.A.F.) has performed over 250 temporal lobectomies since 1952 and these seriously disturbed patients have been followed annually for up to ten years. Yet no patient of ours has yet been charged with a crime performed during or immediately after a seizure. Walker, however, recorded an instance where a man, apparently inexplicably, killed his wife with numerous stab wounds. He was found drenched in blood and indicated the whereabouts of the body to the police. He strongly protested that he was 'being framed', claimed total amnesia for the event, and denied that his wife was dead. He was committed to a mental hospital where later a left temporal lobectomy was performed. Eventually he died and a post-mortem revealed a superficial angioma of the right temporal lobe. Walker reviewed a number of murders where the question of epilepsy was raised, and concluded that there are six criteria to consider in assessing such a case: (1) the patient was subject to *bona fide* epilepsy; (2) the spontaneous attacks were similar to the attacks which allegedly occurred at the time of the crime; (3) the period of loss of consciousness was commensurate with the type of fit the patient had; (4) the degree of assumed unconsciousness was commensurate with that noted in previous attacks; (5) the EEG findings are compatible with the type of clinical disorder assumed to be present—this usually means that spike discharges are required; and (6) the circumstances of the crime are compatible with the assumption of lack of awareness of the individual at the time of the crime. If several of these criteria are absent Walker believes that the case should be regarded with suspicion. The homicide reported by Fenton and Udwin[28] was regarded by them as probably the result of depressed mood occurring in association with temporal lobe epilepsy rather than a seizure itself. So far no report has yet contradicted the view of Alström[1] that crimes of violence are not a significant part of ictal behaviour.

Temporal Lobe Epilepsy in Childhood

Pond and Bidwell[75] emphasized that it is those adults whose epilepsy starts in childhood who provide the hard core of serious problems of management. Most studies of temporal epilepsy suggest that about half the cases start before the age of ten years. Thus epilepsy must often be seen not merely as a current problem, but also as one that has exercised its effect over a long time and at critical periods in the life history.

Considering temporal lobe epilepsy in children, the age of onset is again unevenly spread over the first decade; in both our own study[96] and that of Ounsted, Lindsay and Norman[65] the median age of onset for children starting before the age of ten years was about two years. From what is known of the functions of the temporal structures in learning, memory, autonomic control, and affect, it will be realized that damage sustained to these structures early in life will critically influence development. On top of this come the secondary handicaps, the effects of social rejection, over-protection, and family discord triggered off by the presence of the damaged child[94].

Nearly half our surgical cases of temporal lobe epilepsy have been found to exhibit mesial temporal sclerosis which was strongly associated with a history of febrile convulsions or status epilepticus in early infancy. In the series of Ounsted, Lindsay and Norman[65] one-third of the children with epilepsy had had a status epilepticus, lasting 30 minutes or more, before the age of four years, with a median age of onset of 16 months. Thus, although there may be many years before the habitual epilepsy develops, the structural damage is often sustained early. Nevertheless, seizures of obviously psychomotor type do occur in very young children. Their recognition and distinction from petit-mal type and other generalized seizures has therapeutic implications since ethosuximide (Zarontin) will not influence them, while recourse to phenobarbitone may exacerbate abnormal behaviour to a degree which may be more troublesome than the fits themselves. Careful history-taking and observation are often the sole source of diagnosis, since the EEG may show little or nothing to support the clinical diagnosis until many years later.

Psychomotor seizures in childhood tend to be autonomic in their manifestations, and it is on the recognition of these autonomic components that the diagnosis may depend. A child reacting to an epigastric aura may clutch his belly and flex his hips with pain. Some vasomotor change in the form of pallor or flushing may occur, while a cry is also a frequent accompaniment. Fear may cause a child to flee suddenly to the security of its mother's arms. Tachycardia, borborygmi, drooling and minor motor twitching may be evident to the mother. A few older children will vouchsafe their auras, but often only in the security and trust of a long therapeutic relationship. In short, it is these little actions, like clutching the belly or fleeing to the mother, that distinguish a minor psychomotor seizure in a child from a 'petit mal'.

To some extent the behavioural abnormalities of an epileptic child may themselves suggest to the clinician the possibility that it is suffering from temporal lobe seizures. The emergence of psychomotor epilepsy after a seizure-free interval is sometimes mistaken as an hysterical phenomenon since, although clear-cut clonic convulsions may have occurred in the past, perhaps in association with a febrile illness, recent attacks are bizarre, sometimes related to recent emotional disturbance, and accompanied by changes of mood and demeanour. In children they may not be supported by EEG evidence. Ounsted's original 'hyperkinetics' formed eight per cent of a large population of early onset epileptics, whereas hyperkinetics form 26 per cent of his population of temporal lobe epileptics[64, 65]. Likewise, 36 per cent of his sample suffered attacks of catastrophic rage. Aggression is a feature which both James[47] and Serafetinides[85] found to be associated with early onset epilepsy. In our experience both these features are frequently aggravated by medication with phenobarbitone and its close analogues.

Hyperkinesis in particular leads to social isolation and exclusion from school. It is the most serious sequel of the epileptic state in childhood. The end point of hyperkinesis seems to be the classic ixophrenia of early adult life.

Mental deficiency is the most serious sequel to the brain damage with which temporal lobe epilepsy is so often associated. The earlier in life that brain damage is sustained, the greater the defect tends to be. Serious intellectual retardation is almost certainly directly due to the insult to the brain, whether by anoxia, trauma, or infection, and not to the epileptic process itself. Progressive mental deterioration in an epileptic therefore strongly suggests that the pathological basis of the epilepsy is itself progressive.

The child with epilepsy is, however, at risk for failure to learn in a variety of ways. Hyperkinesis, characterized by an increased and fixed level of motor activity, shortened span of attention, distractability, and loss of fear and affection render a child almost impossible to educate. Very large discrepancies within the Wechsler profiles and between verbal and performance subtests are often found, and the discrepant abilities bring serious educational problems in their wake. Further, subclinical paroxysms seem to interfere with the child's ability to deal with the material presented to it.

Most series of temporal lobe epilepsies which have been studied clinically have been adults from whom the defective have been excluded by various processes. Thus the serious complication of mental defect is often overlooked. In a recently published series, however, no less than 23 per cent of the children had I.Q.s below 70[65].

PATHOLOGY

Temporal lobe epilepsy is essentially a 'focal' epilepsy, and with increasing interest in it attention has been turning more and more to its underlying pathological substrata. Various lesions, both macroscopic and microscopic, found within the temporal lobes removed from epileptic patients, can trigger it. Among the former are cerebral tumours of various types, arteriovenous malformations, depressed fractures, gun-shot wounds, scars from intracerebral abscesses, and other such tangible causes. The part played by closed head injuries, however, is open to some doubt. Courville[10] concluded that 'pure' psychomotor seizures are only rarely produced by such means. In autopsy material, as in surgical material, traumatic scars are quite often found, but it is often impossible to say whether they are primary to the epilepsy or secondary to head injuries sustained during seizures.

The fact remains that these gross lesions account for only a minority of cases of temporal lobe epilepsy. For too long it has been taught that most cases of temporal lobe epilepsy are of idiopathic origin. Fortunately, through a correlation of autopsy studies in epileptic patients who have died a natural death with the pathological findings in the resected temporal lobes of patients submitted to operation, we are beginning to realize that there is usually a pathological substrate to the condition.

In a series of 100 consecutive patients submitted by us to an anterior temporal lobectomy performed in such a fashion that the mesial temporal structures, including the hippocampus, amygdala, and uncus, were included with the rest of the temporal lobe in the resected specimen, the pathological findings listed in Table 2 were found[25]. A similar distribution of lesions has since been reported in another series of 100 patients[26].

TABLE 2

Pathological findings in 100 Patients with Temporal Lobe Epilepsy

Mesial temporal sclerosis	47
Hamartomas (small cryptic 'tumours')	24*
Miscellaneous focal lesions	13*
Non-specific lesions	22
	106

* Includes three cases with mesial temporal sclerosis

Mesial Temporal Sclerosis

The development of this concept has recently been described by us[21, 26]. It originated in 1825 with the observation by two Frenchmen[7] that smallness and induration of Ammon's horn (hippocampus) had been observed by naked eye in the brains of nine out of 18 epileptics who had a natural death. Further post-mortem studies in recent times[57, 82, 88] have shown that this lesion is present in the brains of slightly more than half the adult epileptics who die a natural death. Our colleagues[25] introduced the term 'mesial temporal sclerosis' because usually the process also involves other mesial structures within the temporal lobe, such as the amygdala and uncus. Evidence is now forthcoming that mesial temporal sclerosis is commonly the result of an asphyxial episode in infancy, such as prolonged febrile convulsions or status epilepticus, occurring at a period of life when the hippocampus and other mesial structures are particularly vulnerable to anoxia. Birth trauma appears to play little part. The damage then caused in infancy subsequently develops into a sclerosing process that develops into an epileptogenic lesion, and which is the most common single cause of habitual temporal lobe epilepsy of grand mal, psychomotor, and absence types originating within the first two decades of life. In our own material a history of habitual epilepsy in first degree relatives was more commonly associated with mesial temporal sclerosis. Ounsted, Lindsay and Norman[65] showed that children who suffered status epilepticus had a far greater incidence of febrile convulsions in their siblings than those who developed temporal lobe epilepsy from any other cause. No satisfactory explanation has yet been put forward to account for why the lesion is commonly unilateral in autopsy studies.

Hamartomas

These occur in a quarter to a fifth of surgical cases and comprise a wide range of benign indolent lesions which are not definitely neoplastic and should be regarded more as congenital malformations. More common are glial malformations, but occasionally tuberose sclerosis, small capillary angiomas, or even small dermoid cysts are found[25]. These lesions are now being described by others, but they were not found in the brains of adult epileptics who came to autopsy and were studied[57].

Miscellaneous Lesions

These include scars and infarcts, lesions which, as has already been discussed, may be secondary to head injuries sustained during seizures rather than their cause. Their precise significance in relation to the epilepsy is often not known.

Equivocal or Non-specific Lesions

These do not show definite pathological changes affecting neurones. Some cases show subpial and white matter gliosis, but these lesichs are so common in non-epileptic material that they cannot be regarded as a cause. In the surgical material this subgroup comprised about a quarter to a fifth of the cases. Although they do not respond to surgical extirpation of the temporal lobe as well as do cases of mesial temporal sclerosis and hamartoma, a few patients are benefited. The explanation for this may be that the resection of the temporal lobe has interrupted neuronal circuits responsible for the propagation of seizure discharges and that the lesion responsible for the epilepsy is situated outside the temporal lobe at a distance from the hippocampus and the amygdala. For instance, two such cases, each due to a small calcified hamartoma in the occipital region, have been relieved by removal of the hamartomas[24].

DIAGNOSIS

Clinical Examination

The diagnosis of temporal lobe epilepsy depends primarily upon the interpretation of the fit-patterns, coupled with information gathered from the neurological examination, the neuroradiological studies, the psychometric tests and the EEG findings. The extent to which the various investigations should be pushed depends upon the frequency and the severity of the epilepsy, the possibility that it is an expression of a progressive neoplasm, or that it is a focal form of a generalized disease such as hypoglycaemia, phenylketonuria, Schilder's disease or one of the encephalitides.

It is most important that the patient's seizure-patterns be thoroughly worked out. Descriptions of these should be obtained not only from the patient but also from as many reliable eye-witnesses as possible. In specialized units the nursing staff should be trained to observe seizures and to subsequently record them on a 'fit chart' which itemizes the various features at the onset of the attack, during its course, and at its conclusion. Most of the patients have a re-membered aura of the type listed in Table 1 and many have more than one aura. We have already discussed the relative frequency of such auras and given a comment on their significance. In our experience none of them have lateralizing value, not even déjà vu, which Penfield once listed as coming predominantly from the minor hemisphere[22].

With gross lesions, such as tumours, there may be on neurological examination such signs as papilloedema, an upper quadrantic homonymous hemianopia, and a speech disturbance if the major hemisphere is involved. However, in other cases there may be little or nothing in the way of neurological signs. When examining our patients we look for such slight inequalities in limb and hand size that might indicate some cerebral damage or lesion dating from early life. Speech disturbances accompany many seizures and may prove of localizing value. Thus dysphasia in relation to the ictus strongly points to the major (usually left) hemisphere, whereas ictal speech automatisms may arise from either hemisphere, although slightly more often from the minor than from the major hemisphere[15, 23]. It is therefore of great importance to check the handedness of the patient and so determine which cerebral hemisphere is likely to be dominant. Indeed it may sometimes be necessary to proceed to the intracarotid sodium amytal test to determine cerebral dominance[86, 102].

Psychological Testing

When epilepsy arises in one temporal lobe its laterality can often be indicated by the accompanying intellectual and cognitive changes. A detailed psychometric assessment can therefore sometimes be of help. Review of the cognitive deficits associated with temporal lobe disease suggest that they are closely related to the laterality of the affected lobe. When deficits in verbal abilities occur, the dominant temporal lobe is more likely to be involved, while non-verbal deficits tend to occur with lesions of the non-dominant temporal lobe[12, 59] (*also* Blakemore, 1968. Personal communication). These phenomena are similar to those found with localized pathology elsewhere in the cerebral hemispheres. Indeed with temporal lobe epileptics a discrepancy of as little as eight points between the verbal and the performance scales of the Wechsler Intelligence Tests correlates with EEG evidence of laterality of the discharging focus, such that when the verbal scale is higher than the performance scale the non-dominant temporal lobe tends to be implicated, while when the performance scale is higher than the verbal scale the dominant lobe is usually involved (Blakemore, 1968. Personal communication). Such a small discrepancy is, of course, not significant in the general population.

Defects of long-term retention have also been found to correlate with the laterality of the affected temporal lobe. Thus, when the logical memory subtest of the Wechsler Memory Scale is used, patients with abnormalities of the non-dominant temporal lobe usually retain one hour later more than 50 per cent of the items recalled immediately after the presentation, while in patients with lesions of the dominant temporal lobe this quotient usually falls to below 30 per cent. These intellectual and cognitive deficits associated with temporal lobe epilepsy remain essentially unchanged by temporal lobectomy, even though the epilepsy is benefited.

Following operation patients whose dominant temporal lobe has been removed usually show a differential but transient impairment of learning abilities. Thus, after removal of the dominant temporal lobe, the patient usually shows a marked impairment of verbal learning ability, particularly for verbal material presented in the auditory modality. No similar impairment of learning and retention occurs following excision of the non-dominant lobe. The learning impairments which occur after dominant temporal lobectomy persist for some time, but we now know that these impairments do recover within three to five years of operation[4]. In this respect they are similar to the intellectual changes following temporal lobectomy, for often after operation there is a sharp decline in the intellectual abilities associated with the side of the resected temporal lobe, namely, a decline in verbal I.Q. after dominant temporal lobectomy and of performance I.Q. scores after non-dominant lobectomies. However, these usually recover to their preoperative level within one year of operation. There is also suggestion that if an adult patient happens to develop late-onset epilepsy from a tumour, he may develop an auditory learning deficit and have difficulty in such actions as taking messages over the telephone (*also* Falconer, 1969. Unpublished observations).

Radiological Investigations

X-rays of the skull are usually normal, but if one middle cranial fossa is slightly smaller than the other, this suggests a lesion on that side, which may be mesial temporal sclerosis or may be a glial hamartoma[22, 26]. Likewise, the air encephalogram may show relative smallness or enlargement of the temporal horn. Occasionally a glial abnormality is sufficiently calcified to show in skull x-rays[24, 25, 34].

EEG Investigations

The EEG diagnosis of temporal lobe epilepsy is dealt with in Chapter 13. Suffice it to say here that when considering patients with drug-resistant temporal lobe epilepsy for operation, we select only those in whom repeated EEG investigations have shown a spike-discharging focus located consistently within a temporal lobe. We like to see that this focus is unilateral, but often we find that there are spike foci affecting both temporal lobes independently. We then select for operation only those patients in whom the spike-discharging activity is four times as great or more on the side to be resected[23]. If both sides appear equally involved we do not operate, assuming that the pathological changes involve both temporal lobes. Also, it has been pointed out[5] that a unilateral temporal lobectomy seldom benefits a patient in whom the preoperative EEG abnormalities involve both temporal lobes equally.

In all cases we employed 'sphenoidal' electrodes together with the regular scalp montages and used intravenous barbiturate (usually thiopentone) narcosis as an activating agent[67]. We found that Metrazol or Megimide activations could give misleading information. The reduction of thiopentone-induced fast activity first described by Kennedy and Hill[49] is reliable evidence of a lesion, but this lesion may be either mesial temporal sclerosis or a hamartoma[19, 26]. On a few occasions we have studied patients in whom indwelling electrodes with multiple pick-up points were implanted into various parts of the temporal lobe as well as into other parts of the cerebrum for a period of about two weeks, but the wealth of data thus obtained usually did not clarify the problem.

TREATMENT

All forms of treatment should be based on adequate diagnosis and the exclusion of general factors in the causation of focal epilepsy. The therapist will need to bear constantly in mind the possible sequelae of temporal lobe epilepsy and to guard against them. These include status epilepticus, which may cause death or serious morbidity, the risks of accidents due to seizures, the emergence of psychosis and possible suicide, and morbid effects of stigma and social failure[95].

Medical Treatment

Medical treatment takes three broad lines: pharmacological, psychological, and social. It is often taken as a *sine qua non* that drug treatment is always indicated to eradicate the attacks, but there must be some qualifications to this point of view. Firstly, some late-onset epilepsies are due to developing tumours, and over-zealous treatment may indeed inhibit the attacks and lead to a false sense of security with failure to observe the development of sinister signs. Secondly, premature treatment may mean a patient with a single attack being unnecessarily medicated and socially stigmatized. Thirdly, children with epilepsy need to be sufficiently alert and well behaved to be able to acquire social learning and intellectual training. It is sometimes impossible to achieve full control of epilepsy by medication and yet retain behavioural normality.

Similarly, the seriously incapacitated patient who reaches the psychiatrist may be more incapacitated by his secondary than by his primary handicaps. There is at times an antithetical relationship between seizures and mental state[52] while epileptic psychoses tend to emerge out of a period when major seizures are subsiding[30, 72]. Gibbs[35] found that drugs such as phenurone may eliminate temporal lobe seizures and yet cause psychosis. In fact, the psychiatrist may find that attention to the secondary handicaps will reduce the stress and so lessen seizure frequency. Minor tranquillizers of the benzo-diazepine group, particularly chlordiazepoxide(Librium) are often useful in this regard. Lastly, recent evidence suggests that some chronic epileptic patients taking phenobarbitone or phenytoin are depleted of folic acid, and that this deficiency may lead to the emergence of psychological symptoms[80]. Excellent summaries of the various anticonvulsants and their actions, indications, and unwanted effects are available[8, 81]. The best course seems to be to use a few drugs such as phenobarbitone, phenytoin and primidone thoroughly, and to medicate with as small an amount as possible.

Psychiatrists naturally tend to have referred to them patients who have a mental disorder as well as epilepsy. Further, they are more prone to perceive the psychopathology in any case. This biases their view of the frequency of the association. Nevertheless the existence of severe personality disorder or psychopathology, to-gether with epilepsy, need not imply a causal relationship either way. Thus the psychiatric aspects may be treated independently of the epilepsy although they may originate in reaction to it. The secondary handicaps are more likely to be modifiable. Conventional psycho-therapy often proves singularly unrewarding and arduous on account of the slow thought processes, low intelligence, and ruminative obsessionality which so many patients show. Yet the therapist may mobilize some of the patient's resources through his relationship until the external rewards achieved form a more secure inducement. Sympathetic management by a physician able to understand the psychodynamics of chronic illness and cope with the reactions within the family is of course necessary.

For a proportion of patients a period of time spent in an ordered, disciplined and yet sympathetic environment in company with similarly incapacitated persons allows an opportunity to escape from unsatisfying domestic situations and deteriorating family relation-ships. Certainly the provision of special schools or colonies for epi-leptic children allows the family to recognize that their relative is being sympathetically dealt with, while their own exposure to the patient is reorganized into acceptably brief intervals. Such a provision allows the family to adopt better attitudes when they are in contact.

Surgical Treatment

There have been several approaches to problems of surgical treatment of drug-resistant temporal lobe epilepsy. The one with which we are most familiar is that of resecting as much as possible of the affected lobe, preferably in one piece, so that an adequate histological study of it can be made.

However, in recent years several surgeons have attempted to relieve temporal lobe epilepsy by various stereotactic means, such as interruption of the fornix system[99, 100], destruction of the amygdala[62, 90], or of certain thalamic nuclei[61, 63]. As none of these authors have yet reported their results in more than a few cases, and then only for short periods of time, it is as yet impossible to assess adequately the long-term value of procedures of this sort.

The largest series of cases treated by unilateral temporal lobectomy so far recorded is that reported by Rasmussen and Branch[78]. Out of a grand total of 389 patients submitted to an anterior temporal lobectomy and followed up for periods ranging from one to 25 years, 43 per cent came within the 'success' group. The criterion of success which they used, however, concerned only the relief of epilepsy, and not the patient's social adaptation[70]. Furthermore, their technique of temporal lobe excision involved piecemeal removal of the mesial temporal structures and hence they were not able to report on the detailed histological changes in their resected specimens.

Realizing also that the narrow parameter of relief or amelioration of seizures is not a sufficient criterion on which to judge the 'worthwhileness' of operation (although this is usually the only criterion employed in drug trials), we[96] have recently reported studies upon 100 consecutive English-speaking patients who were operated upon without mortality and with very little morbidity, and subsequently followed up for from two to ten years. In these patients we also investigated the effects of operation on social adjustment. Furthermore, all the resected lobes were examined histologically by Dr J. A. N. Corsellis, and so we were able to make many clinico-pathological correlations[21, 26, 96].

Prior to operation all these patients suffered from drug-resistant epilepsy, had no clinical or radiological evidence of a neoplasm or a vascular malformation, and had a spike-discharging EEG focus on the affected side. Many of our patients had an associated psychiatric illness. Indeed 45 of them had been at one time or another confined to an institution for three months or longer, such as a mental hospital, epileptic colony or a prison. We tended to reject patients whose I.Q. was below 70. Only 13 patients were judged mentally normal before operation and 16 patients were psychotic. We operated on these patients primarily for the relief of epilepsy, and if in so doing we obtained an improvement in social adaptation we regarded this as fortunate. The operation cannot be viewed as 'psychosurgery' since the favourable modifications of personality are not the objective nor the immediate sequel of surgery, but are dependent on substantial relief of epilepsy.

After operation 42 of our patients became completely seizure-free, while allowing for one or two seizures in any one year the 'success rate' was 62 per cent. The highest cure rate was seen in the group of patients with mesial temporal sclerosis, for 50 per cent of these were rendered completely seizure-free. We also found that if the epilepsy were relieved or lessened, there was also often an improvement in social adaptation as judged by the above parameters; 32 instead of 13 persons were now considered normal psychiatrically, while 51 on balance showed a good social adjustment after operation compared with 34 before operation.

Again, 16 patients were psychotic immediately prior to operation. Those with a confusional psychosis responded, but 12 of them had a psychosis of schizophrenic or severe paranoid type, and these psychoses tended to persist after operation, even though the epilepsy had been relieved. Not one of these 12 patients had mesial temporal sclerosis, but had either hamartomas, scars, or non-specific lesions in their resected specimens. We have reason to believe that as regards their seizures, patients with hamartomas respond to surgery as well as do patients with mesial temporal sclerosis, but not as regards their psychological and personality traits. We do not understand this although Malamud[56] recently reported a series of patients with neoplasms of the limbic system and schizophrenic symptomatology. The worst results as regards surgery were where no 'specific' lesion was disclosed, although some of these were benefited.

Most of our operations have been performed under local analgesia enabling us to simulate the exposed cortex in conscious patients. We did this at first because of the recommendation of the Montreal school, but as our experience has grown we agree with Walker[104] that general anaesthesia can be substituted. The impression now appears widespread that electrical stimulation of the temporal cortex in conscious patients will evoke past memories, but the evidence for this lacks detailed confirmation. The notion stems largely from observations made by Penfield over the course of 25 years in epileptic patients in whom the temporal lobe had been exposed. These observations were summarized by Penfield and Perot[71] who reported having elicited memory responses from the temporal cortex in 40 out of 520 patients operated upon under local analgesia, an incidence of 7·7 per cent. Yet we ourselves have never encountered these phenomena in close on 200 patients operated upon under comparable conditions. Only rarely have these phenomena been reported by other neurosurgeons (Walker 1968. Personal communication) and therefore it is hoped that those who have will report them. Our only instance of these phenomena occurred in one patient whose hippocampus had been stimulated[66]. A possible explanation of our differing experiences is that Penfield's patients had been off all medication for several days (Baldwin. Personal communication).

We concluded from our studies that mesial temporal lobe sclerosis is the most common single cause of drug-resistant epilepsy arising in the first two decades of life. It seems to be an acquired rather than an inherited lesion, although family susceptibility to infantile convulsions probably plays an important part. The chief cause appears to be an asphyxial episode in early childhood, and this results in nerve cell damage or less in the mesial temporal structures, which then develops into an epileptogenic lesion. In its classical form the lesion is usually unilateral, a fact which no one has satisfactorily explained. The best results of surgical treatment of drug-resistant temporal lobe epilepsy, not only as regards seizure-improvement but also as regards social adaptation, occur whenever this lesion is encountered.

SUMMARY

Temporal lobe epilepsy is thus of special interest to the psychiatrist, for it is common and often associated with psychiatric illness or disability. It can occur at all age periods but is particularly common in children. There is often an unsuspected and hitherto largely ignored pathological substrate. Most cases can probably be relieved by drug-therapy and some patients may spontaneously lose their seizures. We, however, have endeavoured to consider the problem as confronted by the psychiatrist called upon to deal with the psychiatric aspects. Much research into these various aspects is still required.

REFERENCES

1. Alström, C. H. (1950). 'A Study of Epilepsy in its Clinical, Social and Genetic Aspects'. *Acta psychiat. neurol. scand.* Suppl. 63
2. Bailey, P. and Gibbs, F. A. (1951). 'The Surgical Treatment of Psychomotor Epilepsy'. *J. Am. med. Ass.* **145,** 365

3. Bengzon, A. R. A., Rasmussen, T., Gloor, P., Dussault, J. and Stephens, M. (1968). 'Prognostic Factors in the Surgical Treatment of Temporal Lobe Epileptics'. *Neurology* **18, 7**17

4. Blakemore, C. B. and Falconer, M. A. (1967). 'Long-term Effects of Anterior Temporal Lobectomy on Certain Cognitive Functions'. *J. Neurol. Neurosurg. Psychiat.* **30,** 364

5. Bloom, D., Jasper, H. and Rasmussen, T. (1960). 'Surgical Therapy on Patients with Temporal Lobe Seizures and Bilateral EEG Abnormalities'. *Epilepsia* **1,** 35

6. Blumer, D. and Walker, A. E. (1967). 'Sexual Behaviour in Temporal Lobe Epilepsy'. *Archs Neurol., Chicago* **16,** 37

7. Bouchet, and Cazauvieilh, (1825 and 1826). 'De l'épilepsie considérée dans ses rapports avec l'aliénation mentale'. *Archs gén. méd.* **9,** 510; **10,** 5

8. British Medical Journal (1968). 'Today's Drugs: Drugs for Epilepsy'. **2,** 350

9. College of General Practitioners (1960). 'A Survey of the Epilepsies in General Practice'. *Br. med. J.* **2,** 416

10. Courville, C. B. (1958). 'Traumatic Lesions of the Temporal Lobe as the Essential Cause of Psychomotor Epilepsy'. In *Temporal Lobe Epilepsy*. Ed. by M. Baldwin and P. Bailey. Springfield, Ill.: Charles C. Thomas

11. De Jong, R. N. (1957). ' "Psychomotor" or "Temporal Lobe" Epilepsy: A Review of the Development of our Present Concepts'. *Neurology* **7,** 1

12. Dennerll, R. P. (1964). 'Cognitive Deficits and Lateral Brain Dysfunction in Temporal Lobe Epilepsy'. *Epilepsia* **5,** 177

13. Dostoievsky, F. (1953). *The Possessed*, published as *The Devils*. Harmondsworth, Middlesex: Penguin

14. — (1955). *The Idiot*. Harmondsworth, Middlesex: Penguin

15. Driver, M. V., Falconer, M. A. and Serafetinides, E. A. (1964). 'Ictal Speech Automatism Reproduced by Activation Procedures: A Case Report with Comments on Pathogenesis'. *Neurology* **14,** 455

16. Esquirol, E. Quoted by Falret (1860–61)

17. Falconer, M. A. (1954). 'Clinical Manifestations of Temporal Lobe Epilepsy and their Recognition in Relation to Surgical Treatment'. *Br. med. J.* **2,** 939

18. — (1959). 'Discussion on the Anatomy of Temporal Lobe Seizures'. In *First International Congress of Neurological Sciences*, Vol. 3, p. 532. Ed. by L. van Bogaert and J. Rademaker. London: Pergamon Press

19. — (1966). 'Problems in Neurosurgery: Temporal Lobe Epilepsy'. *Trans. med. Soc. Lond.* **82,** 111

20. — (1967). 'Some Functions of the Temporal Lobes with Special Regard to Affective Behaviour in Epileptic Patients'. *J. psychosom. Res.* **9,** 25

21. — (1968). 'The Significance of Mesial Temporal Sclerosis (Ammon's Horn Sclerosis) in Epilepsy'. *Guy's Hosp. Rep.* **117**, 1

22. — and Cavanagh, J. B. (1959). 'Clinico-pathological Con siderations of Temporal Lobe Epilepsy due to Small Foca-Lesions'. *Brain* **82**, 483

23. — and Serafetinides, E. A. (1963). 'A Follow-up Study of Surgery in Temporal Lobe Epilepsy'. *J. Neurol. Neurosurg. Psychiat.* **26**, 154

24. — Driver, M. V. and Serafetinides, E. A. (1962). 'Temporal Lobe Epilepsy due to Distant Lesions: Two Cases Relieved by Operation'. *Brain* **85**, 521

25. — Serafetinides, E. A. and Corsellis, J. A. N. (1964). 'Etiology and Pathogenesis of Temporal Lobe Epilepsy'. *Archs Neurol., Chicago* **10**, 233

26. — and Taylor, D. C. (1968). 'Surgical Treatment of Drug-resistant Temporal Lobe Epilepsy due to Mesial Temporal Sclerosis: Etiology and Significance'. *Archs Neurol., Chicago* **19**, 353

27. Falret, J. (1860 and 1861). 'De l'état mental des épileptiques'. *Archs gén. Méd.* **16**, 666; **17**, 461; **18**, 423

28. Fenton, G. W. and Udwin, E. L. (1965). 'Homicide, Temporal Lobe Epilepsy and Depression: A Case Report'. *Br. J. Psychiat.* **111**, 304

29. Ferguson, S. M. (1962). 'Temporal Lobe Epilepsy: Psychiatric and Behavioural Aspects'. *Bull. N.Y. Acad. Med.* **38**, 668

30. Flor-Henry, P. (1969). 'Psychosis and Temperal Lobe Epilepsy—A Controlled Investigation'. *Epilepsia* **10**, 362

31. Frantz, R. (1947). 'The Psychiatric Manifestations of Temporal Lobe Lesions'. *Bull. Los. Ang. neurol. Soc.* **12**, 150

32. Gastaut, H. (1953). 'So-called "Psychomotor" and "Temporal" Epilepsy'. *Epilepsia* **2**, 59

33. — and Colomb, H. (1954). 'Etude du comportement sexuel chez les Épileptiques Psychomoteurs'. *Annls méd.-psychol.* **112**, 657

34. Geyelin, H. R. and Penfield, W. (1929). 'Cerebral Calcification Epilepsy: Endarteritis Calcificans Cerebri'. *Archs Neurol. Psychiat., Chicago* **21**, 1020

35. Gibbs, F. A. (1950). 'Psychiatric Disorders Temporal Lobe Epilepsy'. In *The Biology of Mental Health and Disease*. Milbank Memorial Fund. New York: Holber

36. — Gibbs, E. L. and Lennox, W. G. (1937). 'Epilepsy: A Paroxysmal Cerebral Dysrhythmia'. *Brain* **60**, 377

37. Gloor, P. Tsat, C. and Haddad, F. (1958). 'An Assessment of the Value of Sleep-encephalography in the Diagnosis of Temporal Lobe Epilepsy'. *Electroenceph. clin. Neurophysiol.* **10**, 633

38. Gowers, R. W. (1964). 'Epilepsy and other Chronic Convulsive Diseases: Their Causes, Symptoms and Treatment'. In *American Academy of Neurology Reprint Series 1881*, p. 165. New York: Dover Publications

39. Graham, P. and Rutter, M. (1968). 'Organic Brain Dysfunction and Child Psychiatric Disorder'. *Br. med. J.* **3**, 695

40. Hierons, R. and Saunders, M. (1966). 'Impotence in Patients with Temporal Lobe Lesions'. *Lancet* **2**, 761

41. Hill, D. (1953). 'Discussion on the Surgery of Temporal Lobe Epilepsy'. *Proc. R. Soc. Med.* **46**, 965

42. — (1953). 'Psychiatric Disorders of Epilepsy'. *Med. Press* **20**, 473

43. — Pond, D. A., Mitchell, W. and Falconer, M. A. (1957). 'Personality Changes Following Temporal Lobectomy for Epilepsy'. *J. ment. Sci.* **103**, 18

44. Horsley, V. (1886). 'Brain Surgery'. *Br. med. J.* **2**, 670

45. Hunter, R., Logue, V. and McMenemy, W. H. (1963). 'Temporal Lobe Epilepsy Supervening on Longstanding Transvestism and Fetishism'. *Epilepsia* **4**, 60

46. Jackson, J. H. (1888). 'On a Particular Variety of Epilepsy ("Intellectual Aura"). One Case with Symptoms of Organic Brain Disease'. *Brain* **9**, 179

47. James, I. P. (1960). 'Temporal Lobectomy for Psychomotor Epilepsy'. *J. ment. Sci.* **106**, 543

48. Johnson, J. (1965). 'Sexual Impotence and the Limbic System'. *Br. J. Psychiat.* **111**, 300

49. Kennedy, W. A. and Hill, D. (1958). 'Surgical Prognostic Significance of the Electroencephalographic Prediction of Ammon's Horn Sclerosis in Epileptics'. *J. Neurol. Neurosurg. Psychiat.* **21**, 24

50. Keschner, M., Bender, M. B. and Strauss, I. (1936). 'Mental Symptoms in Cases of Tumour of the Temporal Lobe'. *Archs Neurol. Psychiat., Chicago* **35**, 572

51. Klüver, H. and Bucy, P. C. (1939). 'Preliminary Analysis of the Functions of Temporal Lobes in Monkeys'. *Archs Neurol. Psychiat., Chicago* **42**, 979

52. Landolt, H. (1958). 'Serial Electroencephalographic Investigations during Psychotic Episodes in Epileptic Patients and during Schizophrenic Attacks'. In *Lectures on Epilepsy*. Ed. by A. M. Lorentz de Haas. Amsterdam: Elsevier

53. Lennox, W. (1951). 'Phenomena and Correlates of the Psychomotor Triad'. *Neurology* **1**, 357

54. Lishman, W. A. (1968). 'Brain Damage in Relation to Psychiatric Disability after Head Injury'. *Br. J. Psychiat.* **114**, 373

55. Maeder, A. (1909). 'Sexualität und Epilepsie'. *Jb. psychoanalyt. psychopath. Forsch.* **1**, 119

56. Malamud, N. (1967). 'Psychiatric Disorder with Intracranial Tumours of the Limbic System'. *Archs Neurol., Chicago* **17**, 113

57. Margerison, J. H. and Corsellis, J. A. N. (1966). 'Epilepsy and the Temporal Lobes; A Clinical, Electroencephalographic and Neuropathological Study of the Brain in Epilepsy, with Particular Reference to the Temporal Lobes'. *Brain* **89**, 499

58. Meyer, V. and Falconer, M. A. (1966). 'Defects of Learning Ability with Massive Lesions of the Temporal Lobe'. *J. ment. Sci.* **106,** 472

59. Milner, B. (1962). 'Laterality Effects in Audition'. In *Inter-hemispheric Relations and Cerebral Dominance,* p. 177. Ed. by V. B. Hardcastle. Baltimore: Johns Hopkins Press

60. Mitchell, W., Falconer, M. A. and Hill, D. (1954). 'Epilepsy with Fetishism Relieved by Temporal Lobectomy'. *Lancet* **2,** 626

61. Mullen, S., Vailati, G., Karasick, J. and Mailis, M. (1967). 'Thalamic Lesions for the Control of Epilepsy'. *Archs Neurol., Chicago* **16,** 277

62. Narabayashi, H., Nagao, T., Saito, V., Yoshida, M. and Nagahata, M. (1963). 'Stereotaxic Amygdalotomy for Behaviour Disorders'. *Archs Neurol., Chicago* **9,** 1

63. Orthor, H. and Lohmann, R. (1966). 'Erfahrungen mit Stereotaktischen Eingriffen bei Epilepsie'. *Dt. med. Wschr.* **91,** 981

64. Ounsted, C. (1955). 'The Hyperkinetic Syndrome in Epileptic Children'. *Lancet* **2,** 303

65. — Lindsay, J. and Norman, R. Eds. (1966). In *Biological Factors in Temporal Lobe Epilepsy.* Clinics in Developmental Medicine, No. 22. London: Heineman

66. Pampiglione, G. and Falconer, M. A. (1962). 'Phénomènes subjectifs et objectifs provoqués par la stimulation de l'hippocampe chez l'homme', p. 399. Paris: Editions du Centre National de la Recherche Scientifique

67. — and Kerridge, J. (1956). 'EEG Abnormalities from the Temporal Lobe Studied with Sphenoidal Electrodes'. *J. Neurol. Neurosurg. Psychiat.* **19,** 117

68. Penfield, W. (1957). 'Thoughts on the Function of the Temporal Cortex'. *Clin. Neurosurg.* **4,** 21

69. — (1959). 'The Interpretive Cortex: The Stream of Consciousness in the Human Brain can be Electrically Reactivated'. *Science* **129,** 1719

70. — and Steelman, H. (1947). 'The Treatment of Focal Epilepsy by Cortical Excision'. *Ann. Surg.* **126,** 740

71. — and Perot, P. (1963). 'The Brain's Record of Auditory and Visual Experience'. *Brain* **86,** 595

72. Pond, D. A. (1957). 'Psychiatric Aspects of Epilepsy'. *J. Indian med. Prof.* **3,** 1441

73. — (1961). 'Psychiatric Aspects of Epileptic and Brain-damaged Children'. *Br. med. J.* **2,** 1377, 1454

74. — (1963). 'Maturation, Epilepsy and Psychiatry'. *Proc. R. soc. Med.* **56,** 710

75. — and Bidwell, B. H. (1960). 'A Survey of Epilepsy in Fourteen General Practices II (Social and Psychological Aspects)'. *Epilepsia* **1,** 285

76. — — and Stein, L. (1960). 'A Survey of Epilepsy in Fourteen General Practices I (Demographic and Medical Data)'. *Psychiat. Neurol. Neurochir.* **63,** 217

77. Preston, D. W. and Attack, E. A. (1964). 'Temporal Lobe Epilepsy: A Clinical Study of 97 Cases'. *Canad. med. Ass. J.* **9,** 1256

78. Rasmussen, T. and Branch, C. (1962). 'Temporal Lobe Epilepsy: Indications for and Results of Surgical Therapy'. *Postgrad. Med.* **31,** 9

79. Rey, H., Pond, D. A. and Evans, C. (1949). 'Clinical and Electro-encephalographic Studies of Temporal Lobe Function'. *Proc. R. soc. Med.* **42,** 891

80. Reynolds, E. H., Chanarin, I. and Matthews, D. M. (1968). 'Neuropsychiatric Aspects of Anticonvulsant Megaloblastic Anaemia'. *Lancet* **1,** 394

81. Robb, P. (1965). 'Epilepsy: A Review of Basic and Clinical Research'. NINDB Monograph No. 1. *Publ. Hlth Serv. Publs, Wash.* No. 1357

82. Sano, K. and Malamud, N. (1953). 'Clinical Significance of Sclerosis of the Cornu Ammonis'. *A.M.A. Archs Neurol. Psychiat.* **70,** 40

83. Schneider, R. C., Crosby, E. C., Bagchi, B. K. and Calhoun, R. D. (1961). 'Temporal or Occipital Lobe Hallucinations Triggered from Frontal Lobe Lesions'. *Neurology* **11,** 172

84. Schreiner, L. and Kling, A. (1953). 'Behavioural Changes Following Rhinencephalic Injury in the Cat'. *J. Neurophysiol.* **16,** 643

85. Serafetinides, E. A. (1965). 'Aggressiveness in Temporal Lobe Epilepsies and its Relation to Cerebral Dysfunction and Environmental Factors'. *Epilepsia* **6,** 33

86. — Hoare, R. D. and Driver, M. V. (1965). 'Intracarotid Sodium Amylobarbitone and Cerebral Dominance for Speech and Consciousness'. *Brain* **88,** 107

87. Slater, E., Beard, A. W. and Glitheroe, E. (1963). 'The Schizophrenia-like Psychoses of Epilepsy'. *Br. J. Psychiat.* **109,** 95

88. Stauder, H. K. (1936). 'Epilepsie und Schläfenläppen'. *Arch. Psychiat. NervKrankh.* **104,** 181

89. Symonds, C. P. (1954). 'Classification of the Epilepsies with Particular Reference to Psychomotor Seizures'. *A.M.A. Archs Neurol. Psychiat.* **72,** 631

90. Talairach, J. and Szikla, G. (1965). 'Particular Amygdalo Hippocampal Destruction by Yttrium[90] in Treatment of Rhinencephalic Epilepsies'. *Neurochirurgie* **11,** 233

91. Taylor, D. C. (1967). 'Factors Related to Mental State in Patients with Temporal Lobe Epilepsy Treated by Temporal Lobectomy'. *M. D. Thesis. University of London*. Gowers Memorial Prize Essay. International League against Epilepsy, British Branch.

92. — (1969). 'Sexual Behaviour and Temporal Lobe Epilepsy'. *Archs Neurol.* **21**, 510

93. — (1969). 'Aggression and Epilepsy'. *J. psychosom. Res.* **13**, 229

94. — (1968). 'Some Psychiatric Aspects of Epilepsy'. In *Current Problems in Neuropsychiatry*. Ed. by R. N. Herrington, British Journal of Psychiatry Special Publication No. 4, 106. London: Royal Medico-Psychological Association

95. — (1968). 'Treatment of Epilepsy'. In *Practical Treatment in Psychiatry*. Ed. by J. Crammer and D. Watt. Oxford: Blackwell

96. — and Falconer, M. A. (1968). 'Clinical, Socio-economic, and Psychological Changes after Temporal Lobectomy for Epilepsy'. *Br. J. Psychiat.* **114**, 1247

97. Terzian, H. (1958). 'Observations on the Clinical Symptomatology of Bilateral Partial or Total Removal of the Temporal Lobes in Man'. In *Temporal Lobe Epilepsy*, p. 510. Ed. by M. Baldwin and P. Bailey. Springfield, Ill.: Charles C. Thomas

98. Tizard, B. (1962). 'The Personality of Epileptics: A Discussion of the Evidence'. *Psychol. Bull.* **59**, 196

99. Turner, E. (1963). 'A New Approach to Unilateral and Bilateral Lobectomies for Psychomotor Epilepsy'. *J. Neurol. Neurosurg. Psychiat.* **26**, 285

100. Umbach, W. (1966). 'Elektrophysiologische und Vegetative Phänomene bei Stereotaktischen Hirnoperationen', p. 108. Berlin: Springer

101. Vasquez, J. (1952). 'Epilepsies Temporales et Manifestations Mentales'. *Un. méd. Can.* **81**, 1062

102. Wada, J. and Rasmussen, T. (1960). 'Intracarotid Injection of Sodium Amytal for the Lateralization of Cerebral Speech Dominance. Experimental and Clinical Observations'. *J. Neurosurg.* **27**, 266

103. Walker, A. (1961). 'Murder or Epilepsy'. *J. nerv. ment. Dis.* **133**, 430

104. — (1967). 'Temporal Lobectomy'. *J. Neurosurg.* **26**, 642

105. Williams, D. (1956). 'The Structure of Emotions Reflected in Epileptic Experience'. *Brain* **79**, 29

106. — (1966). 'Temporal Lobe Epilepsy'. *Br. med. J.* **1**, 1439

INDEX